Epigenetic Targets in Drug Discovery

Edited by
Wolfgang Sippl and Manfred Jung

Methods and Principles in Medicinal Chemistry

Edited by R. Mannhold, H. Kubinyi, G. Folkers

Previous Volumes of this Series:

Langer, T./Hoffmann, R. D. (eds.)

Pharmacophores and Pharmacophore Searches

Vol 32

2006, ISBN: 978-3-527-31250-4

Francotte, Eric/Lindner, Wolfgang (eds.)

Chirality in Drug Research

Vol. 33

2006, ISBN: 978-3-527-31076-0

Jahnke, Wolfgang/Erlanson, Daniel A. (eds.)

Fragment-based Approaches in Drug Discovery

Vol. 34

2006, ISBN: 978-3-527-31291-7

Hüser, Jörg (ed.)

High-Throughput Screening in Drug Discovery

Vol. 35

2006, ISBN: 978-3-527-31283-2

Wanner, Klaus/Höfner, Georg (eds.)

Mass Spectrometry in Medicinal Chemistry

Applications in Drug Discovery

Vol. 36

2007, ISBN: 978-3-527-31456-0

Mannhold, Raimund (ed.)

Molecular Drug Properties

Measurement and Prediction

Vol. 37

2007, ISBN: 978-3-527-31755-4

Vaz, Roy J./Klabunde, Thomas (eds.)

Antitargets

Prediction and Prevention of Drug Side Effects

Vol. 38

2008, ISBN: 978-3-527-31821-6

Ottow, Eckhard/Weinmann, Hilmar (eds.)

Nuclear Receptors as Drug Targets

Vol. 39

2008, ISBN: 978-3-527-31872-8

van de Waterbeemd, Han/Testa, Bernard (eds.)

Drug Bioavailability

Estimation of Solubility, Permeability, Absorption and Bioavailability

2., completely revised edition

Vol. 40

2008, ISBN: 978-3-527-32051-6

Todeschini, Roberto/Consonni, Viviana

Molecular Descriptors for Chemoinformatics

Volume I: Alphabetical Listing / Volume II: Appendices, References

Vol. 41

2009, ISBN: 978-3-527-31852-0

Epigenetic Targets in Drug Discovery

Edited by
Wolfgang Sippl and Manfred Jung

WILEY-VCH

WILEY-VCH Verlag GmbH & Co. KGaA

Series Editors

Prof. Dr. Raimund Mannhold
Molecular Drug Research Group
Heinrich-Heine-Universität
Universitätsstraße 1
40225 Düsseldorf
Germany
mannhold@uni-duesseldorf.de

Prof. Dr. Hugo Kubinyi
Donnersbergstrasse 9
67256 Weisenheim am Sand
Germany
kubinyi@t-online.de

Prof. Dr. Gerd Folkers
Collegium Helveticum
STW/ETH Zurich
8092 Zurich
Switzerland
folkers@collegium.ethz.ch

Volume Editors

Prof. Dr. Wolfgang Sippl
Institut für Pharmazie
Martin-Luther-Universität
Wolfgang-Langenbeck-Straße 4
06120 Halle
Germany

Prof. Dr. Manfred Jung
Institut für Pharmazeutische Wissenschaften
Albert-Ludwigs-Universität
Albertstraße 25
79104 Freiburg
Germany

Library of Congress Card No.: applied for

British Library Cataloguing-in-Publication Data
A catalogue record for this book is available from the British Library.

Bibliographic information published by the Deutsche Nationalbibliothek
The Deutsche Nationalbibliothek lists this publication in the Deutsche Nationalbibliografie; detailed bibliographic data are available on the Internet at http://dnb.d-nb.de.

Composition Thomson Digital, Noida, India
Printing Strauss GmbH, Mörlenbach
Bookbinding Litges & Dopf GmbH, Heppenheim
Cover design Schulz Grafik-Design, Fußgönheim

Printed in the Federal Republic of Germany
Printed on acid-free paper

ISBN: 978-3-527-32355-5

Contents

Epigenetic Targets in Drug Discovery. Edited by Wolfgang Sippl and Manfred Jung

ISBN: 978-3-527-32355-5

List of Contributors

Antonio Bedalov
Fred Hutchinson
Cancer Research Center
1100 Fairview Ave. N.
Seattle, WA 98109
USA

Jean Cavarelli
IGBMC (Institut de Génétique et de
Biologie Moléculaire et Cellulaire
UMR7104 CNRS-UDS, INSERM U964)
Département de Biologie et
Génomique Structurales
1 rue Laurent Fries
67404 Illkirch
France

Rasmus P. Clausen
University of Copenhagen
Department of Medicinal Chemistry
Faculty of Pharmaceutical Sciences
2100 Copenhagen
Denmark

John M. Denu
University of Wisconsin
Department of Biomolecular Chemistry
Madison, WI 53706
USA

Adam L. Garske
University of Wisconsin
Department of Chemistry
Madison, WI 53706
USA

Athanassios Giannis
University of Leipzig
Institute for Organic Chemistry
Johannisallee 29
04103 Leipzig
Germany

Alexander-Thomas Hauser
University of Freiburg
Institute of Pharmaceutical Sciences
Albertstr. 25
79104 Freiburg
Germany

Kristian Helin
University of Copenhagen
Biotech Research and Innovation Centre
(BRIC) and Centre for Epigenetics
2200 Copenhagen
Denmark

Epigenetic Targets in Drug Discovery. Edited by Wolfgang Sippl and Manfred Jung

ISBN: 978-3-527-32355-5

Ralf Heinke
Martin-Luther University of Halle-Wittenberg
Department of Pharmaceutical Chemistry
Wolfgang-Langenbeck-Str. 4
06120 Halle/Saale
Germany

Axel Imhof
Ludwig-Maximilians University of Munich
Histone Modifications Group
Adolf-Butenandt Institute
Schillerstr 44
80336 Munich
Germany

Philip Jones
IRBM/Merck Research Labs Rome
Via Pontina KM 30 600
00040 Pomezia
Italy

Manfred Jung
University of Freiburg
Institute of Pharmaceutical Sciences
Albertstr. 25
79104 Freiburg
Germany

Mira Jung
Georgetown University
Department of Radiation Medicine
Lombardi Comprehensive Cancer Center
Division of Radiation Research
Washington, DC 20057
USA

Sung Lee
Georgetown University
Department of Radiation Medicine
Lombardi Comprehensive Cancer Center
Division of Radiation Research
Washington, DC 20057
USA

Hongzhe Li
Fred Hutchinson Cancer Research Center
1100 Fairview Ave. N.
Seattle, WA 98109
USA

Marianne T. Pedersen
University of Copenhagen
Biotech Research and Innovation Centre (BRIC) and Centre for Epigenetics
2200 Copenhagen
Denmark

Jean-Paul Renaud
IGBMC (Institut de Génétique et de Biologie Moléculaire et Cellulaire UMR7104 CNRS-UDS, INSERM U964)
Département de Biologie et Génomique Structurales
1 rue Laurent Fries
67404 Illkirch
France

Christophe Romier
IGBMC (Institut de Génétique et de Biologie Moléculaire et Cellulaire UMR7104 CNRS-UDS INSERM U964)
Département de Biologie et Génomique Structurales
1 rue Laurent Fries
67404 Illkirch
France

Robert Schneider
MPI of Immunbiology
Stübeweg 51
79108 Freiburg
Germany

Martin Seifert
Genomatix GmbH
Bayerstr. 85a
80335 Munich
Germany

Wolfgang Sippl
Martin-Luther University of
Halle-Wittenberg
Department of Pharmaceutical
Chemistry
Wolfgang-Langenbeck-Str. 4
06120 Halle/Saale
Germany

Julian Simon
Fred Hutchinson
Cancer Research Center
1100 Fairview Ave. N.
Seattle, WA 98109
USA

Urszula Uciechowska
Martin-Luther University of
Halle-Wittenberg
Department of Pharmaceutical
Chemistry
Wolfgang-Langenbeck-Str. 4
06120 Halle/Saale
Germany

Ana Villar-Garea
Ludwig-Maximilians University of
Munich
Histone Modifications Group
Adolf-Butenandt Institute
Schillerstr 44
80336 Munich
Germany

Alfredo Velena
Georgetown University
Department of Radiation Medicine
Lombardi Comprehensive Cancer
Center
Division of Radiation Research
Washington, DC 20057
USA

Margarete von Wantoch Rekowski
Institute for Organic Chemistry
University of Leipzig
Johannisallee 29
04103 Leipzig
Germany

Jean-Marie Wurtz
IGBMC (Institut de Génétique et de
Biologie Moléculaire et Cellulaire
UMR7104 CNRS-UDS
INSERM U964)
Département de Biologie et
Génomique Structurales
1 rue Laurent Fries
67404 Illkirch
France

Kwon-Jeong Yong
Georgetown University
Department of Radiation Medicine
Lombardi Comprehensive Cancer
Center
Division of Radiation Research
Washington, DC 20057
USA

Preface

Sir Peter Medawar, Nobel laureate in 1960, thought that the book *On Growth and Form* by D'Arcy Wentworth Thompson is "the finest work of literature in all the annals of science that have been recorded in the English tongue" [1].

The central theme of D'Arcy Wentworth Thompson's work is a critical reframing of the theory of evolution, where he deplored overemphasis of evolution in terms of pure Darwinism and the widespread underestimation of the impact of physical laws and the rules of simple mechanics on "growth and form" of all organisms. He wrote in 1917:

> An organism is so complex a thing, and growth so complex a phenomenon, that for growth to be so uniform and constant in all the parts as to keep the whole shape unchanged would indeed be an unlikely and an unusual circumstance. Rates vary, proportions change, and the whole configuration alters accordingly.

D'Arcy Wentworth Thompson may thus have given a very early definition of epigenetics,[1)] while historically this honor is attributed to the renowned biologist Conrad Hal Waddington, who coined the word epigenetics. In 1942, he defined epigenetics as "the branch of biology which studies the causal interactions between genes and their products which bring the phenotype into being" [2].

Epigenetics has since then been used in most different contexts. Derived from the Greek prefix *epi-*, the term had acquired different meanings such as "after", "post", or "additionally". Nowadays, in the molecular realm, epigenetics has borne out nearly all these meanings, dealing with all processes in a cell that are considered "additional" to classical genetic processes and sources of genetic information like the DNA sequence.

Most recent research in cell biology gives a spectacular confirmation of D'Arcy Wentworth Thompson's visionary hypotheses: Physical forces within and bound to

1) In his pioneering work *On Growth and Form* published in 1917, the biologist D'Arcy Thompson (1860–1948) laid the foundations of what is now called biomathematics.

Epigenetic Targets in Drug Discovery. Edited by Wolfgang Sippl and Manfred Jung

ISBN: 978-3-527-32355-5

the 3D geometries of the locations where the cells grow and transmitted by the cytoskeleton are (in part) responsible for the future functionality of the cell [3–5]. The cellular matrix consisting of collagen and proteoglycans serves as a point of fixation and stabilizes the growing and developing cell. Depending on the geometry offered and influences from neighboring tissue, either an adipocyte or a hepatocyte is generated from a stem cell.

The focus of interest of today's epigenetic research is on linking the phenomenon to molecular evidence [6]. Giving care to a baby may fundamentally alter gene expression profiles due to "simple" cellular chemistry such as methylation and acylation of DNA and histones, which regulates transcription. The levels of glucocorticoid receptors in the hippocampus are higher in groups of rats that give their offspring more maternal care. Obviously, giving care induced a protein involved in the promotion of glucocorticoid receptors in the brain, by attracting methylating and acetylating enzymes to its gene location [7]. This is an example of what the book of Sippl and Jung is about.

After an introduction to the topic, the volume is divided into two large parts, each comprising six chapters. The first part introduces the methodology, ranging from computational approaches to structural biology aspects to cell biology and biochemistry. The second part is devoted to targets. Here, several classes of epigenetic targets and their ligands are presented and discussed in detail.

With this book, the editors, who also contributed chapters of their own, have succeeded to convene leading experts in the growing new field of "epigenetic drug design" and have thus made it possible for everyone entering the field to start off with a sound base of knowledge.

The series editors would like to thank Wolfgang Sippl and Manfred Jung for their excellent work presented in this book. We also want to express our gratitude to Nicola Oberbeckmann-Winter, Waltraud Wüst, and Frank Weinreich from Wiley-VCH for their valuable contributions to this project.

January 2009

Raimund Mannhold, Düsseldorf
Hugo Kubinyi, Weisenheim am Sand
Gerd Folkers, Zürich

References

1 Bretscher, O. (2005) Linear Algebra with Applications, 3rd edn, Pearson Education, Inc., p. 66.

2 Waddington, C.H. (1942) The epigenotype. *Endeavour*, **1**, 18–20.

3 Yilgor, P., Sousa, R.A., Reis, R.L., Hasirci, N. and Hasirci, V. (2008) 3D plotted PCL scaffolds for stem cell based bone tissue engineering. *Macromolecular Symposia*, **269**, 92–99.

4 Graziano, A., d'Aquino, R., Cusella-De Angelis, M.G., De Francesco, F., Giordano, A., Laino, G., Piattelli, A., Traini, T., De Rosa, A. and Papaccio, G. (2008) Scaffold's surface geometry significantly affects human stem cell bone tissue engineering. *Journal of Cellular Physiology*, **214**, 166–172.

5 Chaubey, A. and Burg, K.J.L. (2008) Extracellular matrix components as modulators of adult stem cell differentiation in an adipose system. *Journal of Bioactive and Compatible Polymers*, **3**, 20–37.

6 McGowan, M.S.P. and Meaney, M.J. (2008) The social environment and the epigenome. *Environmental and Molecular Mutagenesis*, **49**, 46–60.
7 Weaver, I.C.G., Cervoni, N., Champagne, F.A., D'Alessio, A.C., Sharma, S., Seckl, J.R., Dymov, S., Szyf, M. and Meaney, M.J. (2004) Epigenetic programming by maternal behavior. *Nature Neuroscience*, **7**, 847–854.

A Personal Foreword

"*Silence like a cancer grows...*" Paul Simon, in "The Sounds of Silence," released on Columbia Records, 1965.

"The role of histone becomes, thus, part of the problem of how the environment affects gene activity. Biology has by now outgrown the abstract and rigid limitations of classical genetics; for now it is clear that the chromosome, like other centres of vital activity, is subject to regulation by feed-back of the periphery." A. E. Mirsky, 1965 (sic !) [1]

Some 40 years later we basically stand in awe when reading those matter-of-factly spoken but definitely at that time prophetic words from Dr. Mirsky. Already in 1950 Stedman had discussed the role of histones in differentiation [2] and in 1964 Allfrey reported on the acetylation of histones [3]. The words of Mirsky are the concluding remarks of a Ciba Foundation symposium on histones and their role in transfer of genetic information. There it was discussed that "chromatin represents a ... metabolically active region of the nucleus" (p. 48). Many "fine bands" had been resolved in electrophoretic analysis of the histones but of course many details of the processes involved totally eluded the scientific knowledge of these days. But already then, a "functional correlation between histone acetylation and the RNA-synthetic capacity of the chromatin" was suggested.

Today we know that DNA methylation and posttranslational modification of histones such as acetylation are the biochemical manifestations of the impact of the environment on the cell and constitute the basis of what we call today "epigenetics". In other words, epigenetics is defined now as inheritable changes on gene expression and hence the proteome that are not based upon changes in the DNA sequence. A prominent example is the silencing of genetically intact tumor suppressor genes that are involved in the pathogenesis of cancer. Although the basic concepts were conceived and the term epigenetics was introduced around 60 years ago [4], epigenetic research (at least in terms of the underlying molecular determinants) remained mostly "silent" until the mid-1990s. Then, the seminal discoveries of Allis [5] and Schreiber [6] introduced histone-modifying enzymes as defined biochemical entities with a role in transcriptional regulation. Later, the first links

Epigenetic Targets in Drug Discovery. Edited by Wolfgang Sippl and Manfred Jung

ISBN: 978-3-527-32355-5

of those enzymes to cancer on a molecular level [7, 8] were identified and the role of further modifications was discovered and described, for example histone methylation [9]. New ground-breaking discoveries like histone demethylation [10] and its link to cancer [11] are not older than five years, so we are still in the infancy of epigenetics; nevertheless the first epigenetic drugs are already approved for the treatment of patients and a number of additional compounds are in clinical trials. So we will continue to listen to the sounds of epigenetic silence and hope that new epigenetic drugs will be able to break the silence and we will be able not to write only scientific monographs but also be able to write the histone code with small molecules.

In this volume we want to present the state of the art of epigenetics with regard to drug discovery. The chapters are divided into two major sections; one series of articles deals with the methodology that is available and the other presents the targets, their link to human diseases and available inhibitors. We apologize to all scientists whose efforts in the field were not duly cited in this book. We thank our authors, the publishers at Wiley-VCH and our families for support.

December 2008

Wolfgang Sippl, Halle (Saale)
Manfred Jung, Freiburg

References

1 Mirsky, A.E. (1966) in *Histones – Their Role in the Transfer of Genetic Information* (eds Ciba Foundation Study Group, Nr. 24), Churchill Ltd, London, p. 112.
2 Stedman, E. (1950) Cell specificity of histones. *Nature*, **166**, 780–781.
3 Allfrey, V.G., Faulkner, R. and Mirsky, A.E. (1964) Acetylation and methylation of histones and their possible role in the regulation of RNA synthesis. *Proceedings of the National Academy of Sciences of the United States of America*, **51**, 786–794.
4 Gottschling, D.E. (2004) Summary: epigenetics – from phenomenon to field. *Cold Spring Harbor Symposia on Quantitative Biology*, **69**, 507–519.
5 Brownell, J.E., Zhou, J., Ranalli, T., Kobayashi, R., Edmondson, D.G., Roth, S.Y. and Allis, C.D. (1996) Tetrahymena histone acetyltransferase A: a homolog to yeast Gcn5p linking histone acetylation to gene activation. *Cell*, **84**, 843–851.
6 Taunton, J., Hassig, C.A. and Schreiber, S.L. (1996) A mammalian histone deacetylase related to the yeast transcriptional regulator Rpd3p. *Science*, **272**, 408–411.
7 Lin, R.J., Nagy, L., Inoue, S., Shao, W., Miller, V.H. and Evans, R.M. (1998) Role of the histone deacetylase complex in acute promyelocytic leukaemia. *Nature*, **391**, 811–814.
8 Grignani, F., De Matteis, S., Nervi, C., Tomassoni, L., Gelmetti, V., Cioce, M., Fanelli, M., Ruthardt, M., Ferrara, F.F., Zamir, I., Seiser, C., Grignani, F., Lazar, M.A., Minucci, S. and Pelicci, P.G. (1998) Fusion proteins of the retinoic acid receptor-alpha recruit histone deacetylase in promyelocytic leukaemia. *Nature*, **391**, 815–818.
9 Rea, S., Eisenhaber, F., O'Carroll, D., Strahl, B.D., Sun, Z.W., Schmid, M., Opravil, S., Mechtler, K., Ponting, C.P., Allis, C.D. and Jenuwein, T. (2000) Regulation of chromatin structure by site-specific histone H3 methyltransferases. *Nature*, **406**, 593–599.
10 Shi, Y., Lan, F., Matson, C., Mulligan, P., Whetstine, J.R., Cole, P.A. and Casero, R.A. (2004) Histone

demethylation mediated by the nuclear amine oxidase homolog LSD1. *Cell*, **119**, 941–953.

11 Metzger, E., Wissmann, M., Yin, N., Muller, J.M., Schneider, R., Peters, A.H., Gunther, T., Buettner, R. and Schule, R. (2005) LSD1 demethylates repressive histone marks to promote androgen-receptor-dependent transcription. *Nature*, **437**, 436–439.

Part One
General Aspects and Methodologies

Epigenetic Targets in Drug Discovery. Edited by Wolfgang Sippl and Manfred Jung

ISBN: 978-3-527-32355-5

1
New Frontiers in Epigenetic Modifications

Adam L. Garske and John M. Denu

1.1
Introduction

The basic packaging unit of the genome, the nucleosome, consists of ~146 bp of DNA wound around an octamer of histone proteins. The histone octamer is composed of an H3/H4 tetramer and two H2A/H2B dimers. The unstructured N-terminal regions (tails) of histones protrude outward from the nucleosomal core through superhelical gyres of DNA. While genetic information is encoded in the DNA sequence, processes such as transcription, recombination, DNA replication and DNA repair are controlled by the "epigenome" (*epi* is Greek for upon or in addition to). The epigenome is often characterized by heritable or long-term alteration in gene expression patterns that cannot be ascribed to changes in DNA sequence [1]. At the molecular level, epigenetics involves the dynamic regulation of covalent modifications to DNA and the histone proteins. Epigenetics is implicated in processes such as gene expression and silencing, apoptosis, maintenance of stem cell pluripotency, X-chromosome inactivation and genomic imprinting [2]. Therefore, epigenetics can be viewed as the conduit from genotype to phenotype. This chapter provides a framework for our current understanding of molecular epigenetics with particular emphasis on the histone code and it examines the utility of small molecule inhibitors of enzymes that modify DNA and histones.

1.2
DNA Methylation

In multicellular eukaryotes, DNA methylation is associated with transcriptional silencing [3]. In these organisms, DNA methylation has been observed exclusively on the C5 position of the cytosine ring and is frequently found in CpG-rich regions. This process is attributed to the action of DNA methyltransferases (DNMTs), which utilize the cofactor, *S*-adenosyl-L-methionine. Approximately half of all human genes have CpG islands in their promoter regions but these stretches of DNA are typically

Epigenetic Targets in Drug Discovery. Edited by Wolfgang Sippl and Manfred Jung

ISBN: 978-3-527-32355-5

hypomethylated and transcriptionally permissive. Methylation in the proximity of the transcription start site or within a gene is associated with transcriptional repression [1, 4, 5].

DNA methyltransferases can be classified in two categories: (1) *de novo* DNMTs and (2) maintenance DNMTs [3]. *De novo* DNMTs methylate previously unmodified cytosines in CpG islands, while maintenance DNMTs duplicate existing DNA methylation patterns onto newly synthesized DNA strands during replication. DNMT3a and 3b are examples of *de novo* DNMTs and are capable of methylating both unmethylated and hemimethylated (only one strand in the DNA duplex is methylated) sites of DNA. Another protein, DNMT3-like (DNMT3L), acts as a regulatory factor in *de novo* methylation of DNA despite lacking a catalytic domain. This protein is involved in genetic imprinting [6] and methylation (indirectly) of retrotransposons in pre-meiotic spermatogonial stem cells [7]. In the case of genomic imprinting, DNMT3L was found to collaborate with DNMT3a to achieve DNA methylation by localizing the latter to unmodified K4 of histone H3 via a plant homeodomain (PHD)-like domain [8]. DNMT1, which has a catalytic preference for hemimethylated DNA, is an example of a maintenance DNA methyltransferase [3]. DNMT1 is localized to replication foci by interaction with proliferating cell nuclear antigen (PCNA) [9]. Recently, an accessory protein, UHRF1, was shown to target DNMT1 to hemimethylated DNA during S phase [10, 11]. UHRF1 is known to bind methylated DNA in the context of CG, CXG (X = A, T or C) or an asymmetrical sequence using a SET and RING associated (SRA) domain [12]. Furthermore, UHRF1 was found to be required for stable association of DNMT1 with chromatin [10]. Therefore, DNMT1 appears to regulate epigenetic inheritance in a mechanism that involves a complex with UHRF1 and PCNA in regions of replicating heterochromatin (tightly packed, transcriptionally repressive chromatin) that contain hemimethylated DNA [11].

Several other means for targeting DNMTs have been identified. In a sequence-dependent manner, DNMTs bind directly to DNA by virtue of a conserved proline and tryptophan (PWWP) domain [13]. For both *de novo* methyltransferases, DNMT3a and DNMT3b, a PWWP domain is essential for chromatin targeting [14]. Missense mutation of the PWWP domain in the *DNMT3B* gene triggers centromeric heterochromatin instability, pericentromeric instability and facial anomalies (ICF) syndrome [14]. A second mechanism for DNMT targeting is through recruitment by site-specific transcriptional repressors [3]. The oncogenic fusion protein, promyelocytic leukemia–retinoic acid receptor (PML-RAR), localizes methylation to specific genes in cancer cells by recruitment of DNMTs [15]. More recently, the polycomb group protein, enhancer of Zeste homolog 2 (EZH2), was found to target DNMTs to EZH2-repressed genes [16]. Finally, small RNA molecules have been implicated in DNMT targeting [3].

Transcriptional repression by DNA methylation is achieved by various modes of action. In one such mechanism, DNA methylation simply inhibits the binding of a transcription factor [17]. By a more complex means of action, a number of DNA methyl-binding proteins potentiate transcriptional silencing. In some cases, binding is accompanied by the action of an associated histone-modifying enzyme.

For example, one DNA methyl-binding protein, MBD1, associates with SET domain bifurcated 1 (SETDB1), a histone methyltransferase (HMT). During DNA replication, SETDB1 associates with MBD1 in addition to chromatin assembly factor-1 and catalyzes methylation of histone H3 at lysine 9. Trimethylation at H3K9 is associated with heterochromatin [18]. A second example that links DNA methylation to a histone modification state involves PML-RARα [19]. MBD1 can form a repressor complex with N-CoR, DNMTs, HDAC3 and PML-RARα to silence PML-RARα-dependent promoters. This aberrant gene silencing is manifested by HDAC-mediated histone deacetylation, DNA methylation, as well as time-dependent spreading of MBD1 outside of the promoter region. The spreading of MBD1 along regions of methylated DNA is thought to recruit additional repressor enzymes [19].

1.3
Histone Modifications and the Histone Code Hypothesis

A vibrant area in epigenetic research involves covalent modifications of histones [20]. The most commonly observed histone modifications include acetylation, methylation and phosphorylation. However, other modifications such as citrullination, ubiquitination, SUMOlyation, prolyl isomerization, ADP-ribosylation and biotinylation are being increasingly recognized. These modifications are primarily located on the unstructured N-terminal tails of histones (Figure 1.1), yet an increasing number of modifications in the α-helical histone fold domains have been documented. In this chapter, we limit our detailed discussion to histone acetylation and methylation. One interpretation of the epigenetic consequences of histone modification is the histone code hypothesis, which predicts that combinatorial histone modification states result in unique biological outcomes [21]. This molecular "code" is regulated by alteration of histone–histone interactions, histone–DNA interactions and histone–nonhistone protein interactions. While there is some dispute whether each histone modification state results in a unique downstream function, it is generally agreed that histone modifications can lead to differences in binding and selectivity and that these differences can propagate a variety of epigenetic outcomes.

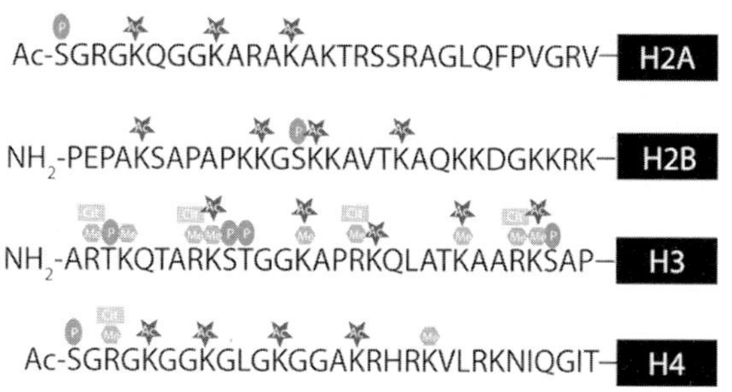

Ac-SGRGKQGGKARAKAKTRSSRAGLQFPVGRV- H2A
NH2-PEPAKSAPAPKKGSKKAVTKAQKKDGKKRK- H2B
NH2-ARTKQTARKSTGGKAPRKQLATKAARKSAP- H3
Ac-SGRGKGGKGLGKGGAKRHRKVLRKNIQGIT- H4

Figure 1.1 PTMs found on the first 30 residues of the human histone proteins. Only acetylation, methylation, deimination (formation of citrulline) and phosphorylation are shown.

A number of strategies have emerged for characterizing histone modifications and understanding their significance. The workhorses of histone modification mapping have been modification-specific antibodies and mass spectrometry [20] (see the requisite chapters in this book for more details). In the ChIP on chip approach, DNA is crosslinked to DNA-binding proteins, digested and immunoprecipitated with an antibody for the histone modification of interest. Following PCR amplification of the associated DNA, the histone modification can be linked to particular gene regions using microarray technology. This methodology was used extensively in a large-scale human and mouse epigenome study [22]. While this method was extremely powerful for mapping locations of histone modification on genes, it is limited by the specificity of available antibodies and cannot be used to determine the modification status of histones within the same nucleosome. Mass spectrometry, in contrast, is capable of determining the modification status of individual histone proteins. A recent study identified 74 unique histone H4 modification patterns in differentiating human embryonic stem cells [23]. Several chemically driven strategies have found utility in studying the effects of histone posttranslational modifications. For example, native chemical ligation/expressed protein ligation [24–26], chemical incorporation of methyl-lysine mimetics [27] and genetic incorporation of modified amino acids (such as acetyl lysine) [28] have enabled the generation of site-specifically modified histones. In one study employing semisynthetic histones, acetylation of H4K16 was shown to modulate chromatin compaction and its ability to form cross-fiber interactions [25]. Recently, we developed a method for assaying the specificity of enzymes and proteins that read the histone modification patterns using combinatorial peptide libraries based on the modification patterns of N-terminal histone tails [29].

Reversible lysine acetylation of histones is regulated by the opposing activity of histone acetyltransferases (HATs) and histone deacetylases (HDACs). Acetylation of the lysine ε-amino group results in neutralization of a positive charge, while deacetylation reestablishes the presence of a primary amine. Hypoacetylation typically facilitates formation of highly condensed chromatin (heterochromatin) and transcriptional repression, while hyperacetylation tracks with chromatin that is more "loosely" associated with DNA (euchromatin) and transcriptional activity. HATs employ an acetyl-CoA cofactor, operate in large multiprotein complexes and can be classified as members of the GNAT, MYST or CBP/p300 families of enzymes [30]. However, a recently identified HAT in yeast, Rtt109, appears to belong to an entirely different family due to lack of homology with other HATs [31]. HDACs are responsible for the removal of acetyl groups from histone lysines. These protein deacetylases are categorized as class I, II, III and IV HDACs [32]. Class I, II and IV HDACs are metal-dependent acetyl hydrolases that yield acetate as a product. Class III HDACs, or sirtuins, utilize an NAD^+ cofactor and couple deacetylation with the formation of *O*-acetyl-ADP-ribose (*O*AADPr) and nicotinamide. Sirtuins have been postulated to link epigenetics to metabolic processes and act on a number of nonhistone proteins [33].

Reversible histone methylation is a highly specific process that is catalyzed by the action of histone methyltransferases (HMTs) and histone demethylases on lysine and arginine residues. Like DNMTs, HMTs employ a SAM cofactor. Lysine can be mono-, di- or trimethylated and arginine can be monomethylated and symmetrically or asymmetrically dimethylated. The consequences of histone methylation appear to be largely context-dependent. For example, trimethylation of H3K4 is a mark of transcriptionally active chromatin, while trimethylation of H3K9 tracks with transcriptionally repressive chromatin. Lysine HMTs are divided into the SET and Dot1 families [30]. Members of the SET family contain a SET domain and representative examples include mixed-lineage leukemia (MLL) and EZH2 proteins, which are specific for methylation of H3K4 and H3K27, respectively. Dot1 lacks a SET domain and is responsible for mono- and dimethylation of H3K79 [30]. Protein arginine methyltransferases (PRMTs) usually act on glycine-arginine-rich regions within their substrates. Following N^{ω}-monomethylation, type I PRMTs can catalyze a subsequent methylation on the same atom (asymmetric dimethylation), while type II PRMTs methylate the other ω-nitrogen (symmetric dimethylation) [30].

The discovery of LSD1, the first histone demethylase to be characterized, invalidated the notion that histone methylation was a permanent mark [34]. LSD1 is an FAD-dependent amine oxidase that catalyzes mono- and di- demethylation of H3K4. Interestingly, a byproduct of LSD1 catalyzed demethylation, hydrogen peroxide, is thought to link local DNA oxidation to estrogen-induced gene expression [35]. The Jumonji C (JmjC) hydroxylases, another class of histone demethylases, require iron and α-ketoglutarate and produce formaldehyde as a byproduct. While LSD1 only demethylates mono- and dimethyl lysine residues in proteins, members of the JmjC family such as JMJD2A and JARID1A are specific for di- and trimethyl lysines. JMJD6 demethylates both symmetric and asymmetric arginine to their monomethylated counterparts at H3R2 and H4R3 [36]. Protein arginine deiminases (PADs) have been suggested to catalyze methylated arginines demethylimination to furnish citrulline [37], yet *in vitro* evidence for this transformation suggests that methylarginine is a very poor substrate, if at all [38]. Further studies are needed to resolve these issues. Deimination of arginine to citrulline, however, has been widely characterized [39]. Currently, there is no evidence that protein deimination is a reversible modification. See the relevant chapters of this book for more information on reversible histone aceylation and methylation.

1.4
Origins of Specificity in Histone Binding Proteins/Modifying Enzymes

The primary readers of the histone code are histone binding domains (HBDs). HBDs are often found in histone-modifying enzymes, ATP-dependent chromatin remodeling factors and transcription factors. In this chapter, we focus on domains with the ability to recognize acetylation and methylation. The observation that bromodomains function as histone acetyl-lysine binding modules [40] set the stage for discovery of a number of specialized HBDs. The specificity of the these binding modules appear to be dictated by both the type of modification and the context of the modified amino acid [41]. For example, although both heterochromatin protein 1 (HP1) and polycomb protein PC2 both contain chromodomains (methyl-lysine binding modules), the former binds trimethylated H3K9 while the latter binds trimethylated H3K27 despite an identical sequence surrounding each lysine (ARKS). The binding specificity is achieved by means of an extended recognition groove in polycomb that recognizes residues 20–24 [42]. Another mechanism for discriminating among potential binding partners is by the extent of a particular modification state (e.g. mono-, di- or trimethylation).

Bromodomains, which are composed of approximately 110 amino acids, fold into a left-handed antiparallel four-helix bundle. They contain a hydrophobic tunnel, which accommodates binding of acetylated lysine. Relative to other histone binding domains, bromodomains are promiscuous with regard to the sequence to which they bind and typically have dissociation constants in the $\sim$50–350 μM range [2]. These targeting modules are frequently found in HATs. It has been suggested that bromodomains enable a mechanism whereby HATs can propagate acetylation along a histone or a nucleosome. Other proteins that harbor bromodomains include members of the HMT family and ATP-dependent remodeling enzymes. One such example, the SWI/SNF ATP-dependent remodeling complex employs a bromodomain to associate with acetylated promoter nucleosomes [43]. Using the energy liberated from ATP hydrolysis, the SWI/SNF complex mobilizes nucleosomes. The bromodomain binding activity of SWI/SNF is essential for displacing the SAGA HAT complex, as well as facilitating octamer transfer on H3-acetylated nucleosomes [44].

The tudor domain royal superfamily includes the chromodomain, double chromodomain, chromo barrel, tudor, double/tandem tudor and MBT domains [45, 46]. Tudor and chromo domains bind to di- and trimethylated lysine while MBT domains prefer mono- and dimethylated lysine. Tudor domains are also capable of recognizing symmetrically dimethylated arginine. Increasing lysine methylation results in reduced hydrogen bonding potential and solvation properties, as well as greater hydrophobicity and a larger cation radius. Because many methyl binding modules engage in cation-π interactions [46], the degree of methylation is critical in conferring specificity. Domains that preferentially bind to higher lysine methylation states can accommodate a diffuse and hydrophobic cation. In contrast, hydrogen bonding and steric exclusion are dominant factors in regulating specificity for lower methylation states (or unmethylated lysine) [46]. It was noted that the chromodomain of HP1 binds specifically to di- and trimethylated H3K9. HP1 recognizes methylation catalyzed by the action of the suppressor of variegation 3–9 homologue 1 (SUV39H1) methyltransferase [30]. Structural analysis revealed that a H3K9 trimethylated histone peptide was immobilized in an induced β-strand sandwich with the protein [46]. Since the original HP1 structures, a similar induced β-strand fit was observed for the interaction between other methyl-recognizing proteins and their methylated peptide binding partners. An example of a double tudor domain is that of the histone demethylase and transcriptional repressor, JMJD2A. The JMJD2A double tudor domain preferentially binds to di- and trimethylated H3K4 and H4K20 [47–49].

With regard to specificity, plant homeodomain (PHD) fingers constitute the most diverse class of histone binding modules. These modules recognize lysine in unmodified, mono-, di- and trimethylated states. Although not structurally related,

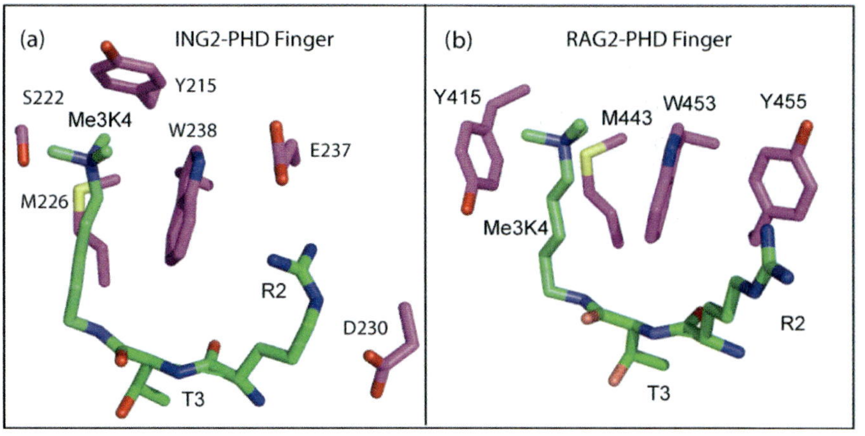

Figure 1.2 Structural comparison of (a) the ING2 [50] (PDB entry 2G6Q) and (b) the RAG2 [52] (PDB entry 2V89) PHD fingers bound to H3 peptides. The ING2-PHD finger binds Me_3K4 in an "aromatic cage," which is adjacent to an R2 binding pocket comprised of W238, E237 and D230. In the RAG2-PHD finger structure, Me_3K4 is enclosed in an "aromatic tunnel," while R2 is splayed outward due to the presence of Y455 and lack of a hydrogen bonding partner.

PHD fingers do share a few salient features with members of the tudor domain royal superfamily: most engage methyllysine through cation-π interactions and induce their peptide binding partners to adopt a complementary β-strand [46]. One of the first PHD fingers to be biochemically and structurally enumerated was that of inhibitor of growth 2 (ING2) [50]. ING2 is a member of the mSin3a-HDAC1 complex and, in response to DNA damage, stabilizes this complex at promoters of proliferation genes via interaction with trimethylated H3K4 [51]. The ING2-PHD finger binds trimethylated lysine by virtue of a two-residue aromatic cage. One of these residues, W238, forms the boundary for an adjacent groove to the H3K4 binding site that accommodates H3R2, which interacts with D230 and E237 (Figure 1.2). A homologous tryptophan has been observed in almost all methyl-binding PHD fingers characterized to date. Unlike the ING2-PHD finger, the RAG2-PHD finger (another trimethylated H3K4 binding module) binds in a conformation in which R2 is twisted out of plane with K4 [52, 53]. Interestingly, this difference in orientation and lack of interaction with a carboxylate permits methylation of R2 without a defect in binding. In fact, it has been suggested that symmetric dimethylation of R2 yields a very modest increase in affinity for peptides trimethylated at H3K4 – an added level of sophistication for the histone code reading capacity of the RAG2-PHD finger [53]. Furthermore, unlike the ING2-PHD finger, the RAG2-PHD finger does not engage trimethylated H3K4 in an aromatic cage (aromatic residues above and adjacent to the quaternary amine) but rather in what is dubbed an "aromatic tunnel" (aromatic residues are only adjacent to the quaternary amine; Figure 1.2). Functional evidence demonstrates that binding at trimethylated H3K4 by the RAG2-PHD finger is necessary for V(D)J recombination *in vivo* [52]. This finding provided the first evidence for involvement of H3K4 trimethylation in a process other than regulation of gene expression. Interestingly, a W453R mutation in the RAG2-PHD finger disrupts this interaction [52] and results in Omenn's syndrome, a rare human immunodeficiency. In contrast to both the ING2 and RAG2-PHD fingers, the PHD finger of BHC80, a member of the LSD1 co-repressor complex, shows a preference for unmethylated H3K4 [54]. Binding of unmethylated H3K4 by the BHC80-PHD finger is characterized by an electrostatic interaction and hydrogen bonding in addition to steric exclusion of methyl groups. Also, unlike the RAG2 and ING2 PHD fingers, the BHC80-PHD finger-induced β-strand extends to R8 of a histone H3 peptide. Binding activity of the BHC80-PHD finger is essential for LSD1-mediated gene repression and appears to function downstream of H3K4 demethylation by retaining LSD1 at target promoters [54]. A recent study revealed that the autoimmune regulator (AIRE)-PHD finger also recognizes unmethylated lysine and links this process to transcription of tissue-restricted antigens [55].

Perhaps most intriguing are proteins capable of reading a histone code with multiple histone binding domains. Multivalent engagement results in a more favorable Gibbs free energy (ΔG) of binding relative to monovalent association. This is because multivalent binding increases the heat liberated upon association (enthalpy) with minimal entropic penalty due to pre-organization of the domains [2]. An example of a protein that utilizes multiple domains for histone binding is TAF1 (formerly $TAF_{II}250$), the largest subunit of the TFIID complex, which is responsible for initiation of transcription. In this protein, the binding pockets of two bromodomains are separated by ~25 Å, making them ideally situated to simultaneously recognize and bind acetylated lysines 5 and 12 or 8 and 16 of histone H4 [56] (Figure 1.3). H4 peptides diacetylated at these positions bind ~28 and ~7 times more

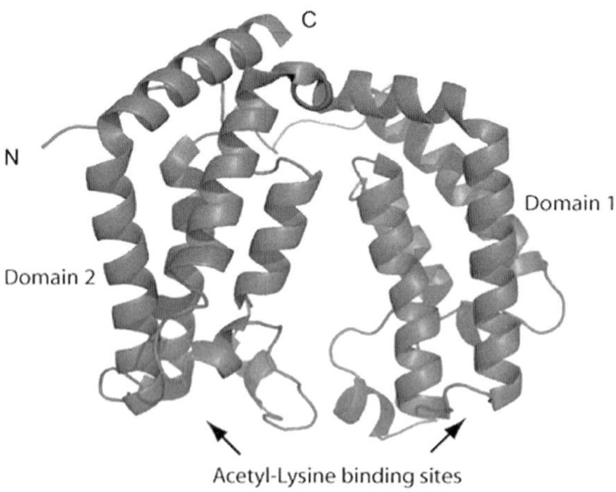

Figure 1.3 Structure of double bromodomain of TAF1 [56] (PDB entry 1EQF). Because the TAF1 bromodomains are separated by ~25 Å, they are proposed to simultaneously bind acetylated lysines 5 and 12 or 8 and 16 of histone H4.

tightly (respectively) than a peptide monoacetylated at lysine 16. A second example of a histone binding protein with the potential for combinatorial histone code reading is the bromodomain and PHD domain transcription factor (BPTF), the largest subunit of the ATP-dependent chromatin remodeling complex, nucleosome remodeling factor (NURF) [57]. BPTF is of particular interest because it bears two different histone-reading modules: a bromodomain and a PHD finger domain, which are appended by an α-helical linker. The PHD finger binds di- and trimethylated H3K4 but the role of the bromodomain is unclear. Recognition of H3K4 by the BPTF subunit may be involved in NURF-mediated ATP-dependent chromatin remodeling and *Hox* gene expression during development [58]. While TAF1 and BPTF are individual proteins with the capacity to recognize dual covalent histone modifications, the yeast Rpd3S HDAC complex contains two proteins with domains that collaborate to recognize methylated H3K36 [59]. The Rpd3S HDAC complex is responsible for suppressing cryptic initiation of transcription within coding regions of a gene by histone deacetylation. This is achieved when the Rpd3S complex is targeted to active sites of transcription by association of the chromodomain of the Eaf3 subunit and the PHD finger of the Rco1 subunit with methylated H3K36. In this cooperative binding event, the Rco1-PHD finger is primarily responsible for providing affinity for nucleosomes, while the Eaf3 chromodomain contributes specificity for the methylated H3K36 mark [59, 60]. These examples demonstrate how multiple domains can cooperate to read a histone code with high fidelity and enhanced affinity.

1.5
Histone Modification Cross-talk

The crux of the histone code is manifested by a variety of cross-regulation or "cross-talk" mechanisms, which serve to regulate the activities of histone binding proteins/modifying enzymes [61]. The most obvious form of regulation is the mutual exclusivity of some modifications. For example, a di- or trimethylated lysine residue cannot be acetylated by a HAT. The occurrence of regularly spaced modifiable amino acids on histones can facilitate antagonistic or agonistic effects on the activities of histone binding proteins/modifying enzymes. An intriguing example involves the interplay between asymmetric trimethylation of H3R2 and trimethylation of H3K4 [62–64] (Figure 1.4). A quantitative chromatin immunoprecipitation study revealed that while H3K4 trimethylation occurs at the 5′ region of actively transcribed genes, asymmetric dimethylation of H3R2 is found within the body of genes or at inactive promoters in a mutually exclusive manner [62]. After identifying PRMT6 as the methyltransferase responsible for asymmetric methylation of R2 *in vivo*, Guccione *et al.* demonstrated that immunoprecipitated PRMT6 can methylate an unmodified H3 peptide but not an H3K4 trimethylated version [63]. An ASH2/WDR5/MLL family methyltransferase complex, which is responsible for H3K4 trimethylation *in vivo*, can methylate an unmodified H3 peptide, but does not tolerate asymmetric dimethylation at R2. This finding was ascribed to

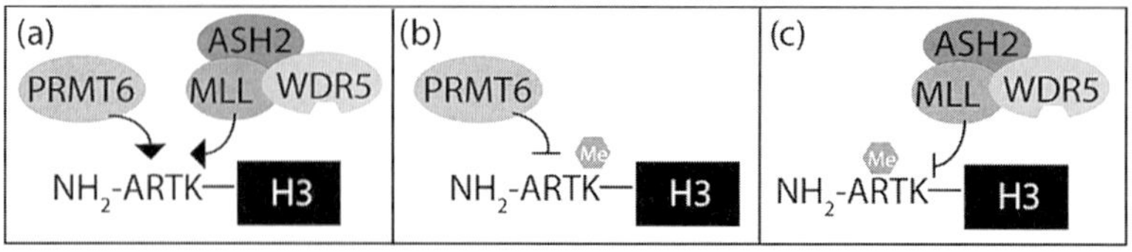

Figure 1.4 Example of histone cross-talk on histone H3. PRMT6 and the ASH2/WDR5/MLL complex are capable of methylation of H3R2 and H3K4, respectively (a). PRMT6 cannot methylate R2 in the presence of H3K4 trimethylation (b). Asymmetric dimethylation of R2 prevents interaction of WDR5 with the H3 tail and subsequent methylation by the MLL complex (c). Trimethylation of H3K4 is a hallmark of active promoters, while asymmetric dimethylation of H3R2 is typically associated with inactive promoters.

disruption of binding of the WDR5-WD40 repeats with H3K4 when H3R2 was dimethylated, a previously observed interaction [46]. A similar study in yeast found that trimethylation of H3K4 by the Set1 methyltransferase complex was abrogated in the presence of asymmetrically dimethylated H3R2. Ablation of enzymatic activity was attributed to disruption of the interaction of the Spp1-PHD finger with H3K4, a component of the Set1 complex that is necessary for trimethylation [64]. These studies reveal how modification cross-talk can be leveraged to achieve transcriptional regulation.

A recent study illustrates the complex interplay of histone modifications in regulation of the interaction with the transcription factor, TFIID [65]. The TFIID complex, which consists of several subunits, is involved in initiation of transcription. Genome-wide surveys [22, 66] revealed that TAF1, the largest TFIID subunit, was frequently found in regions with high distributions of H3K4 trimethylation as well as H3K9 and H3K14 acetylation. Using a quantitative mass spectrometry approach, Vermeulen *et al.* discovered that selective anchoring of TFIID to the nucleosome was facilitated in a trimethylated H3K4-dependent manner [65]. This was ascribed to interaction of the TAF3-PHD finger with trimethylated H3K4. *In vitro* binding assays with H3 peptides revealed that the TAF3-PHD finger has ~10-fold increased affinity for trimethylated H3K4 relative to dimethylated H3K4. Furthermore, asymmetric dimethylation of H3R2 resulted in a >25-fold loss in binding affinity for peptides that were trimethylated at H3K4. Interestingly, acetylation of H3K9 and H3K14 enhanced the affinity of TFIID for H3K4 trimethylated peptides in a pull-down assay. Vermeulen *et al.* suggest that the stronger interaction is due to the combined binding of the TAF3-PHD finger and the TAF1 tandem bromodomain. However, the superior affinity of the TAF3-PHD finger for trimethylated H3K4 is thought to be the dominant driving force behind the interaction. In support of this hypothesis, ablation of the PHD finger interaction reduced the mRNA levels of a variety of genes [65].

The examples of cross-talk in the histone code noted thus far involve events occurring on a single histone, or *in cis*. Cross-talk also occurs *in trans*, that is, between histone molecules. A good example of histone cross-talk *in trans* involves the link between H2B monoubiquitination at H2BK120 (H2BK123 in *Saccharomyces cerevisiae*) and methylation at H3K4 and H3K79, both of which are hallmarks of transcriptionally poised chromatin. During transcription in budding yeast, mono-ubiquitination of H2B precedes di- and trimethylation of H3K4 and trimethylation of H3K79 [61]. Mechanistic insight for the requirement of H2B ubiquitination came with the recent discovery that ubiquitination of H2BK123 in yeast mediates interaction with Cps35, a subunit necessary for the H3K4 methyltransferase activity of COMPASS, the yeast homology of the MLL complex [67]. Interestingly, monomethylation of these residues is not linked to ubiquitination of H2B [68, 69]. Another instance that highlights cross-talk *in trans* involves the activity of UTX, a JmjC-domain containing protein. UTX mediates H3K27 demethylation, which is linked to H3K4 trimethylation and downregulation of H2A ubiquitination [70, 71]. During retinoic acid signaling, a UTX/MLL complex is recruited to *HOX* genes and facilitates transcription by methylating H3K4 and demethylating H3K27. Demethylation of H3K27 blocks chromodomain-mediated interaction with polycomb repressive complexes (PRCs) and subsequent ubiquitination of H2A. The combined action enables transcription of *HOX* genes.

1.6
Inhibitors of DNMTs and HDACs

Because proper epigenetic regulation is essential for normal functioning of the genome, there is burgeoning interest in the development of drugs that target epigenetic misregulation. A dynamic epigenetic model for complex disease suggests that a pre-epimutation (epigenetic occurrence that predisposes one to disease) is compounded by a variety of factors that occur over time [72]. These factors may include the effects of tissue differentiation, hormones and environment. The model predicts that a critical threshold is reached at some point and this results in a disease phenotype. Most studies of epigenetic misregulation involve its role in carcinogenesis and tumor progression. Increasing evidence suggests that epigenetic dysfunction is associated with several types of cancer [72]. Unlike genetic information, epigenetic marks are potentially reversible and therefore represent an opportunity to ameliorate the disease phenotype.

Aberrant DNA methylation can be manifested in two ways: genome-wide hypomethylation and promoter-specific hypermethylation. Genomic hypomethylation is associated with instability as well as the formation of abnormal chromosome structures [1]. In contrast, promoter-specific hypermethylation leads to transcriptional inactivation of genes (notably tumor suppressors). Examples of genes inactivated by inappropriate DNA methylation include those of the cell cycle inhibitor, $p16^{INK4a}$, and the DNA repair proteins BRCA1 and hMLH1 [73]. Because aberrant DNA hypermethylation is often associated with cancer, there have been significant efforts to develop therapeutic agents to target DNMTs. Small molecule inhibitors of DNMTs fall into two classes: nucleoside analogs and non-nucleoside analogs (Figure 1.5). Nucleoside analogs are cytidine mimics that become phosphorylated and incorporated into DNA and/or RNA once inside the cell. These molecules function as irreversible inhibitors in which a covalent DNMT intermediate is trapped

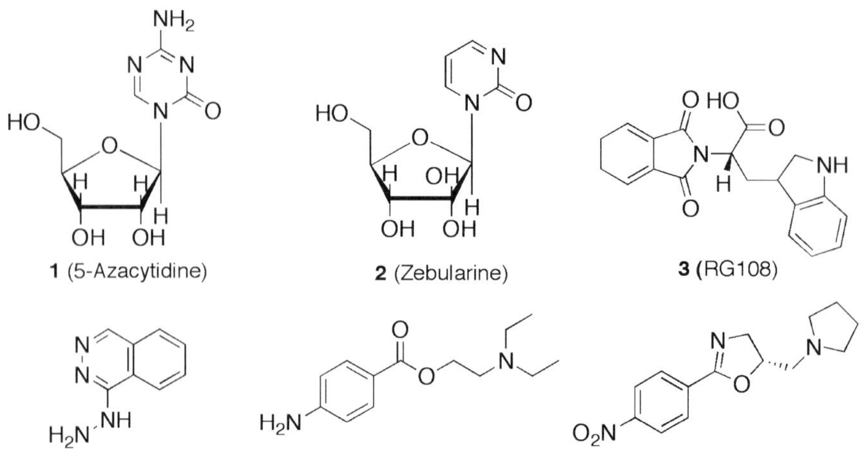

1 (5-Azacytidine) **2** (Zebularine) **3** (RG108)

4 (Hydralazine) **5** (Procaine) **6**

Figure 1.5 Selected small molecule inhibitors of DNMTs. **1** and **2** are irreversible nucleoside inhibitors while **3**, **4**, **5** and **6** are reversible small molecule inhibitors.

at the 6-position of the cytosine ring. In the case of 5-azacytidine (5-Aza-CR; **1**), β-elimination cannot release the DNMT intermediate due to the absence of an acidic hydrogen atom at the 5-position. Zebularine (**2**), which lacks an exocyclic amino group at the 4-position of the ring, does not undergo β-elimination for reasons that are not completely understood. Unfortunately, nucleoside analogs are frequently pleiotropic, often exhibit significant toxicity and have limited stability in aqueous solution. Although zebularine is stable in aqueous solution, it has poor bioavailability [74]. It is unclear whether the effects of nucleoside analog inhibitors are due to decreasing DNA methylation or DNMT depletion [72].

Due to the limitations of nucleoside-mimic DNMT inhibitors, there is considerable interest in developing non-nucleoside inhibitors. For example, RG108 (**3**), a phthaloyl tryptophan derivative was identified in a small molecule screen as a DNMT1 active site inhibitor [75]. RG108 inhibits methyltransferase activity *in vitro* and reduces global methylation levels in human cancer cells [76]. Hydralazine (**4**), a vasodilating drug, is reported to inhibit DNA methylation [77]. Surprisingly, in a recent Phase I study, hydralazine reactivated tumor suppressor genes in cervical cancer patients without altering global methylation levels [78]. Treatment with procaine (**5**), an anesthetic drug, afforded a 40% decrease in cystosine methylation in MCF-7 breast cancer cells [79]. However, *in vitro*, procaine does not exhibit DNMT inhibitory activity [76]. Recently, constrained analogs of the procaine scaffold were developed to increase potency [80]. One pyrrolidine derivative of procaine (**6**) exhibited modest inhibitory activity against DNMT1, but did not appear to decrease global DNA methylation levels in human myeloid leukemia cells relative to treatment with procaine [80]. Natural products such as psammaplin A and

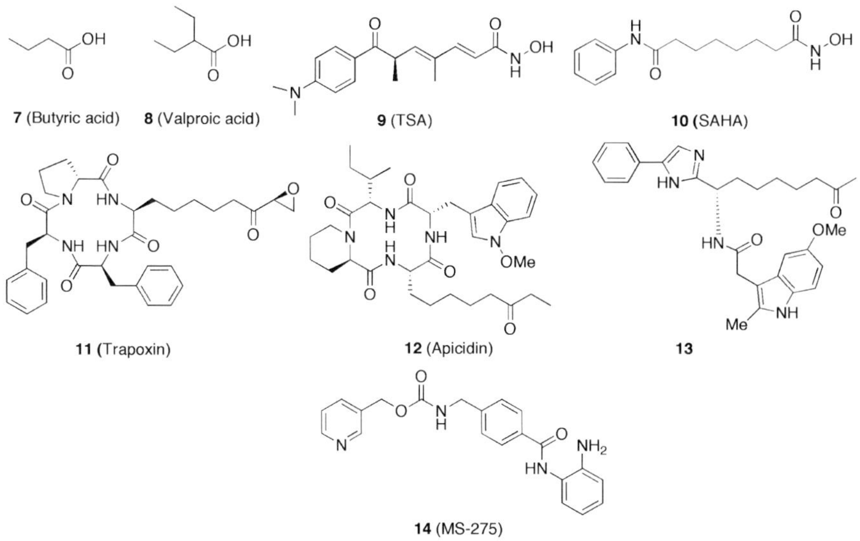

Figure 1.6 Selected small molecule inhibitors of HDACs. Compounds **7** and **8** are short-chain fatty acids, compounds **9** and **10** are hydroxamic acids, compounds **11** and **12** are cyclic tetrapeptides, compound **13** is cyclic tetrapeptide analog and compound **14** is a benzamide.

(−)-epigallocatechin-3-gallate (EGCG) are being evaluated as DNMT inhibitors [1]. Finally, MG98, an antisense oligonucleotide designed to repress expression of *DNMT1* has shown mixed results in clinical trials [72].

HDACs represent another class of epigenetic therapeutic targets. As with aberrant DNA methylation, inappropriate HDAC activity is linked to transcriptional misregulation. At the cellular level, HDAC inhibitors facilitate apoptosis of tumor cells and may control host immune responses and tumor vasculature [32]. To date, the Zn^{2+}-dependent Class I and II HDACs have received the most attention. Inhibitors of Class I and II HDACs include short-chain fatty acids, hydroxamic acids, benzamides and cyclic tetrapeptides [1] (Figure 1.6). Short-chain fatty acids such as butyrate (**7**) and valproic acid (**8**) were the first HDAC inhibitors to be identified. However, these compounds elicit inhibition in the millimolar range, suffer from poor bioavailability and are non-specific. Hydroxamic acids such as the natural product, trichostatin A (TSA) (**9**) and suberoyl anilide hydroxamic acid (SAHA; also known as Vorinostat and Zolinza) (**10**) are among the most successful HDAC inhibitors. TSA is a low-nanomolar Class I and II HDAC inhibitor that antagonizes the growth of non-small-cell lung cancer (NSCLC) at micromolar concentrations [81]. While SAHA is ~30-fold less potent than TSA as an HDAC inhibitor, it has had considerable therapeutic success [72]. SAHA has shown anticancer activity in Phase I studies of refractory hematologic and solid tumors and a partial response in Phase II refractory cutaneous T cell lymphoma (CTCL) studies. Recently, SAHA received FDA approval for the treatment of CTCL-induced skin lesions [72]. The therapeutic success of

SAHA may be due to its ability to inhibit multiple HDACs with moderate efficiency. Cocrystal structures of the HDAC core with TSA and SAHA have been useful in dissecting the molecular details that confer HDAC inhibition [82]. In these structures, the inhibitors coordinate to an active site zinc and engage in a series of hydrogen bonds via their hydroxamic acid moieties. The hydroxamic acids are tethered to an aromatic capping group by an aliphatic linker that participates in multiple van der Waals contacts throughout a tubular pocket. The identity of the capping group appears to confer specificity. For example, HDAC6 is not inhibited by compounds with cyclic tetrapeptide capping groups [30].

Cyclic tetrapeptide natural products such as trapoxin (**11**) and apicidin (**12**) are potent HDAC inhibitors. Trapoxin is an irreversible inhibitor that features an electrophilic α-epoxyketone linked to a peptide capping group. Apicidin, in contrast, exploits an ethyl ketone as its zinc-binding group. Apicidin shows antiproliferative activity against a variety of cancer cell lines by a mechanism that appears to involve induction of the $p21^{WAF1/Cip1}$ gene [72]. Recently, nonpeptidic analogs of apicidin were developed to improve potency and selectivity in HDAC inhibition [83, 84]. A 4-phenylimidazole derivative (**13**) with a methyl ketone zinc-binding group selectively inhibits HDACs 1, 2, 3 (IC_{50} values ~100 nM) and HDAC 6 (IC_{50} ~300 nM). HDACs 4, 5, 7 are not inhibited by **13** at levels as high as 10 μM. The 4-phenylimidazole derivative displayed submicromolar IC_{50} antiproliferation activity against cervical, colon and kidney cell lines [84]. This compound also inhibits tumor growth in a xenograft model.

Benzamides constitute a fourth class of HDAC inhibitors. One example, MS-275, is a phenylenediamine derivative that exhibits robust HDAC inhibition in patients with advanced myeloid leukemia as well as refractory solid tumors or lymphoma in Phase I studies [72]. MS-275 is currently in Phase II trials. In a recent study aimed at optimizing the benzamide scaffold, several bis-(aryl) type analogs were synthesized and evaluated for their activity against a panel of HDACs [85]. Moradei *et al.* found that a thienyl substitution para to the free amino group in the phenylenediamine core rendered inhibitors specific for HDACs1, 2 with potency superior to that of MS-275. Isoform-specific inhibitors should aid in dissecting the roles of HDACs in normal cellular functioning and cancer.

What does the future hold for pharmacological epigenetic modulators? While there will undoubtedly be improvements in HDAC and DNMT inhibitor design, there is increasing interest in using epigenetic modulators in combination therapy (e.g. to sensitize tumors to cytotoxic agents or radiation) [72]. HDAC and DNMT inhibitors might be used together to achieve gene reactivation. Combination therapy has had some success in the case of patients with myelodysplastic syndrome and acute myeloid leukemia (AML) [86]. Another direction in epigenetic drug discovery might be to target interactions between histone binding modules and their cognate binding partners. There have already been reports of small molecules that block the interaction between bromodomains and nonhistone proteins such as HIV-1 Tat [87, 88] and p53 [89]. Further study of the biological modes of action of epigenetic modulators and the continued identification of new epigenetic biomarkers will be essential.

1.7 Conclusions

In this postgenomic era, the ultimate step in understanding how genotype translates to phenotype will require unraveling the language of epigenetics. This pursuit will involve the development and implementation of new technologies to map the epigenome with increasing resolution as well as improving our understanding of the dynamic interplay that represents the histone code. Deciphering the molecular basis for epigenetic regulation will facilitate the development of new drugs and therapies and provide a fertile area of research for years to come.

Acknowledgments

We thank Josh Coon for helpful comments. Epigenetic research in the Denu laboratory is supported by NIH grants GM065386 and GM059785.

References

1 Yoo, C.B. and Jones, P.A. (2006) Epigenetic therapy of cancer: past, present and future. *Nature Reviews. Drug Discovery*, **5**, 37–50.

2 Ruthenburg, A.J., Li, H., Patel, D.J. and Allis, C.D. (2007) Multivalent engagement of chromatin modifications by linked binding modules. *Nature Reviews. Molecular Cell Biology*, **8**, 983–994.

3 Klose, R.J. and Bird, A.P. (2006) Genomic DNA methylation: the mark and its mediators. *Trends in Biochemical Sciences*, **31**, 89–97.

4 Hsieh, C.L. (1997) Stability of patch methylation and its impact in regions of transcriptional initiation and elongation. *Molecular and Cellular Biology*, **17**, 5897–5904.

5 Lorincz, M.C., Dickerson, D.R., Schmitt, M. and Groudine, M. (2004) Intragenic DNA methylation alters chromatin structure and elongation efficiency in mammalian cells. *Nature Structural & Molecular Biology*, **11**, 1068–1075.

6 Bourc'his, D., Xu, G.L., Lin, C.S., Bollman, B. and Bestor, T.H. (2001) Dnmt3L and the establishment of maternal genomic imprints. *Science*, **294**, 2536–2539.

7 Bourc'his, D. and Bestor, T.H. (2004) Meiotic catastrophe and retrotransposon reactivation in male germ cells lacking Dnmt3L. *Nature*, **431**, 96–99.

8 Ooi, S.K. *et al.* (2007) DNMT3L connects unmethylated lysine 4 of histone H3 to de novo methylation of DNA. *Nature*, **448**, 714–717.

9 Chuang, L.S., Ian, H.I., Koh, T.W., Ng, H.H., Xu, G. and Li, B.F. (1997) Human DNA-(cytosine-5) methyltransferase-PCNA complex as a target for p21WAF1. *Science*, **277**, 1996–2000.

10 Bostick, M., Kim, J.K., Esteve, P.O., Clark, A., Pradhan, S. and Jacobsen, S.E. (2007) UHRF1 plays a role in maintaining DNA methylation in mammalian cells. *Science*, **317**, 1760–1764.

11 Sharif, J. *et al.* (2007) The SRA protein Np95 mediates epigenetic inheritance by recruiting Dnmt1 to methylated DNA. *Nature*, **450**, 908–912.

12 Unoki, M., Nishidate, T. and Nakamura, Y. (2004) ICBP90, an E2F-1 target, recruits

HDAC1 and binds to methyl-CpG through its SRA domain. *Oncogene*, **23**, 7601–7610.
13 Qiu, C., Sawada, K., Zhang, X. and Cheng, X. (2002) The PWWP domain of mammalian DNA methyltransferase Dnmt3b defines a new family of DNA-binding folds. *Nature Structural Biology*, **9**, 217–224.
14 Ge, Y.Z., Pu, M.T., Gowher, H., Wu, H.P., Ding, J.P., Jeltsch, A. and Xu, G.L. (2004) Chromatin targeting of de novo DNA methyltransferases by the PWWP domain. *The Journal of Biological Chemistry*, **279**, 25447–25454.
15 Di Croce, L. *et al.* (2002) Methyltransferase recruitment and DNA hypermethylation of target promoters by an oncogenic transcription factor. *Science*, **295**, 1079–1082.
16 Vire, E. *et al.* (2006) The Polycomb group protein EZH2 directly controls DNA methylation. *Nature*, **439**, 871–874.
17 Watt, F. and Molloy, P.L. (1988) Cytosine methylation prevents binding to DNA of a HeLa cell transcription factor required for optimal expression of the adenovirus major late promoter. *Genes and Development*, **2**, 1136–1143.
18 Sarraf, S.A. and Stancheva, I. (2004) Methyl-CpG binding protein MBD1 couples histone H3 methylation at lysine 9 by SETDB1 to DNA replication and chromatin assembly. *Molecular Cell*, **15**, 595–605.
19 Villa, R. *et al.* (2006) The methyl-CpG binding protein MBD1 is required for PML-RARalpha function. *Proceedings of the National Academy of Sciences of the United States of America*, **103**, 1400–1405.
20 Kouzarides, T. (2007) Chromatin modifications and their function. *Cell*, **128**, 693–705.
21 Strahl, B.D. and Allis, C.D. (2000) The language of covalent histone modifications. *Nature*, **403**, 41–45.
22 Bernstein, B.E. *et al.* (2005) Genomic maps and comparative analysis of histone modifications, in human and mouse. *Cell*, **120**, 169–181.
23 Phanstiel, D. *et al.* (2008) Mass spectrometry identifies and quantifies 74 unique histone H4 isoforms in differentiating human embryonic stem cells. *Proceedings of the National Academy of Sciences of the United States of America*, **105**, 4093–4098.
24 He, S. *et al.* (2003) Facile synthesis of site-specifically acetylated and methylated histone proteins: reagents for evaluation of the histone code hypothesis. *Proceedings of the National Academy of Sciences of the United States of America*, **100**, 12033–12038.
25 Shogren-Knaak, M., Ishii, H., Sun, J.M., Pazin, M.J., Davie, J.R. and Peterson, C.L. (2006) Histone H4-K16 acetylation controls chromatin structure and protein interactions. *Science*, **311**, 844–847.
26 McGinty, R.K., Kim, J., Chatterjee, C., Roeder, R.G. and Muir, T.W. (2008) Chemically ubiquitylated histone H2B stimulates hDot1L-mediated intranucleosomal methylation. *Nature*, **453**, 812–816.
27 Simon, M.D., Chu, F., Racki, L.R., de la Cruz, C.C., Burlingame, A.L., Panning, B., Narlikar, G.J. and Shokat, K.M. (2007) The site-specific installation of methyl-lysine analogs into recombinant histones. *Cell*, **128**, 1003–1012.
28 Neumann, H., Peak-Chew, S.Y. and Chin, J.W. (2008) Genetically encoding N(epsilon)-acetyllysine in recombinant proteins. *Nature Chemical Biology*, **4**, 232–234.
29 Garske, A.L., Craciun, G. and Denu, J.M. (2008) A combinatorial H4 tail library to explore the histone code. *Biochemistry*, **47**, 8097–8102.
30 Biel, M., Wascholowski, V. and Giannis, A. (2005) Epigenetics–an epicenter of gene regulation: histones and histone-modifying enzymes. *Angewandte Chemie (International Edition in English)*, **44**, 3186–3216.
31 Schneider, J., Bajwa, P., Johnson, F.C., Bhaumik, S.R. and Shilatifard, A. (2006)

Rtt109 is required for proper H3K56 acetylation: a chromatin mark associated with the elongating RNA polymerase II. *The Journal of Biological Chemistry*, **281**, 37270–37274.

32 Bolden, J.E., Peart, M.J. and Johnstone, R.W. (2006) Anticancer activities of histone deacetylase inhibitors. *Nature Reviews. Drug Discovery*, **5**, 769–784.

33 Michan, S. and Sinclair, D. (2007) Sirtuins in mammals: insights into their biological function. *The Biochemical Journal*, **404**, 1–13.

34 Shi, Y., Lan, F., Matson, C., Mulligan, P., Whetstine, J.R., Cole, P.A., Casero, R.A. and Shi, Y. (2004) Histone demethylation mediated by the nuclear amine oxidase homolog LSD1. *Cell*, **119**, 941–953.

35 Perillo, B. *et al.* (2008) DNA oxidation as triggered by H3K9me2 demethylation drives estrogen-induced gene expression. *Science*, **319**, 202–206.

36 Chang, B., Chen, Y., Zhao, Y. and Bruick, R.K. (2007) JMJD6 is a histone arginine demethylase. *Science*, **318**, 444–447.

37 Wang, Y. *et al.* (2004) Human PAD4 regulates histone arginine methylation levels via demethylimination. *Science*, **306**, 279–283.

38 Kearney, P.L., Bhatia, M., Jones, N.G., Yuan, L., Glascock, M.C., Catchings, K.L., Yamada, M. and Thompson, P.R. (2005) Kinetic characterization of protein arginine deiminase 4: a transcriptional corepressor implicated in the onset and progression of rheumatoid arthritis. *Biochemistry*, **44**, 10570–10582.

39 Thompson, P.R. and Fast, W. (2006) Histone citrullination by protein arginine deiminase: is arginine methylation a green light or a roadblock? *ACS Chemical Biology*, **1**, 433–441.

40 Dhalluin, C., Carlson, J.E., Zeng, L., He, C., Aggarwal, A.K. and Zhou, M.M. (1999) Structure and ligand of a histone acetyltransferase bromodomain. *Nature*, **399**, 491–496.

41 Mellor, J. (2006) It takes a PHD to read the histone code. *Cell*, **126**, 22–24.

42 Fischle, W., Wang, Y., Jacobs, S.A., Kim, Y., Allis, C.D. and Khorasanizadeh, S. (2003) Molecular basis for the discrimination of repressive methyl-lysine marks in histone H3 by Polycomb and HP1 chromodomains. *Genes and Development*, **17**, 1870–1881.

43 Hassan, A.H., Prochasson, P., Neely, K.E., Galasinski, S.C., Chandy, M., Carrozza, M.J. and Workman, J.L. (2002) Function and selectivity of bromodomains in anchoring chromatin-modifying complexes to promoter nucleosomes. *Cell*, **111**, 369–379.

44 Hassan, A.H., Awad, S. and Prochasson, P. (2006) The Swi2/Snf2 bromodomain is required for the displacement of SAGA and the octamer transfer of SAGA-acetylated nucleosomes. *The Journal of Biological Chemistry*, **281**, 18126–18134.

45 Maurer-Stroh, S., Dickens, N.J., Hughes-Davies, L., Kouzarides, T., Eisenhaber, F. and Ponting, C.P. (2003) The Tudor domain "Royal Family": Tudor, plant Agenet, Chromo, PWWP and MBT domains. *Trends in Biochemical Sciences*, **28**, 69–74.

46 Taverna, S.D., Li, H., Ruthenburg, A.J., Allis, C.D. and Patel, D.J. (2007) How chromatin-binding modules interpret histone modifications: lessons from professional pocket pickers. *Nature Structural & Molecular Biology*, **14**, 1025–1040.

47 Kim, J., Daniel, J., Espejo, A., Lake, A., Krishna, M., Xia, L., Zhang, Y. and Bedford, M.T. (2006) Tudor, MBT and chromo domains gauge the degree of lysine methylation. *EMBO Reports*, **7**, 397–403.

48 Huang, Y., Fang, J., Bedford, M.T., Zhang, Y. and Xu, R.M. (2006) Recognition of histone H3 lysine-4 methylation by the double tudor domain of JMJD2A. *Science*, **312**, 748–751.

49 Lee, J., Thompson, J.R., Botuyan, M.V. and Mer, G. (2007) Distinct binding modes specify the recognition of methylated histones H3K4 and H4K20 by

JMJD2A-tudor. *Nature Structural & Molecular Biology*, **15**, 109–111.

50 Pena, P.V., Davrazou, F., Shi, X., Walter, K.L., Verkhusha, V.V., Gozani, O., Zhao, R. and Kutateladze, T.G. (2006) Molecular mechanism of histone H3K4me3 recognition by plant homeodomain of ING2. *Nature*, **442**, 100–103.

51 Shi, X. *et al.* (2006) ING2 PHD domain links histone H3 lysine 4 methylation to active gene repression. *Nature*, **442**, 96–99.

52 Matthews, A.G. *et al.* (2007) RAG2 PHD finger couples histone H3 lysine 4 trimethylation with V(D)J recombination. *Nature*, **450**, 1106–1110.

53 Ramon-Maiques, S., Kuo, A.J., Carney, D., Matthews, A.G., Oettinger, M.A., Gozani, O. and Yang, W. (2007) The plant homeodomain finger of RAG2 recognizes histone H3 methylated at both lysine-4 and arginine-2. *Proceedings of the National Academy of Sciences of the United States of America*, **104**, 18993–18998.

54 Lan, F. *et al.* (2007) Recognition of unmethylated histone H3 lysine 4 links BHC80 to LSD1-mediated gene repression. *Nature*, **448**, 718–722.

55 Org, T. *et al.* (2008) Peterson, The autoimmune regulator PHD finger binds to non-methylated histone H3K4 to activate gene expression. *EMBO Reports*, **9**, 370–376.

56 Jacobson, R.H., Ladurner, A.G., King, D.S. and Tjian, R. (2000) Structure and function of a human TAFII250 double bromodomain module. *Science*, **288**, 1422–1425.

57 Li, H., Ilin, S., Wang, W., Duncan, E.M., Wysocka, J., Allis, C.D. and Patel, D.J. (2006) Molecular basis for site-specific read-out of histone H3K4me3 by the BPTF PHD finger of NURF. *Nature*, **442**, 91–95.

58 Wysocka, J. *et al.* (2006) A PHD finger of NURF couples histone H3 lysine 4 trimethylation with chromatin remodelling. *Nature*, **442**, 86–90.

59 Li, B., Gogol, M., Carey, M., Lee, D., Seidel, C. and Workman, J.L. (2007) Combined action of PHD and chromo domains directs the Rpd3S HDAC to transcribed chromatin. *Science*, **316**, 1050–1054.

60 Joshi, A.A. and Struhl, K. (2005) Eaf3 chromodomain interaction with methylated H3-K36 links histone deacetylation to Pol II elongation. *Molecular Cell*, **20**, 971–978.

61 Latham, J.A. and Dent, S.Y. (2007) Cross-regulation of histone modifications. *Nature Structural & Molecular Biology*, **14**, 1017–1024.

62 Guccione, E. *et al.* (2006) Myc-binding-site recognition in the human genome is determined by chromatin context. *Nature Cell Biology*, **8**, 764–770.

63 Guccione, E., Bassi, C., Casadio, F., Martinato, F., Cesaroni, M., Schuchlautz, H., Luscher, B. and Amati, B. (2007) Methylation of histone H3R2 by PRMT6 and H3K4 by an MLL complex are mutually exclusive. *Nature*, **449**, 933–937.

64 Kirmizis, A. *et al.* (2007) Arginine methylation at histone H3R2 controls deposition of H3K4 trimethylation. *Nature*, **449**, 928–932.

65 Vermeulen, M. *et al.* (2007) Selective Anchoring of TFIID to Nucleosomes by Trimethylation of Histone H3 Lysine 4. *Cell*, **131**, 58–69.

66 Heintzman, N.D. *et al.* (2007) Distinct and predictive chromatin signatures of transcriptional promoters and enhancers in the human genome. *Nature Genetics*, **39**, 311–318.

67 Lee, J.S., Shukla, A., Schneider, J., Swanson, S.K., Washburn, M.P., Florens, L., Bhaumik, S.R. and Shilatifard, A. (2007) Histone crosstalk between H2B monoubiquitination and H3 methylation mediated by COMPASS. *Cell*, **131**, 1084–1096.

68 Dehe, P.M. *et al.* (2005) Histone H3 lysine 4 mono-methylation does not require ubiquitination of histone H2B. *Journal of Molecular Biology*, **353**, 477–484.

69 Shahbazian, M.D., Zhang, K. and Grunstein, M. (2005) Histone H2B ubiquitylation controls processive methylation but not monomethylation by Dot1 and Set1. *Molecular Cell*, **19**, 271–277.

70 Lee, M.G., Villa, R., Trojer, P., Norman, J., Yan, K.P., Reinberg, D., Di Croce, L. and Shiekhattar, R. (2007) Demethylation of H3K27 regulates polycomb recruitment and H2A ubiquitination. *Science*, **318**, 447–450.

71 Agger, K. *et al.* (2007) UTX and JMJD3 are histone H3K27 demethylases involved in HOX gene regulation and development. *Nature*, **449**, 731–734.

72 Ptak, C. and Petronis, A. (2008) Epigenetics and complex disease: from etiology to new therapeutics. *Annual Review of Pharmacology and Toxicology*, **48**, 257–276.

73 Esteller, M. (2007) Cancer epigenomics: DNA methylomes and histone-modification maps. *Nature Reviews. Genetics*, **8**, 286–298.

74 Holleran, J.L. *et al.* (2005) Plasma pharmacokinetics, oral bioavailability, and interspecies scaling of the DNA methyltransferase inhibitor, zebularine. *Clinical Cancer Research*, **11**, 3862–3868.

75 Siedlecki, P., Boy, R.G., Musch, T., Brueckner, B., Suhai, S., Lyko, F. and Zielenkiewicz, P. (2006) Discovery of two novel, small-molecule inhibitors of DNA methylation. *Journal of Medicinal Chemistry*, **49**, 678–683.

76 Stresemann, C., Brueckner, B., Musch, T., Stopper, H. and Lyko, F. (2006) Functional diversity of DNA methyltransferase inhibitors in human cancer cell lines. *Cancer Research*, **66**, 2794–2800.

77 Arce, C., Segura-Pacheco, B., Perez-Cardenas, E., Taja-Chayeb, L., Candelaria, M. and Duennas-Gonzalez, A. (2006) Hydralazine target: from blood vessels to the epigenome. *Journal of Translational Medicine*, **4**, 10.

78 Zambrano, P. *et al.* (2005) A phase I study of hydralazine to demethylate and reactivate the expression of tumor suppressor genes. *BMC Cancer*, **5**, 44.

79 Villar-Garea, A., Fraga, M.F., Espada, J. and Esteller, M. (2003) Procaine is a DNA-demethylating agent with growth-inhibitory effects in human cancer cells. *Cancer Research*, **63**, 4984–4989.

80 Castellano, S., Kuck, D., Sala, M., Novellino, E., Lyko, F. and Sbardella, G. (2008) Constrained analogues of procaine as novel small molecule inhibitors of DNA methyltransferase-1. *Journal of Medicinal Chemistry*, **51**, 2321–2325.

81 Mukhopadhyay, N.K., Weisberg, E., Gilchrist, D., Bueno, R., Sugarbaker, D.J. and Jaklitsch, M.T. (2006) Effectiveness of trichostatin A as a potential candidate for anticancer therapy in non-small-cell lung cancer. *The Annals of Thoracic Surgery*, **81**, 1034–1042.

82 Finnin, M.S., Donigian, J.R., Cohen, A., Richon, V.M., Rifkind, R.A., Marks, P.A., Breslow, R. and Pavletich, N.P. (1999) Structures of a histone deacetylase homologue bound to the TSA and SAHA inhibitors. *Nature*, **401**, 188–193.

83 Jones, P. *et al.* (2006) A series of novel, potent, and selective histone deacetylase inhibitors. *Bioorganic & Medicinal Chemistry Letters*, **16**, 5948–5952.

84 Jones, P. *et al.* (2008) A novel series of potent and selective ketone histone deacetylase inhibitors with antitumor activity in vivo. *Journal of Medicinal Chemistry*, **51**, 2350–2353.

85 Moradei, O.M. *et al.* (2007) Novel aminophenyl benzamide-type histone deacetylase inhibitors with enhanced potency and selectivity. *Journal of Medicinal Chemistry*, **50**, 5543–5546.

86 Gore, S.D. *et al.* (2006) Combined DNA methyltransferase and histone deacetylase inhibition in the treatment of myeloid neoplasms. *Cancer Research*, **66**, 6361–6369.

87 Zeng, L., Li, J., Muller, M., Yan, S., Mujtaba, S., Pan, C., Wang, Z. and Zhou, M.M. (2005) Selective small molecules blocking HIV-1 Tat and coactivator PCAF association. *Journal of the American Chemical Society*, **127**, 2376–2377.

88 Pan, C., Mezei, M., Mujtaba, S., Muller, M., Zeng, L., Li, J., Wang, Z. and Zhou, M.M. (2007) Structure-guided optimization of small molecules inhibiting human immunodeficiency virus 1 Tat association with the human coactivator p300/CREB binding protein-associated factor. *Journal of Medicinal Chemistry*, **50**, 2285–2288.

89 Sachchidanand, L., Resnick-Silverman, L., Yan, S., Mutjaba, S., Liu, W.J., Zeng, L., Manfredi, J.J. and Zhou, M.M. (2006) Target structure-based discovery of small molecules that block human p53 and CREB binding protein association. *Chemistry & Biology*, **13**, 81–90.

2
Structural Biology of Epigenetic Targets

Christophe Romier, Jean-Marie Wurtz, Jean-Paul Renaud, and Jean Cavarelli

2.1
Introduction

The dynamic remodeling of chromatin is essential to most DNA-based nuclear processes [1, 2], and it comes as no surprise that epigenetic changes are implicated not only in normal development but also in various diseases, including cancer [3–5]. The intricacy of epigenetic mechanisms is shown by the large number of possible epigenetic marks [6] and the discovery that these marks not only destabilize nucleosomes but help in recruiting other epigenetic effectors to specific locations – information which led to the histone code hypothesis [7, 8]. Consequently, the number of studies in the past two decades dedicated to deciphering these mechanisms and their effectors at the cellular and molecular levels followed an almost exponential growth [9].

This large effort was accompanied by a wealth of structural data on epigenetic effectors in an attempt to understand epigenetic mechanisms at the atomic level. Certainly, the most impressive achievement was the crystallographic structure of the nucleosome [10] that showed not only how the DNA is wrapped around the (H2A/H2B)-$(H3/H4)_2$-(H2A/H2B) histone octamer, but also how histone tails, the main targets of histone-modifying enzymes, interact with DNA. This structure represented a cornerstone in the field of epigenetics as, for the following biochemical and structural studies, it provided a first view on how DNA recognition sites and epigenetic marks might be presented to incoming effectors.

Structural studies also embraced all epigenetic effectors in an effort to understand their structure/function relationships. Thanks to the large progress of structural biology in fields as diverse as biochemistry, molecular biology, nuclear magnetic resonance, X-ray crystallography and computer hardware and software, three-dimensional structures of epigenetic effectors have been obtained, either in a free state or in complex with cofactors and/or peptide substrates from target proteins. So far, most of the structural work has been carried out on individual, defined modules bearing either a catalytic activity, as described in this chapter, or responsible for the specific

Epigenetic Targets in Drug Discovery. Edited by Wolfgang Sippl and Manfred Jung

ISBN: 978-3-527-32355-5

recognition of an epigenetic mark [11]. Clearly, a lot of work remains to be done, but the structural data already collected give a crucial molecular insight into the anatomy that underlies some epigenetic target recognition and binding and the chemistry behind the function of these macromolecules.

This large set of structural knowledge already obtained on epigenetic targets paves the way for drug design studies to act on major biological processes such as development, aging, diseases and notably cancer (see dedicated chapters in this book). Catalytic domains are specifically addressed by many of these studies. In this chapter, we review the structural knowledge gained on catalytic domains of the main DNA- and histone-modifying enzymes: histone acetyl transferases, histone deacetylases/sirtuins, histone methylases, histone demethylases and DNA methylases.

2.2
Histone Acetyltransferases

Histone acetyltransferases (HATs) are enzymes that acetylate specific lysine residues in histones through the transfer of an acetyl group from an acetyl-coenzymeA (AcCoA) molecule, causing profound effects on chromatin structure and assembly as well as gene transcription. HATs are found in most, if not all, eukaryotic organisms as multiprotein complexes, some HAT catalytic subunits even being shared between various complexes that display different substrate specificities based on their subunit composition [12]. Despite their name, HATs do not restrict themselves to the acetylation of histones, since these enzymes have also been shown to act on nonhistone proteins, broadening their scope of action [13].

HAT catalytic subunits are divided into several families based on conserved sequence motifs [14]. The two major families are termed GNAT (Gcn5-related N-acetyltransferases) and MYST (MOZ, Ybf2/Sas3, Sas2, Tip60). Smaller families have also been defined: p300/CBP (CREB-binding protein), nuclear receptor co-activators, ATF-2, Rtt109 and possibly $TAF_{II}1$ [12]. Whereas proteins from the GNAT and MYST families display some sequence similarity in their conserved regions, the other families are much more divergent in terms of sequence [14]. Following the isolation of the first HAT subunits, numerous structural studies were carried out on these enzymes in the past decade and led to a wealth of structural data on the GNAT, MYST and p300/CBP families.

2.2.1
Structures from the GNAT Family

The structures of four HATs (yeast Hat1, Gcn5 from yeast (y) and *Tetrahymena thermophila* (t), human PCAF, yeast Hpa2) from the GNAT family have been solved so far [15–19]. These structures show that the evolutionarily conserved sequences of these proteins – termed motifs A, B, C, D [14] – form a conserved structural core. This core domain is constituted by a central highly curved five-stranded

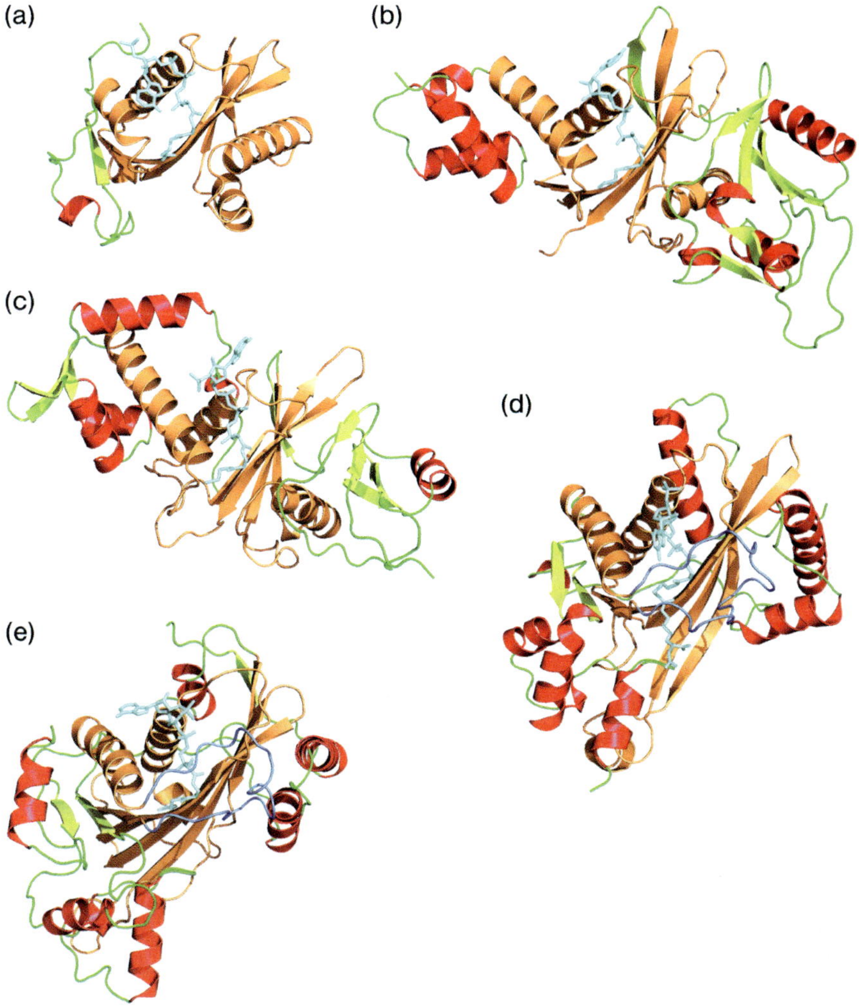

Figure 2.1 Structures of histone acetyltransferases (HATs). Ribbon representation of the structures of the HAT domains of (a) *Tetrahymena thermophila* Gcn5 (PDB code 1qsr), (b) *Saccharomyces cerevisiae* Hat1 (PDB code 1bob), (c) *S. cerevisiae* Esa1 (PDB code 1mja), (d) *Homo sapiens* p300 (PDB code 3biy) and (e) *S. cerevisiae* Rtt109 (PDB code 3d35). The conserved structural core is colored orange, whereas the rest of the structures are colored according to the secondary structure elements. The acetyl-coenzymeA (AcCoA)/coenzymeA (CoA; Gcn5, Hat1, Esa1, Rtt109) or Lysine-coenzymeA (p300) molecules bound to the enzymes are colored cyan. The specific loops of p300 and Rtt109 HATs that cover the AcCoA binding groove are colored blue.

antiparallel β-sheet flanked by three α-helices (Figure 2.1). The highest structural conservation is observed for the three central strands and the helix-linking strands β4 and β5, which correspond to the most conserved sequence motifs, D and A. In contrast, the remaining N- and C-terminal regions of these proteins that flank this conserved structural core show much more structural divergence or are sometimes structurally totally unrelated (Figure 2.1).

Recognition of AcCoA, the cofactor that donates the acetyl group to the lysine substrate, is highly similar in these structures. AcCoA binds to a groove at the surface of the protein that is formed by the structural core (Figure 2.1). The protein/AcCoA interactions imply almost exclusively motifs A and B of the enzymes, many of these interactions being made via hydrogen bonds to the protein backbone, which explains why the mode of recognition of the cofactor is similar despite protein sequence variations. Direct interactions with side-chains as well as water-mediated interactions are also observed [15–21]. Interestingly, these interactions are made predominantly with the acetyl group, the pantetheine arm and the pyrophosphate group of AcCoA. The 3′ phosphate-adenosine moiety, in contrast, makes relatively few or no contacts with the protein, which explains its different conformations observed in the various structures.

2.2.2 Structures of HATs from the MYST Family

For the MYST family, structural data have been described for two proteins: yeast Esa1 and human MOZ (monocytic leukemia zinc finger) [22, 23]. Surprisingly, although sequence conservation between the GNAT and MYST families concerns only motif A, these enzymes display a highly similar structural core as described for the GNAT family (Figure 2.1). Especially, the five-stranded antiparallel β-sheet and the three α-helices are also found in these structures. Overall comparison of Esa1 and MOZ structures reveals relatively little structural difference. However, comparing these enzymes to those of the GNAT family shows a structural divergence for the N- and C-terminal regions of these proteins. In contrast and as expected from the conservation of the structural core between the two families, binding of AcCoA to the MYST and GNAT enzymes is highly similar, with a strong interaction with the acetyl group, the pantetheine arm and the pyrophosphate group of AcCoA, and less with the 3′ phosphate-adenosine moiety. It should be noted that the structures (pdb codes 2giv, 2ou2) of the human MYST enzymes MOF and Tip60 in complex with CoA and AcCoA, respectively, confirm the observations made with the Esa1 and MOZ proteins.

2.2.3 Structure of the p300 and Rtt109 HATs

Structure of a HAT from the p300/CBP family has been long awaited, since these enzymes have no sequence similarity with enzymes of the GNAT and MYST families. The structure of the p300 HAT domain was solved very recently in complex with a Lys-CoA bi-substrate inhibitor, which required a highly intricate expression and purification protocol in order to produce a protein amenable to crystallization studies [24]. Analysis of the structure revealed however that, despite no sequence conservation, a similar structural core is observed as for the GNAT and MYST families (Figure 2.1). This structural core is composed of the five-stranded antiparallel β-sheet and two of the three α-helices. The region encompassing the missing helix is structurally completely divergent from the other HAT enzymes whose structure is known.

Still, the binding of the CoA moiety of the Lys-CoA inhibitor is highly reminiscent of the binding of CoA and AcCoA to enzymes of the GNAT and MYST families. Notably, the location of the acetyl group, the pantetheine arm and the pyrophosphate group is nearly identical. The major difference comes from the 3′ phosphate-adenosine moiety that interacts much more strongly with the enzyme. Further, a large p300-specific loop – formed by an insertion between the fifth strand and the C-terminal helix of the conserved structural core – almost entirely covers the AcCoA binding pocket, increasing the number of interactions made between the protein and the cofactor (Figure 2.1). Finally, comparison of the electrostatic potential at the surface of p300, Gcn5 and Esa1 HATs shows major differences for the former enzyme that may account for its substrate specificity [24].

Yeast Rtt109 HAT acetylates lysine 56 at the end of helix α1 of histone H3. The recently published structure of this enzyme in complex with AcCoA revealed that, despite a lack of sequence similarity, it contains a conserved structural core [25–27] (Figure 2.1). Comparison of the Rtt109 structure to other known HAT structures shows the highest structural similarity with the p300 enzyme, notably with the presence of the specific loop covering the AcCoA-binding pocket, suggesting that they belong to the same family.

2.2.4
Binding of Histone Substrates by HATs of the GNAT Family

The most detailed structural analysis of histone substrate binding by HAT has been carried out on the Gcn5 enzyme from the GNAT family [17, 28–30]. Gcn5 has been shown to acetylate preferentially histone H3 on lysine 14, but it can also acetylate histone H4 and p53 *in vivo* ([28] and references therein). The structures of Gcn5 in complex with CoA and either H3, H4 or p53 19mers has brought specific structural knowledge on substrate recognition by this enzyme [28, 30]. Interestingly, in all structures the lysine to be acetylated is bound to a pocket located in close vicinity of the binding site for the acetyl group of the AcCoA molecule (Figure 2.2). Especially, binding is built up on van der Waals interactions and hydrogen bonding to both the protein and the CoA molecule.

However, whereas lysine recognition is similar, large differences are observed for the rest of the peptides. In the case of the H4 and p53 peptides, electron density is observed for only a few more residues C-terminal to this lysine. The picture is completely different for the H3 peptide since 15 of the 19 residues are observed in density, showing a strong binding of the peptide in a cleft at the surface of the protein (Figure 2.2). Anchoring of the peptide is not only due to the lysine to be modified (K14) but also to several other residues that create an extensive set of interactions with Gcn5 [17, 30]. Strikingly, the use of an identical peptide bearing an additional epigenetic mark, the phosphorylation of serine 10 (S10P) enhances even further

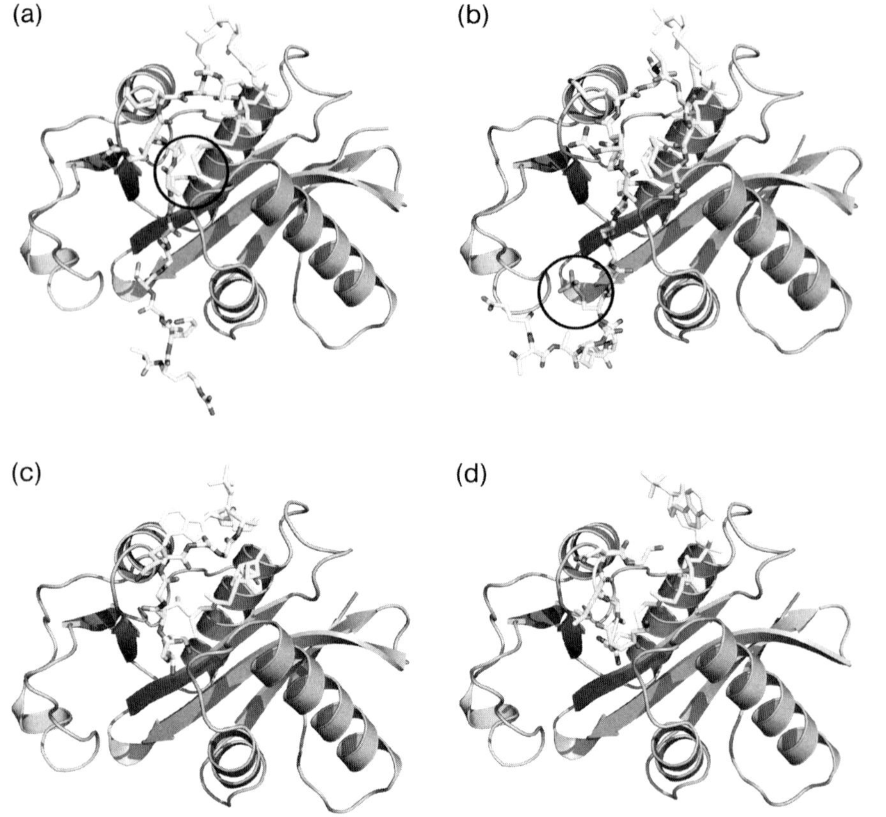

Figure 2.2 Structures of Gcn5 histone acetyltransferase (HAT) bound to coenzymeA and various peptides. Schematic representation of *Tetrahymena thermophila* Gcn5 HAT domain (ribbon representation) bound to coenzymeA and 19mers (both shown as ball and sticks) from (a) histone H3 (PDB code 1pu9), (b) histone H3 phosphorylated on serine 10 (PDB code 1pua), (c) histone H4 (PDB code 1q2c) and (d) p53 (PDB code 1q2d). The black circle in (a) shows the proximity of the lysine to be modified to the coenzymeA molecule. The black circle in (b) indicates the phosphorylated serine 10.

the binding of the H3 peptide to Gcn5 [30]. In this structure, all 19 residues are seen in density, with large rearrangements of the binding of the N-terminal region of the peptide (Figure 2.2). Notably, residues 9, 10 and 11 display a completely new set of interactions with Gcn5.

Altogether these structural studies on Gcn5 bound to various 19mer peptides from H3, H4 and p53 clearly highlight how HATs can display substrate specificity despite the presence of a similar structural core in all these enzymes. In fact, peptide binding is not only carried out by the conserved structural core, which anyway does not display strong sequence conservation, but also by nonconserved structural regions of the protein. This view is further reinforced by the structure of Hat1 bound to AcCoA and a H4 peptide (PDB code 2p0w), where the peptide apparently binds differently relative to the conserved structural core.

2.2.5 Catalytic Mechanism of HATs

In the case of the GNAT family, biochemical and structural studies on yGcn5 led to the proposal of a ternary complex mechanism involving glutamate residue 173 located in strand β4 of the conserved structural core [21, 31]. In this mechanism, deprotonation of the Nε-nitrogen of the target lysine by Glu173 is followed by a direct nucleophilic attack of the deprotonated nitrogen on the acetyl group of the AcCoA molecule [31]. Although this glutamate residue is conserved in the Gcn5 and human PCAF enzymes, different residues are found at this position in other members of the GNAT family. However, comparison with the structure of Hat1 shows that glutamate 255 on strand β5 of the conserved structural core could play an identical role [21]. The picture is less clear when considering the structure of Hpa2 [15], indicating that further experiments should be carried out to characterize more precisely the catalytic mechanism of HATs from the GNAT family.

Understanding of the catalytic mechanism of members from the MYST family also remains unclear. Initial structural and biochemical studies on yeast Esa1 revealed that glutamate residue 338 is structurally conserved at position Glu255 of Hat1 and that catalytic activity is lost upon its mutation in glutamine, leading to the proposal of a ternary complex mechanism as for GNAT enzymes [22]. Further studies showed however that Cys304 is also absolutely required for catalysis and forms an acetyl-cysteine intermediate, indicative of a ping-pong catalytic mechanism for MYST HATs [32]. However, recent studies of yeast Esa1 in the context of the HAT complex Piccolo Nua4 have shown that this complex acts through a ternary complex mechanism involving Glu338 [33]. Clearly, further studies are required to solve these discrepancies.

Finally, the recent structure of the p300 HAT and concomitant biochemical work shed some light on the mechanism of this enzyme. Notably, these experiments appeared to contradict a ternary complex or a ping-pong mechanism. Rather, the authors proposed a Theorell–Chance catalytic mechanism for this HAT [24]. Once again, it is expected that further work will be required to confirm this hypothesis. The mechanism of Rtt109 is still poorly characterized but preliminary data indicate that this enzyme could proceed through a ping-pong mechanism; possibly through the formation of an acetyl-lysine intermediate formed with Rtt109 lysine290 [25–27].

2.3 Histone Deacetylases

Histone deacetylases (HDACs) catalyze the removal of acetyl groups from the Nε atom of histone lysines in a nucleosomal context, ensuring the reversibility of histone acetylation. Histone deacetylation is often associated with transcriptional repression and silencing since it promotes chromatin higher order structures and the recruitment of silencers [34]. As other enzymes involved in chromatin modifications, HDACs also deacetylate nonhistone proteins, mostly transcription factors, but also cytoskeletal proteins, nuclear import factors and molecular chaperones, affecting their biological activity or stability [35].

HDACs belong to the lysine deacetylase superfamily, whose members are found from bacteria to animals. At least 18 protein lysine deacetylases are found in vertebrates, divided into four classes based on phylogeny [36]: class I (HDACs 1–3, 8), homologous to yeast Rpd3, class II (HDACs 4–7, 9, 10), homologous to yeast Hda1, class III (SIRTs 1–7), homologous to yeast Sir2 and class IV (currently containing only HDAC11). Classes I, II and IV HDACs are Zn^{2+}-dependent deacetylases and are now referred to as "classic" HDACs [37], whereas class III HDACs are unrelated, NAD^{+}-dependent deacetylases called sirtuins (see below). Class II is further divided into two subclasses: class IIa (HDACs 4, 5, 7, 9) containing a single catalytic domain and class IIb (HDACs 6, 10) containing two catalytic domains.

Classic HDACs are related to archaeal and eubacterial enzymes, suggesting a common ancestor with nonhistone deacetylase activity [36, 38]. In agreement, not all HDACs use histones as substrates: enzymatically active histone deacetylases belong mostly to class I, whereas class IIa members function as signal transducers involved in nucleocytoplasmic trafficking and class IIb members are cytoplasmic regulators [39]. The HDAC activity attributed to class IIa HDACs would rather function by recruiting pre-existing enzymatically active SMRT/N-CoR complexes containing HDAC3 [40]. In contrast, little is known about the single class IV member, HDAC11. Interestingly, as for HATs, HDACs are mostly functional within multiprotein complexes which target their catalytic activity to specific chromatin sites [9]. This catalytic activity is even more tightly regulated since the sequence-specific DNA-binding proteins which recruit HDACs also contribute to their activation.

2.3.1
Structure of HDACs

Initial structural work led to the structure determination of a bacterial class I HDAC homolog from *Aquifex aeolicus*, HDLP (histone deacetylase-like protein), both apo and in complex with HDAC inhibitors [41]. The structure revealed a single α/β domain, with a central eight-stranded parallel β-sheet sandwiched between two layers of α-helices. Only one half of the residues constitute these secondary structure elements, the other half forming loops. The protein was shown to bind a catalytic Zn^{2+} ion coordinating two conserved aspartates and one conserved histidine, as well as the bidentate hydroxamic acid inhibitor. HDAC8 was the first mammalian HDAC whose structure was solved [42, 43] (Figure 2.3). Despite the low sequence identity between HDAC8 and HDLP, both structures share the same fold, most differences being observed in loops and peripheral regions. HDAC8 binds not only a catalytic Zn^{2+} ion but also two other cations (most probably K^{+}) that appear to play a structural role.

The crystal structure of FB188 HDAH (histone deacetylase-like amidohydrolase from *Bordetella/Alcaligenes* strain FB188), a bacterial class II HDAC homolog,

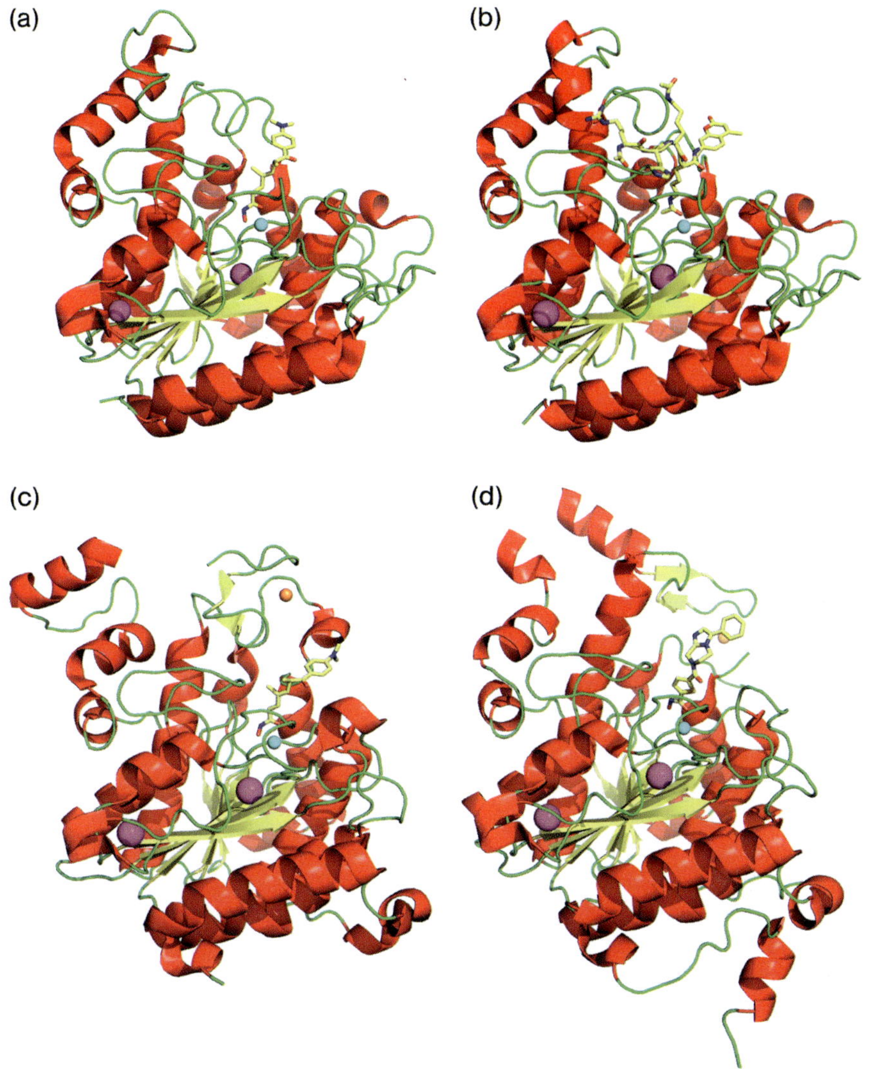

Figure 2.3 Structures of mammalian "classic" histone deacetylases. Ribbon representation of the conserved catalytic domain of: (a) class I human HDAC8 in complex with trichostatin A (TSA; PDB code 1t64), (b) human HDAC8 Tyr306Phe inactive mutant in complex with a peptidic acetyl-lysine substrate (PDB code 2v5w), (c) class IIa human HDAC7 in complex with TSA (PDB code 3C10) and (d) class IIa human HDAC4 in complex with an hydroxamic acid inhibitor (PDB code 2vqm). The proteins are colored according to secondary structure elements, the catalytic Zn^{2+} ions are shown as cyan spheres, the class IIa-specific structural Zn^{2+} ions as orange spheres and the structural K^{+} ions as magenta spheres.

brought a first glimpse into the structure of class II HDACs [44]. Although this enzyme shares only around 20% sequence identity with HDLP and HDAC8, it exhibits a similar fold as class I HDACs and the Zn^{2+}- and proximal cation-binding sites are also conserved. In both cases, major differences are found in the loops surrounding the entrance to the active site, reflecting differences in protein substrates for class I and class II deacetylases. Presumably, the loop variability across all HDACs, especially at the rim of the active site channel, allows substrate protein recognition and specificity.

The first structures of eukaryotic class IIa HDAC catalytic domains appeared very recently: those of human HDAC7 and HDAC4, in the apo form and in complex with different inhibitors [45, 46] (Figure 2.3). Their overall fold is similar to that of the class I HDAC8, the bacterial class I homolog HDLP and the bacterial class II homolog FB188 HDAH. As mentioned for the FB188 HDAH enzyme, the greatest structural variability is found in the loop regions around the active site entrance. One striking feature is a novel, class IIa HDAC-specific zinc-binding motif close to the active site entrance (Figure 2.3). This motif, conserved within and unique to eukaryotic class IIa HDACs, is probably involved in substrate recognition and may provide a site for docking of regulatory factors. Furthermore, this domain in HDAC4 shows some conformational flexibility: it adopts a "closed" conformation in the apo form similar to the one observed in HDAC7 and an "open" conformation in the inhibitor complexes. Curiously, the second Zn^{2+}-binding site coordination is slightly different in the open conformation.

2.3.2
Binding of Acetylated Lysine by HDACs

The structure of an inactive mutant of HDAC8 bound to a diacetylated peptide derived from p53 ((N-acetyl)Arg-His-Lys(ε-acetyl)-Lys(ε-acetyl)(C-amino-7-yl-methyl-4-coumarin)) [47] confirmed the position of the active site that had been inferred from the position of various inhibitors, a 12-Å tunnel-like, hydrophobic cavity with the catalytic Zn^{2+} ion at the end. In the structure, the C-terminal ε-acetyl-lysine is buried in this cavity and coordinates the zinc ion through the carbonyl oxygen of the acetyl group, located approximately as the carbonyl oxygen of hydroxamate inhibitors (Figure 2.3). The structure also highlights the important role of Asp101 in substrate recognition and positioning. This residue, conserved in class I and class II HDACs but not in HDLP, HDAH, and HDAC11, is located at the rim of the active site tunnel, where its side-chain carboxylate interacts with the backbone of the peptidic substrate, imposing a constrained *cis*-conformation. Presumably, this interaction locks the histone tail and correctly positions the acetyl-lysine during the deacetylation reaction. Indeed, the enzymatic activity of mutant HDAC8 Asp101Ala towards purified histones is greatly reduced.

Although no structure of class II HDAC has been solved in complex with an acetylated peptide, the structure of FB188 HDAH bound to an acetate molecule, the deacetylation reaction product, showed that the acetate was bound to the Zn^{2+} ion [48]. A 17-Å long channel was found in FB188 HDAH, leading from the bottom of the active site cavity to the protein surface, and was proposed to function as an exit tunnel for the acetate, as previously proposed for HDLP [41, 44].

2.3.3
Catalytic Mechanism of HDACs

Biochemical and mutagenesis studies and the various structures of HDACs led to the proposal of a catalytic mechanism that would imply the nucleophilic attack by an enzyme-activated water molecule (deprotonated by the His142-Asp176 charge relay system; HDAC8 numbering) on the carbonyl carbon of the ε-acetyl group on the substrate lysine, leading to a tetrahedral intermediate. The breakdown of this tetrahedral intermediate requires the protonation of the amide nitrogen. It is proposed that a proton would be transferred from His142 to the neighboring His143, which would then protonate the amide nitrogen [49]. Another hypothesis suggests that this proton is donated by Tyr306, hence explaining that the Tyr306Phe mutant is inactive against the substrate [47]. However, it is not clear how the tyrosinate anion would be stabilized. At least, Tyr306 is probably involved in enhancing the polarization of the carbonyl bond through a hydrogen bond between Tyr306 OH and the carbonyl oxygen of the acetyl group, making the carbonyl carbon more susceptible to a nucleophilic attack, and in stabilizing the transition state by hydrogen bonding the oxyanion intermediate. Interestingly, Tyr306 is conserved in all other class I HDACs (1, 2, 3), in the class I homolog HDLP, in the class II homolog HDAH, in class IIb HDACs (6, 10) and in class IV HDAC11, but not in class IIa HDACs (4, 5, 7, 9) which all possess a histidine at the corresponding position, in good agreement with their low level of enzymatic activity towards histone acetyl-lysines. In HDAC4, His976 (corresponding to Tyr306 in HDAC8) is rotated away from the active site, making room for a water molecule which makes a hydrogen bond with the carbonyl oxygen of the hydroxamic acid inhibitor. This water molecule could stabilize the oxyanion intermediate as Tyr306, though less efficiently, thus explaining the low activity of class II HDACs against acetylated histones. In HDAC4 His976Tyr/inhibitor structures, the tyrosine is oriented as Tyr306 in HDAC8, at a distance compatible with its participation in catalysis [46], in good agreement with a mutagenesis study which showed that a His-to-Tyr mutation in HDAC4, 5 and 7 strongly increased their catalytic activity; conversely, a Tyr-to-His mutation in class I HDACs drastically reduced their activity [50].

2.3.4
Structural Basis of Inhibition of HDACs

The seminal work on HDLP revealed the mode of binding of two classic inhibitors: trichostatin A (TSA) and suberoylanilide hydroxamic acid (SAHA) [41]. Both show anticancer activities and SAHA was recently approved by the FDA for the treatment of cutaneous T-cell lymphoma. In both cases, the Zn^{2+} ion is coordinated by two aspartates, one histidine and the bidentate hydroxamic acid of the inhibitor through the carbonyl oxygen and the hydroxyl oxygen. Inhibitor binding to HDAC8 is similar [42, 43]. Comparison with the binding of a peptidic substrate to a HDAC8 inactive mutant confirmed that the carbonyl oxygen of the hydroxamic acid mimics the carbonyl oxygen of the acetyl-lysine and that the hydroxyl group mimics the catalytic water [47]. Like the acetyl-lysine side-chain, the various inhibitors make van der Waals contacts in the hydrophobic channel with the conserved Gly151, Phe152, Phe208 of HDAC8. In HDAC7/inhibitor complex structures, the hydroxamic acid binds the Zn^{2+} ion in a monodentate fashion through the hydroxyl oxygen and a water molecule makes a hydrogen bond with the hydroxamic acid carbonyl oxygen. In HDAC4, the situation is also different: the hydroxamic acid binds the Zn^{2+} ion in a monodentate fashion through the carbonyl oxygen, which is also bound to a water molecule. Finally, the recent structure of HDCA4 in complex with a trifluoromethylketone inhibitor revealed that the trifluoromethylketone is in its hydrated form, with both oxygen atoms of the gem-diol binding the catalytic zinc ion [46].

2.4 Sirtuins

The sirtuins (*s*ilent *i*nformation *r*egulator *2*-related prote*ins*; class III HDACs) form a specific class of histone deacetylases. First, they do not share any sequence or structural homology with the other HDACs. Second, they do not require zinc for activity, but rather use the oxidized form of nicotinamide adenine dinucleotide (NAD^+) as cofactor. The reaction catalyzed by these enzymes is the conversion of histones acetylated at specific lysine residues into deacetylated histones, the other products of the reaction being nicotinamide and the metabolite 2′-O-acetyl-adenosine diphosphate ribose (OAADPR) [51, 52]. As HATs and other HDACs, sirtuins not only use acetylated histones as substrates but can also deacetylate other proteins. Intriguingly, some sirtuins do not display any deacetylase activity but act as ADP-ribosyl transferases.

Sirtuins have been conserved from bacteria to eukaryotes. Notably, they all possess a conserved catalytic core domain flanked by sequence-divergent N- and C-terminal regions. If bacteria and archaebacteria generally possess one or two sirtuins, this number is higher in eukaryotes, with five sirtuins in *Saccharomyces cerevisiae* and seven in human. The presence of sirtuins in all phyla of life led to a wealth of structural data, not only on eukaryotic enzymes but also on bacterial and archaebacterial enzymes.

2.4.1 Structure of Sirtuins

The resolution of the structures of a sirtuin homolog from *A. fulgidus* and the catalytic core of human SIRT2 revealed that the core domain of sirtuins is composed of a Rossmann fold domain and a smaller domain composed of an α-helical module and a zinc-binding module, with a large groove between these two domains [53, 54] (Figure 2.4). Initial structural studies showed that the NAD^+ molecule binds in this groove in a so-called "inverted conformation." Three binding pockets (A, B, C) were defined in these studies and NAD was shown to bind to the A and B pockets, although pockets B and C were shown to be required for catalysis [54, 55]. Further studies showed that NAD binding was not efficient in the initial structures, explaining that the nicotinamide moiety could not be seen in density [56, 57]. These new studies refined the view on NAD binding, showing that the nicotinamide moiety binds in pocket C (Figure 2.4).

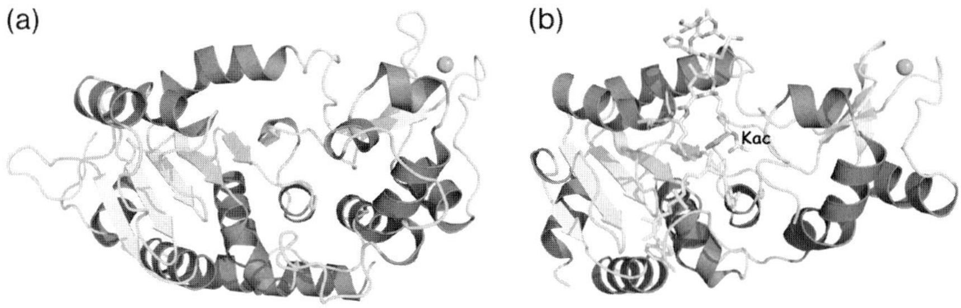

Figure 2.4 Structures of histone deacetylases from the sirtuin family. Ribbon representation of the structures of the conserved catalytic domain of histone deacetylases: (a) *Homo sapiens* SirT2 (PDB code 1j8f) and (b) *Thermotoga maritima* Sir2 bound to NAD^+ and an acetylated p53 peptide (PDB code 2h4f). The secondary structure of the proteins are shown as dark gray helices and the beta strands and coil regions are in light gray. The zinc ions are shown as spheres. (b) The NAD^+ molecule bound to the enzyme and the acetylated peptide of p53 are shown as ball and sticks. The acetylated lysine is labeled.

This mode of binding of the NAD^+ molecule is in agreement with acetylated lysine binding, since the structures of sirtuin/acetylated peptides revealed a binding of the modified peptide in the major groove of sirtuins, the acetylated lysine being found in a tunnel that leads to the NAD^+ binding site [56, 58–61] (Figure 2.4). Two residues are also found in the vicinity: a histidine and an asparagine that have been shown to be important for catalytic activity [54].

2.4.2 Catalytic Mechanism of Sirtuins

Despite the large amount of biochemical and structural studies of sirtuins in complex with various substrates, cofactors and reaction products, the catalytic mechanism of this class of enzymes is still a matter of debate. SN^1-like [56] and SN^2-like [60] mechanisms have been inferred from structural studies but further biochemical and possibly structural studies will be required to clarify which mechanism is used by sirtuins. It should also be noted that another matter of debate concerns the mode of noncompetitive inhibition of sirtuins by the reaction product nicotinamide [62], various structural studies having highlighted different binding pockets for this molecule [63, 64].

2.5 Histone Methylation Enzymes

Protein methylation is one of the most common protein modifications found in a wide range of prokaryotic and eukaryotic proteins that are involved either in regulation of transcription or in translation. Several amino acids can be modified, mainly by either N-methylation or C-methylation. Protein methylation has been reviewed in several recent articles or book chapters [65–67] and therefore in this chapter we only focus on the main trends found in structural modules involved in histone methylation.

Within histones, lysine and arginine residues are abundant and highly posttranslationally modified; and methylation of these two amino acids has been extensively studied during the past several years, as it is correlated with either activation or repression. The state of methylation has been shown to create recognition or binding templates recruiting effectors, resulting in the modification of the chromatin environment or specific chromatin states. Aberrant histone methylation has been linked to a number of developmental disorders and human diseases. Lysine methylation and arginine methylation are catalyzed, respectively, by lysine methyltransferases (KMTs) and protein arginine methyltransferases (PRMTs).

Each nucleosomal histone is extensively posttranslationally modified, particularly in its flexible N-terminal tail. The best characterized sites of histone methylation are mainly located on histones H3 and H4. Histone methylation uses S-adenosyl-L-methionine (AdoMet or SAM), the second most widely used enzyme substrate, as methyl donor group to form different states of methylated lysine or arginine and S adenosyl-L-homocysteine (AdoHcy or SAH). SAM-binding proteins represent an extremely heterogeneous assemblage of 15 different folds [68]. Among them, SAM-dependent methyltransferases are divided into five structurally distinct classes, revealing how an overall similar mechanism of methyl transfer can be achieved with large global and local structural diversities [69].

2.5.1
Histone Lysine Methyltransferases

Histone lysine (K) methyltransferase (HKMTs) may lead to mono, di- and trimethylation of the ε-amino group and the extent of modification at a specific site controls the recruitment of the effector proteins. Two unequally populated folds are presently known: the SET domain-containing family and the Dot1 family (for a recent review, see Ref. [70])

2.5.1.1 SET Domain of HKMTs

The SET domain, originally identified in three *Drosophila* proteins, Su(var)3–9, enhancer of zeste, and trithorax, which are all involved in epigenetic gene regulation, posttranslationally methylate a variety of cellular proteins. This conserved domain, which is approximately 130 amino acids long, is mainly found in a large number of eukaryotic proteins as a general lysine methyltransferase. For this domain, there are currently 1795 sequences from 289 species in the Pfam database (see PFAM PF00856) and 30 structures in the PDB.

SET domain containing HKMTs have been classified according to the presence or absence and the nature of the sequences surrounding the SET domain that are conserved within families [71, 72]. The SET domain has a unique structural fold classified as class V AdoMet-dependent methyltransferase (MTase) [69], characterized by four highly-conserved signature sequences, namely motif I

(GxG), motif II (YxG), motif III (RFINHxCxPN) and motif IV (ELxFDY; where x is any amino acid). The conserved domain folds into several small β-sheets that surround a knot-like structure to which additional domains (pre-SET (or nSET), post-SET (or cSET)) or an insertion domain (i-SET) may be added (Figure 2.5).

HKMTs with SET domains methylate various N-terminal lysine residues of histones H3 and H4. The first SET domains containing histone lysine methylase reported were the mammalian Suv39h1 and its fission yeast homolog Clr4, which methylate histone H3 at Lys 9 [73]. Subsequently, other SET domain-containing proteins (Set1, Set2, Set7/Set9, G9a, ESET) were shown to methylate Lys 4, Lys 9, Lys 27, or Lys 36 of histone H3 tail. More than 15 structures of HKMTs containing a SET domain (either in the free form or in complex with cofactor SAH and/or substrate peptides; and therefore mimicking an enzyme/cofactor/substrate complex) have been solved, including *Neurospora crassa* DIM-5,

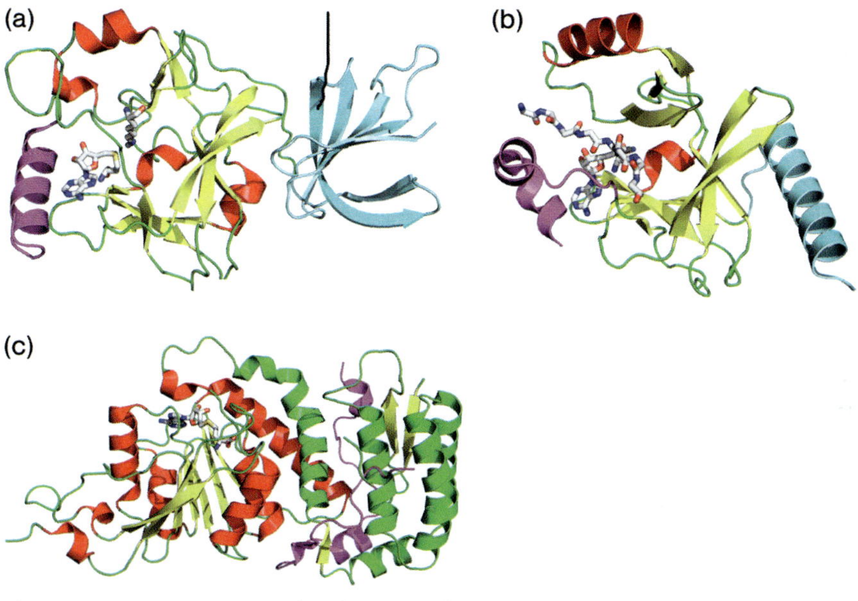

Figure 2.5 Representative examples of two SET domain-containing structures. (a) Human SET7/9 in complex with SAH and a histone peptide cofactor (PDB code 1o9s). The N-SET (shown in light blue), SET (β strands shown in yellow and helices in red) and C-SET (shown in magenta) domains in SET7/9 are indicated. The bound SAH molecule is shown in a stick model, together with the lysine side-chain of the bound histone peptide (the rest of the peptide is not shown). (b) Structure of human SET8 in complex with a histone H4 peptide (PDB code 1zkk). The SET domain is color-coded as in panel A. The bound SAH molecule is shown in a stick model, together with main chain of the bound histone peptide (side-chains are not shown). (c) Structure of yeast Dot1 (PDB code 1u2z). Only one monomer is represented. The C-terminal catalytic domain is shown in yellow (β strands) and red (helices). The bound SAM is shown as shown in a stick model.

Schizosaccharamyces pombe Clr4 and several structures of histone H3 K4-specific methyltransferase SET7/9, SET8/PreSET7 and a viral SET domain protein (referred to as vSET) from *Paramecium bursaria chlorella* virus 1 (for a recent exhaustive review, see Ref. [74]).

Thus, a large amount of structural data has been collected, revealing deep structural insights into the molecular basis of the substrate specificity, methylation multiplicity and catalytic mechanism of histone lysine methylation. The results were recently reviewed in detail (see Refs. [70, 74–76]). The lysine substrate and SAM/SAH cofactor binding sites are located on separate faces of the domain. The U-shaped conformation of the cofactor SAH bound to the SET domain and the geometry of its binding cleft are highly conserved in SET domain lysine methyltransferases, together with a narrow hydrophobic channel that links the substrate lysine or methylated lysine and SAH (Figure 2.5). However, due to their high substrate specificity, SET domain HMTs show overall low sequence similarity and the residues at the active site are not all conserved. Substrate specificity is controlled by a network of polar interactions between the peptide substrate and the SET domain, including residues from the i-SET region. The chemical and geometrical nature of the channel (which creates an idiosyncratic network of molecular interactions between the enzyme, cofactor and the methylated peptide) has been shown to play a crucial role in determining the methylation multiplicity of the SET domain. The structural studies of ternary complexes of several SET domains strongly argue in favor of a SN^2 nucleophilic attack of the ε-amine to transfer the methyl group form SAM and form SAH and methylated lysine. Several possible mechanisms have been proposed and discussed, but no clear consensus in the understanding of the catalytic reaction has emerged.

2.5.1.2 **Dot1 HKMTs**

Dot1, a nuclear protein originally identified in a genetic screen for high-copy disruption of telomeric silencing [77], methylates Lys-79 within the core domain of histone H3. Methylation of histone H3 at lysine 79 is conserved among most eukaryotic species. As suggested by sequence analysis, Dot1 has been shown to contain *SAM*-binding motifs characteristic of class I MTases, similar to those found in PRMTs. Dot1 homologs vary in length from 582 residues in yeast to 2232 in *Drosophila* and contain a conserved core catalytic domain. Structures of Dot1 confirm that the catalytic domain is formed by a seven-stranded β-sheet flanked by α-helices, a characteristic feature of the class I AdoMet-dependent MTases (Figure 2.5). Structures of Dot1 with SAM/SAH cofactors reveal an extended SAM conformation distinct from the U-shaped conformation observed in structures of SET HKMTs [78, 79].

Dot1 proteins and SET HKMTs illustrate how methyl transfer to a protein Lys side-chain can be done with different structural scaffolding and unrelated local active site spatial arrangements. To date, Dot1 proteins are the only nonSET HKMTs and further work and structures are needed to understand the mechanism of methylation of Lys-79, a histone core residue.

2.5.2
Histone Arginine Methyltransferases

Posttranslational methylation of arginine is a widespread epigenetic modification found in eukaryotes that is catalyzed by the protein arginine methyltransferases (PRMTs). At least nine members of PRMTs (PRMT1 to PRMT9) have been identified and classified into two main classes (type I and II PRMTs; for a recent review, see Refs. [80–82]). Both classes catalyze the formation of mono-methylarginine as intermediate. In a second step, type I PRMTs (PRMT1, PRMT3, PRMT4, PRMT6) form asymmetric dimethylarginine, whereas type II enzymes form symmetric dimethylarginine.

PRMTs belong to class I MTases and contain a catalytic core domain of 320 residues that is well conserved in sequence (and therefore in structure) among all PRMTs members (for recent reviews, see Refs. [65, 81]. Idiosyncratic modules may be added to this catalytic domain. Several structures of the catalytic domain of type I PRMTs are known including rat PRMT1 [83], rat PRMT3 [84], yeast PRMT1/Hmt1 [85] and mouse PRMT4/CARM1 [86, 87]. The catalytic module is folded into two domains connected by a conserved *cis*-proline residue (Figure 2.6). The first domain at the N-terminal end contains a typical Rossmann fold and two terminal helices. The second domain is a β-barrel to which an arm containing a four-helix segment is added. This arm has been shown to be involved in the dimerization of PRMTs. The Rossmann fold domain harbors the AdoMet consensus fold conserved in AdoMet-dependent methyltransferases [88]. PRMTs are characterized by four signature sequences, two located in the Rossmann fold-like domain and the other two in the β-barrel. Crystal structures of the catalytic cores of apo and SAH-bound PRMTs revealed induced folding upon cofactor binding and a detailed vision of the cofactor binding site which is surrounded by all four PRMT signature sequences. Based on those structures, a putative arginine-binding pocket can be defined and involvement of several residues in a classic SN^2 type mechanism has been proposed.

Despite this large structural information, the binding mode of substrates prior to methylation or the binding mode of product subsequent to methylation remains to be visualized and understood at the atomic level. Dimer formation has been shown to be a conserved feature in the PRMT family. It is proposed that the dimer structure is necessary to build up the productive SAM binding site and to allow stepwise production of the final methylation product, dimethylarginine. The PRMT family has a wide substrate spectrum and the molecular mechanism by which PRMTs can recognize and methylate so many different protein substrates still remains unclear despite extensive work by many groups. Further insights should come from the structures of binary or ternary complexes including PRMTs domains and peptide substrates.

2.6
Histone Demethylases

Until recently, methylation was considered as a permanent modification of chromatin because of the high thermodynamic stability of the $N–CH_3$ bond. Within recent

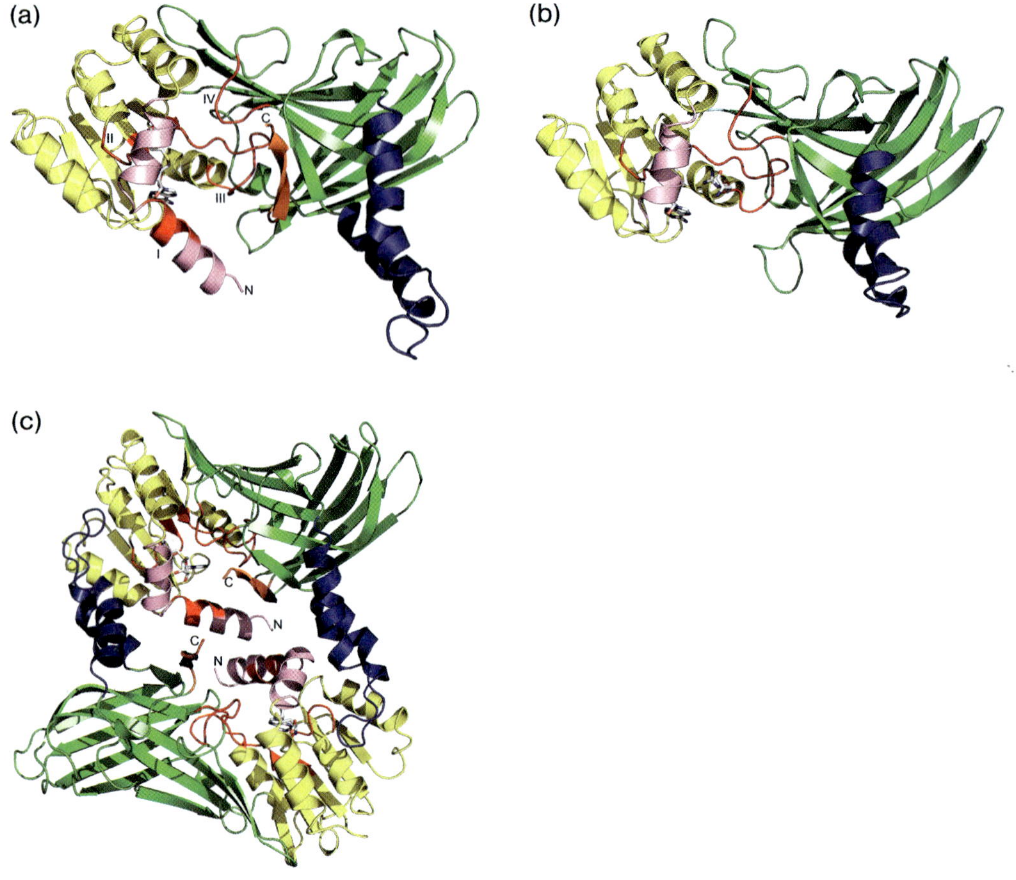

Figure 2.6 (a) Overview of the conserved PRMTs catalytic domain illustrated by the structure of SAH-CARM1$_{140_480}$ at 2.2 Å (PDB code 3b3f). The catalytic module is folded into two domains: SAH/SAM binding domain at the N-terminal end containing a Rossmann fold-like architecture (shown in yellow) and two terminal helices (shown in pink). The second domain is a β-barrel (shown in green) to which a dimerization arm containing helix segments is added (shown in blue). The last C-terminal strand, shown in orange, has not been observed in other known PRMTs structures and is essential for CARM1 activity. The bound SAH molecule is shown in a stick model and the four motifs characteristic of PRMT catalytic domain (labeled I, II, III, IV) are highlighted in red. (b) The 2.35 Å structure of rat SAH-PRMT1 (PDB code 1or8) crystallized with peptides not well ordered in the crystal revealed nevertheless the putative peptide binding site (the side-chain of the arginine to be methylated is shown as stick model). (c) Ribbon representation of PRMT dimer illustrated here by a SAH-CARM1$_{140–480}$ dimer. PRMT dimerization has been shown to be essential for enzymatic activity as it may allow processive production of the final methylation product, asymmetric dimethylarginine for type I PRMTs.

years, several families of histone demethylases have been discovered, revealing the plasticity and the dynamic nature of histone methylation [89, 90]. This discovery led to the identification of proteins that antagonize histone methylation by different enzymatic mechanisms, other than histone exchange or histone tail cleavage.

One type of enzymes removes specifically the methyl group(s) from lysine residues in histones by an oxidative cleavage of the α-carbon bond of the substrate or by the hydrolase of the methyl amine group by the presence of an iron and α-ketoglutarate as cofactor [76, 90, 91].

For methylated arginines two kinds of enzymes have been described. Initially, enzymes catalyzing the demethylimination of the arginine, thus transforming the arginine residue in citrulline, have been isolated [92, 93]. As such these enzymes are not true demethylases as they fail to restore the free arginine residue. More recently, an enzyme catalyzing the demethylation of arginines has been characterized [94].

2.6.1
Lysine Histone Demethylases

Lysine specific demethylases have been classified into seven groups named KDM1 to KDM7 (KDM for Lysine DeMethylase) [90, 91, 95]. The KDM1 group comprises the first enzyme that has been identified as a lysine specific histone demethylase (LSD1). The other six groups (KDM2 to 7) exhibit all a Jumonji-C (JmjC) domain that presents similarities with the AlkB catalytic domain, suggesting that these JmjC-domain containing proteins might have a similar hydrolase activity to function as demethylase [96, 97]. Structural biology studies have been published for several members of these seven groups that reveal key three-dimensional aspects concerning their interaction with different partners or substrates.

2.6.1.1 **LSD1 (KDM1)**

LSD1, also known as BHC110, is the first lysine specific demethylase that was discovered. It has been assigned to group I of lysine demethylases (KDM1) [90, 91]. LSD1 contains an amine oxidase domain responsible of the enzymatic activity and has been isolated as a stable component from several histone modifying complexes. The enzymatic characterization of this protein revealed that FAD (flavine adenine dinucleotide) is required as a cofactor for the removal of the methyl group. Furthermore, LSD1 requires a protonated nitrogen in order to initiate demethylation so that this enzyme is only able to demethylate mono- or dimethylated substrates but not trimethylated substrates [98, 99].

Two independent studies determined the structure of LSD1 alone and showed that this protein is composed of three structural units, comprising a SWIRM N-terminal domain, a six-helix bundle and a C-terminal oxidase domain. All these domains pack closely against each other [98–100] (Figure 2.7). The C-terminal domain contains a large insertion (~100 residues) that forms an additional domain called the tower domain. This last domain protrudes from the compact structure as an antiparallel coiled coil (Figure 2.7). The catalytic domain adopts a two-lobe organization that is also observed in other flavoenzymes. One lobe associates with the FAD cofactor whereas the other lobe is involved in substrate recognition and binding (Figure 2.7).

Further, LSD1 requires Co-REST, a chromatin-associated transcriptional repressor, to demethylate nucleosomal substrates [101, 102]. The structure of this complex

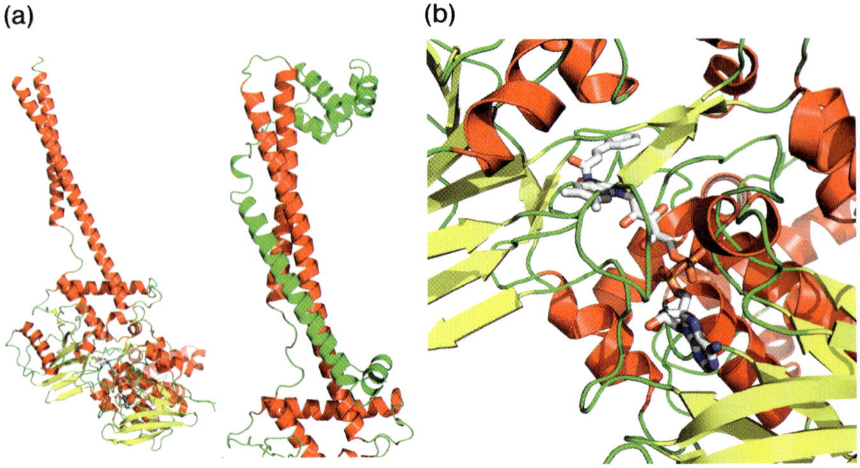

Figure 2.7 Structures of a lysine-specific hystone demethylase 1 (LSD1). In all three pictures, the LSD1 protein is in the same orientation. (a) The human LSD1 structure (PDB code 2HK0) with the tower domain (top two helices), just below the AOL domain, (harboring the FAD cofactor and the substrate-binding subdomain).The protein is represented schematically, with the helices, β-strands and coil regions colored in red, yellow and green, respectively. The FAD cofactor is in stick representation with the carbon, oxygen, phosphorus and nitrogen atoms colored in gray, red, orange and blue, respectively. (b) The human LSD1 complex with a C-terminal fragment of Co-Rest (PDB code 2iw5) comprising the two SANT domains separated by the linker region (helices in green). The picture is a focused view on the Tower domain of human LSD1 and the Co-Rest fragment, as in (a). (c) the histone demethylase LSD1/tranylcypromine complex (PDB code 2z3y). The color code for the protein and the atoms are the same as in (a). The tranylcypromine inhibitor is shown as sticks in the middle of the domain.

reveals that Co-REST wraps around the protruding Tower domain without altering the catalytic domain [103] (Figure 2.7). LSD1/Co-REST was cocrystallized with a peptide of the N-terminal region of H3 with dimethylated K4 that, unfortunately, was not interpretable. More recently, the structure of a similar complex was determined together with a substrate-like peptide inhibitor [104]. This complex reveals that the peptide binds in a funnel-shaped pocket where only 16 out of the 23 residues are visible (Figure 2.7). Other LSD1 complexes have been reported with different substrates that bind intimately to FAD [100, 105, 106].

2.6.1.2 **The JmjC Family: Jumonji-C Domain Containing Proteins**

A large number of histone lysine methylation sites have been characterized, showing that the trimethylated state is prevalent. Given that LSD1 demethylates only mono- and dimethylated lysine substrates, it seemed likely that additional enzymes would catalyze such a reaction. Indeed, the recent discovery of proteins that harbor a JmjC domain and have demethylase activity revealed a novel family of enzymes that also contain other domains associated with chromatin remodeling.

The JmjC-containing histone demethylase (JHDM) family encompasses seven sub-families that comprise approximately 20 members in humans [76, 91, 95]. The first two members JHDM1 (KDM2) and JHDM2 (KDM3) are only able to demethylate mono- or dimethyl lysine residues (H3K36 and H3K9, respectively) [91]. The third group of proteins JHDM3/JMJD2 (KDM4) are true trimethyl demethylases that specifically catalyze the demethylation of H3K9me3 and H3K36me3. The next group is named JARID (KDM5) and is highly similar to JHDM3/JMJD2 but demethylates only H3K4 in either the di- or trimethyl state. Little is known of the last group JMJD3 (KDM6). The catalytic mechanisms of the JmjC domain containing proteins are all hydroxylation reactions that involve iron and α-ketoglutarate as cofactors.

2.6.1.3 Lysine Demethylase JHDM1 (KDM2)

Two JHDM1 genes (JHDM1A and JHDM1B) are present in the human genome. It has been shown that JHDM1A demethylates only mono- and dimethyl lysine of histone H3 (H3K36). This was rather unexpected given that the catalytic mechanism of a JmjC domain does not require a protonated nitrogen, unlike LSD1, and therefore could also have the ability to remove the methyl in all three states. So far, two crystal structures have been deposited in the protein database but without any publication underlining the work. The crystal structures describe two forms of the human JHDM1A lysine demethylase, apo and in a complex with α-ketoglutarate (PDB codes 2yu1 and 2yu2).

2.6.1.4 Lysine Demethylase JHDM3/JMJD2 (KDM4)

The proteins belonging to the JMJD2 subfamilly are specific trimethyl lysine demethylases that comprise four members (JMJD2A-D). The JMJD2 enzymes exhibit a catalytic core in the N-terminal region composed of a JmjN domain and a JmjC domain. JMJD2 enzymes preferentially demethylate H3K9me3, H3K9me2, H3K36me3 and H3K36me2, leading to the accumulation of lysines in the monomethylated state that they are unable to modify. Unlike other members of the JHDM family, the JMJD2 enzyme requires both the JmjN and the JmjC domains to efficiently catalyze the demethylation reaction. The structure of the catalytic core of JMJD2 was recently solved in the absence and presence of α-ketoglutarate [107] (Figure 2.8). These complexes reveal the three-dimensional architecture of the JmjC and JmjN domains that together form most of the catalytic core. The JmjC domain exhibits helices and β-strands that form a jellyroll-like fold typical for metalloenzymes. The JmjC domain provides the scaffold that binds the iron atom that is chelated by three strictly conserved residues, one histidine and two glutamates and is also observed in close contact with the α-ketoglutarate cofactor. Furthermore, the JmjN domain, composed of three helices positioned between two β-strands, is located opposite to the catalytic center and forms extensive interactions with the JmjC domain. The JmjN domain is not present in all JHDM enzymes, suggesting that it may play a particular role in the demethylation reaction as suggested by deletion experiments [91].

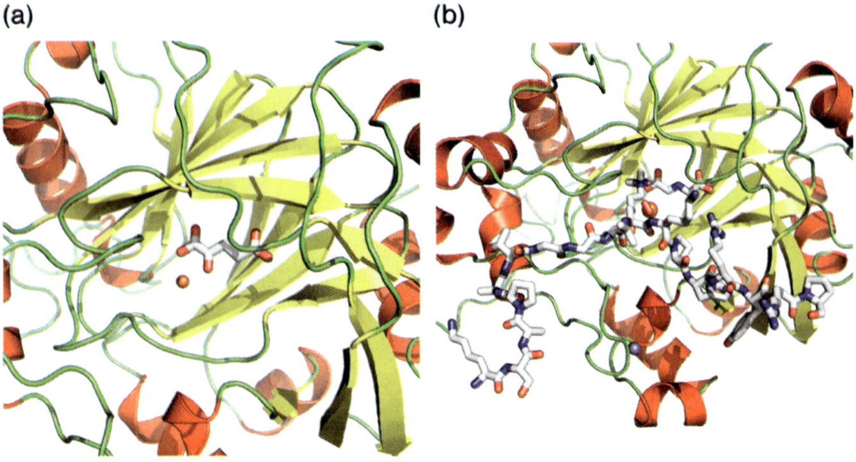

Figure 2.8 Structures of the catalytic core domain of JMJD2A. (a) The catalytic core without substrate (PDB code 2gp3) but in the presence of iron and zinc atoms (spheres in red and blue respectively). (b) The catalytic core in the presence of α-ketoglutarate (pdb code 2gp5). The substrates are shown as sticks with the carbon, oxygen and nitrogen atoms colored in gray, red and blue, respectively. In all pictures the protein is represented schematically, with the helices, β-strands and coil regions colored in red, yellow and green, respectively.

Additional structural elements have been revealed by these three-dimensional structures, such as the presence of a mixed domain between the JmjN and JmjC domains, which is composed of a few helices and coils, and a novel zinc finger following the JmjC domain. The zinc finger motif is unique as it is formed by two cysteine residues from the JmjC domain and a cysteine and histidine residue of the region following the JmjC domain.

Further, different groups crystallized the catalytic core of the JMJD2A enzyme as a complex in the presence of different lysine substrates, iron and an analog of the α-ketoglutarate that mimics the initial coordination of the cofactor, but does not initiate the hydroxylation process (Figure 2.8). Detailed interactions were obtained for different methylated lysine states of histone H3K9 and H3K36 with either two or three methyl groups [108, 109].

2.6.2
Arginine Demethylases

2.6.2.1 Histone Demethylimination

Enzymes that convert peptidyl arginine to citrulline comprise a large family of peptidyl arginine deiminases (PADs). PADs are highly specific for peptidylarginine residues and they belong to a larger superfamily known as guanidine-modifying enzymes, called the amidinotransferase superfamily [93, 110]. Today five homologs have been identified in humans, named PAD1–4 and PAD6. They are multidomain enzymes whose activity is regulated by calcium. The proteins are composed of a

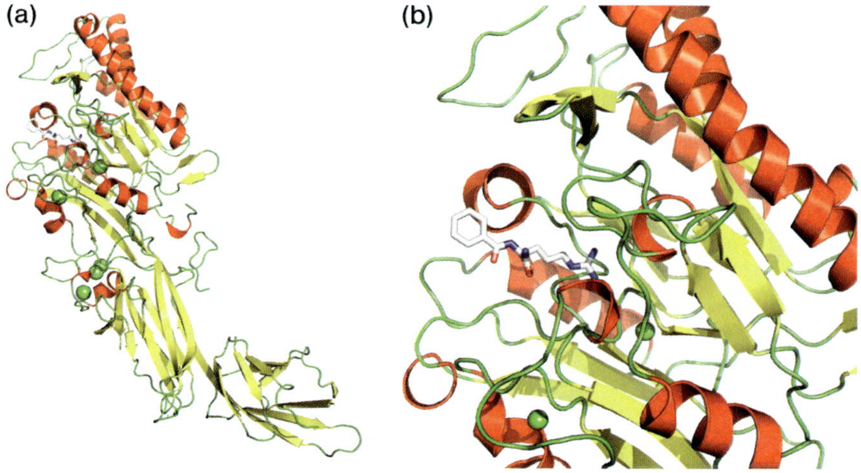

Figure 2.9 Overall structure of Peptidylarginine deiminase 4 (PAD4). PAD4 is a Ca^{2+}-dependent enzyme that catalyzes the conversion of protein arginine residues to citrulline. (a) Ribbon representation of the PAD4/benzoyl-L-arginine amide complex (PDB code 1wda) in the presence of the Ca^{2+} ions (green spheres). (b) Close up view of the substrate benzoyl-L-arginine amide bound to PAD4. The substrate carbon, oxygen, phosphorus and nitrogen atoms are colored in gray, red, orange and blue, respectively. The protein is represented schematically, with the helices, β-strands and coil regions colored in red, yellow and green, respectively.

catalytic domain and the human members exhibit two immunoglobulin-like domains at the N-terminus of the protein that are thought to be involved in protein-protein interactions and/or substrate targeting.

PAD4 is a nuclear protein that has been shown to deiminate histones at multiple arginine sites of histones H2A, H3, and H4. This enzyme is able to modify either nonmethylated histone arginines or monomethylated histone arginines. It has been shown that this enzymatic modification antagonizes the arginine methylation [92, 93, 110]. The structure of PAD4 shows that this enzyme adopts an elongated form, the C-terminal catalytic domain presenting an α/β propeller fold [111] (Figure 2.9). The structure of PAD4 with benzoyl-L-arginine amide further revealed an active site cleft built up by β-strands [111]. Further, structures of an inactive mutant of PAD4 in complex with various peptides provided a deeper insight into how PAD4 recognizes natural target proteins [112] (Figure 2.9).

2.6.2.2 **Histone Arginine Demethylase**

The conversion of arginine into citrulline does not represent the reverse modification of methylation per se. The recent discovery of a histone arginine demethylase containing a JmjC domain (JMJD6) revealed a more direct way for performing arginine demethylation [94]. Structural data are awaited to decipher the catalytic mechanism of this enzyme and the differences that lead to arginine rather than lysine recognition by the JmjC domain.

2.7 DNA Methyltransferases

Methylation of DNA occurs in all phyla of life. In eukaryotes, methylation is dependent upon the kind of organism, some eukaryotes being even devoid of methylated DNA [113]. In mammals, a major mark is the methylation of cytosine at its C5 position (^{5m}C), found mostly in CpG dinucleotides. So far, four enzymes have been implicated in ^{5m}C methylation of DNA in these organisms: Dnmt1, Dnmt3a, Dnmt3b, DnmtL. Dnmt3a and Dnmt3b appear responsible for initial CpG methylation, whereas Dnmt1 seems mostly in charge of maintaining the methylation pattern during chromosome replication, changing hemi-methylated DNA into fully methylated DNA [114]. DnmtL is similar in sequence to the Dnmt3a/b enzymes but is devoid of any activity due to the lack of conserved catalytic residues. However, Dnmt3L is required for the methylase activity of the Dnmt3a/b proteins.

Structural knowledge has long remained scarce on mammalian DNA methyltransferases. If this remains true for Dnmt1, recent studies shed light on the Dnmt3 and Dnmt3L proteins. Notably, structures were obtained of: (1) the complex formed between the C-terminal domains of Dnmt3a and Dnmt3L and the reaction product S-adenosyl-L-homocysteine (AdoHcy) [115] and (2) full-length Dnmt3L bound to a histone H3 peptide unmethylated on lysine 4, methylation of this lysine preventing binding of Dnmt3L to histone H3 [116]. These structures show that both Dnmt3a and Dnmt3L have a fold characteristic of unpermuted, AdoMet-dependent MTases of class I [69]. However, in the ternary complex only Dnmt3a binds an AdoHcy molecule.

The structure of the Dnmt3a/Dnmt3L complex shows a tetrameric arrangement with a central homodimer of Dnmt3a flanked on each side by Dnmt3L molecules [115] (Figure 2.10). Such an arrangement is biologically relevant, as demonstrated by mutational analysis of various residues at protein/protein interfaces. Further, the binding of Dnmt3L appears to lock the catalytic loop of Dnmt3a in an active conformation and to enhance the binding of AdoMet to Dnmt3a, thus providing an explanation for its regulatory role in the methylation reaction. Further, dimerization of Dnmt3a would be in agreement with observations of tandem methylation of CpG dinucleotides [115].

The structure of full-length Dnmt3L bound to an unmethylated peptide from histone H3 N-terminal tail [116] is providing additional information on how the Dnmt3a/b-Dnmt3L complex may act on nucleosomal substrates as well as a structural view on the link between histone and DNA modifications. In this structure, the histone H3 peptide is interacting with the N-terminal zinc-binding domain of Dnmt3L (Figure 2.10). Using both structures, modeling of a full-length Dnmt3a-Dnmt3L complex binding to a single nucleosome provides a structural explanation to the fact that mammalian DNA methyltransferases act on nucleosomes [114].

Neither structure provides a direct view on the catalytic mechanism of these enzymes. However, prior biochemical and structural studies on bacterial MTases in complex with DNA revealed a mechanism involving base-flipping followed by a nucleophilic attack of a conserved cysteine on carbon C6 of the cytosine to be

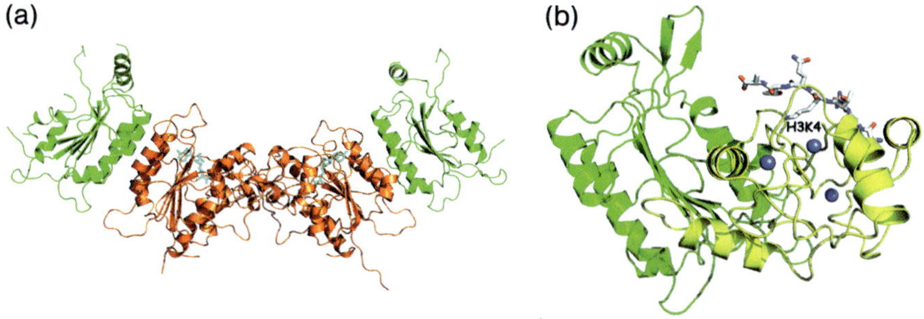

Figure 2.10 Structures of mammalian DNA methylases. (a) Ribbon representation of the structure of the tetrameric complex formed between the C-terminal domain of Dnmt3a2 (orange) and the C-terminal domain of Dnmt3L (green) (PDB code 2qrv). The AdoHcy molecules are colored cyan. (b) Ribbon representation of the structure of full-length Dnmt3L with an unmethylated histone H3 peptide bound (PDB code 2pvc). Dnmt3L is colored green for the C-terminal domain oriented as in (a) and yellow for the N-terminal zinc-binding domain. The peptide is colored according to the atom type. The structural zinc ions of the N-terminal domain of Dnmt3L are shown as blue spheres. The unmethylated lysine is labeled.

modified [117, 118]. In the following step, a C5 nucleophilic displacement of the methyl group of AdoMet leads to the 5-methyl-6-Cys-S-5,6-dihydrocytosine transient intermediate that might be deprotonated into the final ^{5m}C product by a water molecule [119].

It has long been thought that DNA methylation was a long-term epigenetic mark. Recent studies that show a cyclic pattern of DNA methylation and demethylation at promoters are challenging this view [120, 121]. Dnmt3a and Dnmt3b are also suggested to be the enzymes carrying out the demethylation of the DNA, possibly in complex with other proteins, the mechanism for this reaction remaining unknown [120].

2.8
Concluding Remarks: the Challenge of Structural Studies of Epigenetic Targets

Despite the large amount of cellular, biochemical and structural data obtained so far on epigenetic targets, major debates remain on how epigenetic mechanisms are carried out. In the case of structural studies, this is exemplified by the lack of clear understanding of the molecular mechanisms sustaining the catalytic activities of the various enzymes involved in epigenetics, as discussed above. Explanations for this are multiple and highlight the future challenge of structural studies of epigenetic targets as well as major implications for drug design approaches.

First, it should be noted that most of the modules whose structures were determined so far often represent subdomains of epigenetic effectors. Indeed, a landmark of many of these proteins is to be composed of different modules, some responsible for epigenetic marks recognition and others bearing catalytic activities.

The rationale behind this is to be able to recruit an enzymatic activity at specific locations, for instance a histone acetyltransferase being recruited by a bromodomain – recognizing acetylated histone tails – to propagate chromatin decondensation by acetylation at specific gene promoters [122]. Furthermore, many studies have demonstrated that full-length proteins display different recognition properties towards epigenetic marks or modified catalytic activities than their isolated modules, showing an influence of medium- or long-range intramolecular interactions.

Second, many epigenetic effectors are part of macromolecular complexes, as illustrated by HATs [12]. The multiple subunits composing these complexes are also very often composed of multiple modules, thus expanding the capacity of recruiting one or several catalytic activities at specific locations, depending on several different epigenetic marks rather than on a single one and making extended use of the histone code [7, 8, 11]. Additionally, in this context an epigenetic mark recognition or a catalytic activity is not only influenced by intramolecular but also by intermolecular interactions. Another implication for structural analyses is that studies with substrates should not be restricted to small molecules and peptides but should also consider larger substrates, such as full-length transcription factors, nucleosomes – epigenetically modified or not – or even nucleosomal arrays.

Clearly, the use of single modules from epigenetic effectors has opened the way for understanding how these proteins are acting. It has also eased structural studies since many of these modules could be produced in large quantities in *Escherichia coli*, with a few exceptions where the baculovirus expression system was used (CARM1, HDAC7) or in the case of p300 HAT domain that required a complicated expression protocol prior to structural studies, explaining why it took so long to obtain structural data on this module [24]. It can be expected that the intricacy of the biochemical work required prior to structural studies will increase to tackle the challenge of understanding epigenetic mechanisms in molecular terms in the context of full-length proteins and macromolecular complexes. This will require an extended use of existing techniques, for instance applying multiexpression techniques [123] and endogenous purification [124] in complex reconstitution. But the development of new techniques will certainly be also necessary, notably to stabilize and characterize transient interactions. Further, structural studies will not be addressed solely by NMR or crystallography but by a combination of these techniques with others such as small angle X-ray scattering (SAXS) and electron microscopy (EM).

Drug design approaches should definitively benefit from these studies since they will be able to study the effect of their effectors in a context that should be biologically more relevant. Several aspects should however be considered. First, many epigenetic effectors bearing catalytic activity are shared between different macromolecular complexes where their activity might be differently modulated. Second, the composition of these complexes might be influenced by both the cell type and the cell state, varying even further the modulation of the catalytic activity. Integrating these data in drug design studies might be of paramount importance since it could allow the precise design of effectors molecules that would affect a precise pathway leaving others unaffected.

References

1 Li, B., Carey, M. and Workman, J.L. (2007) The role of chromatin during transcription. *Cell*, **128** (4), 707–719.

2 Groth, A., Rocha, W., Verreault, A. and Almouzni, G. (2007) Chromatin challenges during DNA replication and repair. *Cell*, **128** (4), 721–733.

3 Feinberg, A.P. (2007) Phenotypic plasticity and the epigenetics of human disease. *Nature*, **447** (7143), 433–440.

4 Wang, G.G., Allis, C.D. and Chi, P. (2007) Chromatin remodeling and cancer. Part II: ATP-dependent chromatin remodeling. *Trends in Molecular Medicine*, **13** (9), 373–380.

5 Wang, G.G., Allis, C.D. and Chi, P. (2007) Chromatin remodeling and cancer. Part I: Covalent histone modifications. *Trends in Molecular Medicine*, **13** (9), 363–372.

6 Kouzarides, T. (2007) Chromatin modifications and their function. *Cell*, **128** (4), 693–705.

7 Strahl, B.D. (2000) Allis CD: The language of covalent histone modifications. *Nature*, **403** (6765), 41–45.

8 Jenuwein, T. and Allis, C.D. (2001) Translating the histone code. *Science*, **293** (5532), 1074–1080.

9 Yang, X.J. and Seto, E. (2007) HATs and HDACs: from structure, function and regulation to novel strategies for therapy and prevention. *Oncogene*, **26** (37), 5310–5318.

10 Luger, K., Mader, A.W., Richmond, R.K., Sargent, D.F. and Richmond, T.J. (1997) Crystal structure of the nucleosome core particle at 2.8 A resolution. *Nature*, **389** (6648), 251–260.

11 Taverna, S.D., Li, H., Ruthenburg, A.J., Allis, C.D. and Patel, D.J. (2007) How chromatin-binding modules interpret histone modifications: lessons from professional pocket pickers. *Nature Structural & Molecular Biology*, **14** (11), 1025–1040.

12 Lee, K.K. and Workman, J.L. (2007) Histone acetyltransferase complexes: one size doesn't fit all. *Nature Reviews. Molecular Cell Biology*, **8** (4), 284–295.

13 Yang, X.J. and Seto, E. (2008) Lysine acetylation: codified crosstalk with other posttranslational modifications. *Molecular Cell*, **31** (4), 449–461.

14 Neuwald, A.F. and Landsman, D. (1997) GCN5-related histone N-acetyltransferases belong to a diverse superfamily that includes the yeast SPT10 protein. *Trends in Biochemical Sciences*, **22** (5), 154–155.

15 Angus-Hill, M.L., Dutnall, R.N., Tafrov, S.T., Sternglanz, R. and Ramakrishnan, V. (1999) Crystal structure of the histone acetyltransferase Hpa2: A tetrameric member of the Gcn5-related N-acetyltransferase superfamily. *Journal of Molecular Biology*, **294** (5), 1311–1325.

16 Dutnall, R.N., Tafrov, S.T., Sternglanz, R. and Ramakrishnan, V. (1998) Structure of the histone acetyltransferase Hat1: a paradigm for the GCN5-related N-acetyltransferase superfamily. *Cell*, **94** (4), 427–438.

17 Rojas, J.R., Trievel, R.C., Zhou, J., Mo, Y., Li, X., Berger, S.L., Allis, C.D. and Marmorstein, R. (1999) Structure of Tetrahymena GCN5 bound to coenzyme A and a histone H3 peptide. *Nature*, **401** (6748), 93–98.

18 Lin, Y., Fletcher, C.M., Zhou, J., Allis, C.D. and Wagner, G. (1999) Solution structure of the catalytic domain of GCN5 histone acetyltransferase bound to coenzyme A. *Nature*, **400** (6739), 86–89.

19 Clements, A., Rojas, J.R., Trievel, R.C., Wang, L., Berger, S.L. and Marmorstein, R. (1999) Crystal structure of the histone acetyltransferase domain of the human PCAF transcriptional regulator bound to coenzyme A. *The EMBO Journal*, **18** (13), 3521–3532.

20 Dutnall, R.N., Tafrov, S.T., Sternglanz, R. and Ramakrishnan, V. (1998) Structure of the yeast histone acetyltransferase Hat1: insights into substrate specificity and implications for the Gcn5-related

N-acetyltransferase superfamily. *Cold Spring Harbor Symposia on Quantitative Biology*, **63**, 501–507.

21 Trievel, R.C., Rojas, J.R., Sterner, D.E., Venkataramani, R.N., Wang, L., Zhou, J., Allis, C.D., Berger, S.L. and Marmorstein, R. (1999) Crystal structure and mechanism of histone acetylation of the yeast GCN5 transcriptional coactivator. *Proceedings of the National Academy of Sciences of the United States of America*, **96** (16), 8931–8936.

22 Yan, Y., Barlev, N.A., Haley, R.H., Berger, S.L. and Marmorstein, R. (2000) Crystal structure of yeast Esa1 suggests a unified mechanism for catalysis and substrate binding by histone acetyltransferases. *Molecular Cell*, **6** (5), 1195–1205.

23 Holbert, M.A., Sikorski, T., Carten, J., Snowflack, D., Hodawadekar, S. and Marmorstein, R. (2007) The human monocytic leukemia zinc finger histone acetyltransferase domain contains DNA-binding activity implicated in chromatin targeting. *The Journal of Biological Chemistry*, **282** (50), 36603–36613.

24 Liu, X., Wang, L., Zhao, K., Thompson, P.R., Hwang, Y., Marmorstein, R. and Cole, P.A. (2008) The structural basis of protein acetylation by the p300/CBP transcriptional coactivator. *Nature*, **451** (7180), 846–850.

25 Lin, C. and Yuan, Y.A. (2008) Structural insights into histone H3 lysine 56 acetylation by Rtt109. *Structure*, **16** (10), 1503–1510.

26 Stavropoulos, P., Nagy, V., Blobel, G. and Hoelz, A. (2008) Molecular basis for the autoregulation of the protein acetyl transferase Rtt109. *Proceedings of the National Academy of Sciences of the United States of America*, **105** (34), 12236–12241.

27 Tang, Y., Holbert, M.A., Wurtele, H., Meeth, K., Rocha, W., Gharib, M., Jiang, E., Thibault, P., Verrault, A., Cole, P.A. *et al.* (2008) Fungal Rtt109 histone acetyltransferase is an unexpected structural homolog of metazoan p300/CBP. *Nature Structural & Molecular Biology*, **15** (7), 738–745.

28 Poux, A.N. and Marmorstein, R. (2003) Molecular basis for Gcn5/PCAF histone acetyltransferase selectivity for histone and nonhistone substrates. *Biochemistry*, **42** (49), 14366–14374.

29 Poux, A.N., Cebrat, M., Kim, C.M., Cole, P.A. and Marmorstein, R. (2002) Structure of the GCN5 histone acetyltransferase bound to a bisubstrate inhibitor. *Proceedings of the National Academy of Sciences of the United States of America*, **99** (22), 14065–14070.

30 Clements, A., Poux, A.N., Lo, W.S., Pillus, L., Berger, S.L. and Marmorstein, R. (2003) Structural basis for histone and phosphohistone binding by the GCN5 histone acetyltransferase. *Molecular Cell*, **12** (2), 461–473.

31 Tanner, K.G., Trievel, R.C., Kuo, M.H., Howard, R.M., Berger, S.L., Allis, C.D., Marmorstein, R. and Denu, J.M. (1999) Catalytic mechanism and function of invariant glutamic acid 173 from the histone acetyltransferase GCN5 transcriptional coactivator. *The Journal of Biological Chemistry*, **274** (26), 18157–18160.

32 Yan, Y., Harper, S., Speicher, D.W. and Marmorstein, R. (2002) The catalytic mechanism of the ESA1 histone acetyltransferase involves a self-acetylated intermediate. *Nature Structural Biology*, **9** (11), 862–869.

33 Berndsen, C.E., Albaugh, B.N., Tan, S. and Denu, J.M. (2007) Catalytic mechanism of a MYST family histone acetyltransferase. *Biochemistry*, **46** (3), 623–629.

34 Yang, X.J. and Seto, E. (2003) Collaborative spirit of histone deacetylases in regulating chromatin structure and gene expression. *Current Opinion in Genetics & Development*, **13** (2), 143–153.

35 Glozak, M.A., Sengupta, N., Zhang, X. and Seto, E. (2005) Acetylation and deacetylation of non-histone proteins. *Gene*, **363**, 15–23.

36 Gregoretti, I.V., Lee, Y.M. and Goodson, H.V. (2004) Molecular evolution of the histone deacetylase family: functional implications of phylogenetic analysis. *Journal of Molecular Biology*, **338** (1), 17–31.

37 de Ruijter, A.J., van Gennip, A.H., Caron, H.N., Kemp, S. and van Kuilenburg, A.B. (2003) Histone deacetylases (HDACs): characterization of the classical HDAC family. *The Biochemical Journal*, **370** (Pt 3), 737–749.

38 Leipe, D.D. and Landsman, D. (1997) Histone deacetylases, acetoin utilization proteins and acetylpolyamine amidohydrolases are members of an ancient protein superfamily. *Nucleic Acids Research*, **25** (18), 3693–3697.

39 Yang, X.J. and Seto, E. (2008) The Rpd3/Hda1 family of lysine deacetylases: from bacteria and yeast to mice and men. *Nature Reviews. Molecular Cell Biology*, **9** (3), 206–218.

40 Fischle, W., Dequiedt, F., Hendzel, M.J., Guenther, M.G., Lazar, M.A., Voelter, W. and Verdin, E. (2002) Enzymatic activity associated with class II HDACs is dependent on a multiprotein complex containing HDAC3 and SMRT/N-CoR. *Molecular Cell*, **9** (1), 45–57.

41 Finnin, M.S., Donigian, J.R., Cohen, A., Richon, V.M., Rifkind, R.A., Marks, P.A., Breslow, R. and Pavletich, N.P. (1999) Structures of a histone deacetylase homologue bound to the TSA and SAHA inhibitors. *Nature*, **401** (6749), 188–193.

42 Somoza, J.R., Skene, R.J., Katz, B.A., Mol, C., Ho, J.D., Jennings, A.J., Luong, C., Arvai, A., Buggy, J.J., Chi, E. *et al.* (2004) Structural snapshots of human HDAC8 provide insights into the class I histone deacetylases. *Structure (London, England: 1993)*, **12** (7), 1325–1334.

43 Vannini, A., Volpari, C., Filocamo, G., Casavola, E.C., Brunetti, M., Renzoni, D., Chakravarty, P., Paolini, C., De Francesco, R., Gallinari, P. *et al.* (2004) Crystal structure of a eukaryotic zinc-dependent histone deacetylase, human HDAC8, complexed with a hydroxamic acid inhibitor. *Proceedings of the National Academy of Sciences of the United States of America*, **101** (42), 15064–15069.

44 Nielsen, T.K., Hildmann, C., Dickmanns, A., Schwienhorst, A. and Ficner, R. (2005) Crystal structure of a bacterial class 2 histone deacetylase homologue. *Journal of Molecular Biology*, **354** (1), 107–120.

45 Schuetz, A., Min, J., Allali-Hassani, A., Schapira, M., Shuen, M., Loppnau, P., Mazitschek, R., Kwiatkowski, N.P., Lewis, T.A., Maglathin, R.L. *et al.* (2008) Human HDAC7 harbors a class IIa histone deacetylase-specific zinc binding motif and cryptic deacetylase activity. *The Journal of Biological Chemistry*, **283** (17), 11355–11363.

46 Bottomley, M.J., Lo Surdo, P., Di Giovine, P., Cirillo, A., Scarpelli, R., Ferrigno, F., Jones, P., Neddermann, P., De Francesco, R., Steinkuhler, C. *et al.* (2008) Structural and functional analysis of the human HDAC4 catalytic domain reveals a regulatory structural zinc-binding domain. *The Journal of Biological Chemistry*, **283** (39), 26694–26704.

47 Vannini, A., Volpari, C., Gallinari, P., Jones, P., Mattu, M., Carfi, A., De Francesco, R., Steinkuhler, C. and Di Marco, S. (2007) Substrate binding to histone deacetylases as shown by the crystal structure of the HDAC8-substrate complex. *EMBO Reports*, **8** (9), 879–884.

48 Nielsen, S.J., Schneider, R., Bauer, U.M., Bannister, A.J., Morrison, A., O'Carroll, D., Firestein, R., Cleary, M., Jenuwein, T., Herrera, R.E. *et al.* (2001) Rb targets histone H3 methylation and HP1 to promoters. *Nature*, **412** (6846), 561–565.

49 Vanommeslaeghe, K., De Proft, F., Loverix, S., Tourwe, D. and Geerlings, P. (2005) Theoretical study revealing the functioning of a novel combination of catalytic motifs in histone deacetylase.

Bioorganic and Medicinal Chemistry, **13** (12), 3987–3992.

50 Lahm, A., Paolini, C., Pallaoro, M., Nardi, M.C., Jones, P., Neddermann, P., Sambucini, S., Bottomley, M.J., Lo Surdo, P., Carfi, A. *et al.* (2007) Unraveling the hidden catalytic activity of vertebrate class IIa histone deacetylases. *Proceedings of the National Academy of Sciences of the United States of America*, **104** (44), 17335–17340.

51 Hodawadekar, S.C. and Marmorstein, R. (2007) Chemistry of acetyl transfer by histone modifying enzymes: structure, mechanism and implications for effector design. *Oncogene*, **26** (37), 5528–5540.

52 Sauve, A.A., Wolberger, C., Schramm, V.L. and Boeke, J.D. (2006) The biochemistry of sirtuins. *Annual Review of Biochemistry*, **75**, 435–465.

53 Finnin, M.S., Donigian, J.R. and Pavletich, N.P. (2001) Structure of the histone deacetylase SIRT2. *Nature Structural Biology*, **8** (7), 621–625.

54 Min, J., Landry, J., Sternglanz, R. and Xu, R.M. (2001) Crystal structure of a SIR2 homolog-NAD complex. *Cell*, **105** (2), 269–279.

55 Chang, J.H., Kim, H.C., Hwang, K.Y., Lee, J.W., Jackson, S.P., Bell, S.D. and Cho, Y. (2002) Structural basis for the NAD-dependent deacetylase mechanism of Sir2. *The Journal of Biological Chemistry*, **277** (37), 34489–34498.

56 Zhao, K., Harshaw, R., Chai, X. and Marmorstein, R. (2004) Structural basis for nicotinamide cleavage and ADP-ribose transfer by NAD(+)-dependent Sir2 histone/protein deacetylases. *Proceedings of the National Academy of Sciences of the United States of America*, **101** (23), 8563–8568.

57 Avalos, J.L., Boeke, J.D. and Wolberger, C. (2004) Structural basis for the mechanism and regulation of Sir2 enzymes. *Molecular Cell*, **13** (5), 639–648.

58 Zhao, K., Chai, X. and Marmorstein, R. (2003) Structure of the yeast Hst2 protein deacetylase in ternary complex with 2′-O-acetyl ADP ribose and histone peptide. *Structure (London, England: 1993)*, **11** (11), 1403–1411.

59 Avalos, J.L., Celic, I., Muhammad, S., Cosgrove, M.S., Boeke, J.D. and Wolberger, C. (2002) Structure of a Sir2 enzyme bound to an acetylated p53 peptide. *Molecular Cell*, **10** (3), 523–535.

60 Hoff, K.G., Avalos, J.L., Sens, K. and Wolberger, C. (2006) Insights into the sirtuin mechanism from ternary complexes containing NAD+ and acetylated peptide. *Structure (London, England: 1993)*, **14** (8), 1231–1240.

61 Cosgrove, M.S., Bever, K., Avalos, J.L., Muhammad, S., Zhang, X. and Wolberger, C. (2006) The structural basis of sirtuin substrate affinity. *Biochemistry*, **45** (24), 7511–7521.

62 Bitterman, K.J., Anderson, R.M., Cohen, H.Y., Latorre-Esteves, M. and Sinclair, D.A. (2002) Inhibition of silencing and accelerated aging by nicotinamide, a putative negative regulator of yeast sir2 and human SIRT1. *The Journal of Biological Chemistry*, **277** (47), 45099–45107.

63 Sanders, B.D., Zhao, K., Slama, J.T. and Marmorstein, R. (2007) Structural basis for nicotinamide inhibition and base exchange in Sir2 enzymes. *Molecular Cell*, **25** (3), 463–472.

64 Avalos, J.L., Bever, K.M. and Wolberger, C. (2005) Mechanism of sirtuin inhibition by nicotinamide: altering the NAD(+) cosubstrate specificity of a Sir2 enzyme. *Molecular Cell*, **17** (6), 855–868.

65 Cheng, X., Collins, R.E. and Zhang, X. (2005) Structural and sequence motifs of protein (histone) methylation enzymes. *Annual Review of Biophysics and Biomolecular Structure*, **34**, 267–294.

66 Lee, D.Y., Teyssier, C., Strahl, B.D. and Stallcup, M.R. (2005) Role of protein methylation in regulation of transcription. *Endocrine Reviews*, **26** (2), 147–170.

67 Polevoda, B. and Sherman, F. (2007) Methylation of proteins involved in translation. *Molecular Microbiology*, **65** (3), 590–606.

68 Kozbial, P.Z. and Mushegian, A.R. (2005) Natural history of S-adenosylmethionine-binding proteins. *BMC Structural Biology*, **5**, 19.

69 Schubert, H.L., Blumenthal, R.M. and Cheng, X. (2003) Many paths to methyltransfer: a chronicle of convergence. *Trends in Biochemical Sciences*, **28** (6), 329–335.

70 Cheng, X. and Zhang, X. (2007) Structural dynamics of protein lysine methylation and demethylation. *Mutation Research*, **618** (1–2), 102–115.

71 Baumbusch, L.O., Thorstensen, T., Krauss, V., Fischer, A., Naumann, K., Assalkhou, R., Schulz, I., Reuter, G. and Aalen, R.B. (2001) The Arabidopsis thaliana genome contains at least 29 active genes encoding SET domain proteins that can be assigned to four evolutionarily conserved classes. *Nucleic Acids Research*, **29** (21), 4319–4333.

72 Kouzarides, T. (2002) Histone methylation in transcriptional control. *Current Opinion in Genetics & Development*, **12** (2), 198–209.

73 Rea, S., Eisenhaber, F., O'Carroll, D., Strahl, B.D., Sun, Z.W., Schmid, M., Opravil, S., Mechtler, K., Ponting, C.P., Allis, C.D. *et al.* (2000) Regulation of chromatin structure by site-specific histone H3 methyltransferases. *Nature*, **406** (6796), 593–599.

74 Qian, C. and Zhou, M.M. (2006) SET domain protein lysine methyltransferases: Structure, specificity and catalysis. *Cellular and Molecular Life Sciences*, **63** (23), 2755–2763.

75 Dillon, S.C., Zhang, X., Trievel, R.C. and Cheng, X. (2005) The SET-domain protein superfamily: protein lysine methyltransferases. *Genome Biology*, **6** (8), 227.

76 Smith, B.C. and Denu, J.M. (Jun 14 2008) Chemical mechanisms of histone lysine and arginine modifications. *Biochimica et Biophysica Acta* (Epub ahead of print).

77 Singer, M.S., Kahana, A., Wolf, A.J., Meisinger, L.L., Peterson, S.E., Goggin, C., Mahowald, M. and Gottschling, D.E. (1998) Identification of high-copy disruptors of telomeric silencing in Saccharomyces cerevisiae. *Genetics*, **150** (2), 613–632.

78 Min, J., Feng, Q., Li, Z., Zhang, Y. and Xu, R.M. (2003) Structure of the catalytic domain of human DOT1L, a non-SET domain nucleosomal histone methyltransferase. *Cell*, **112** (5), 711–723.

79 Sawada, K., Yang, Z., Horton, J.R., Collins, R.E., Zhang, X. and Cheng, X. (2004) Structure of the conserved core of the yeast Dot1p, a nucleosomal histone H3 lysine 79 methyltransferase. *The Journal of Biological Chemistry*, **279** (41), 43296–43306.

80 Pahlich, S., Zakaryan, R.P. and Gehring, H. (2006) Protein arginine methylation: Cellular functions and methods of analysis. *Biochimica et Biophysica Acta*, **1764** (12), 1890–1903.

81 Krause, C.D., Yang, Z.H., Kim, Y.S., Lee, J.H., Cook, J.R. and Pestka, S. (2007) Protein arginine methyltransferases: Evolution and assessment of their pharmacological and therapeutic potential. *Pharmacology & Therapeutics*, **113** (1), 50–87.

82 Bedford, M.T. (2007) Arginine methylation at a glance. *Journal of Cell Science*, **120** (Pt 24), 4243–4246.

83 Zhang, X. and Cheng, X. (2003) Structure of the Predominant Protein Arginine Methyltransferase PRMT1 and Analysis of Its Binding to Substrate Peptides. *Structure (Camb)*, **11** (5), 509–520.

84 Zhang, X., Zhou, L. and Cheng, X. (2000) Crystal structure of the conserved core of protein arginine methyltransferase PRMT3. *The EMBO Journal*, **19** (14), 3509–3519.

85 Weiss, V.H., McBride, A.E., Soriano, M.A., Filman, D.J., Silver, P.A. and Hogle, J.M. (2000) The structure and oligomerization of the yeast arginine methyltransferase, Hmt1. *Nature Structural Biology*, **7** (12), 1165–1171.

86 Yue, W.W., Hassler, M., Roe, S.M., Thompson-Vale, V. and Pearl, L.H. (2007) Insights into histone code syntax from structural and biochemical studies of CARM1 methyltransferase. *The EMBO Journal*, **26** (20), 4402–4412.

87 Troffer-Charlier, N., Cura, V., Hassenboehler, P., Moras, D. and Cavarelli, J. (2007) Functional insights from structures of coactivator-associated arginine methyltransferase 1 domains. *The EMBO Journal*, **26** (20), 4391–4401.

88 Martin, J.L. and McMillan, F.M. (2002) SAM (dependent) I AM: the S-adenosylmethionine-dependent methyltransferase fold. *Current Opinion in Structural Biology*, **12** (6), 783–793.

89 Anand, R. and Marmorstein, R. (2007) Structure and mechanism of lysine-specific demethylase enzymes. *The Journal of Biological Chemistry*, **282** (49), 35425–35429.

90 Shi, Y. and Whetstine, J.R. (2007) Dynamic regulation of histone lysine methylation by demethylases. *Molecular Cell*, **25** (1), 1–14.

91 Klose, R.J. and Zhang, Y. (2007) Regulation of histone methylation by demethylimination and demethylation. *Nature Reviews. Molecular Cell Biology*, **8** (4), 307–318.

92 Wang, Y., Wysocka, J., Sayegh, J., Lee, Y.H., Perlin, J.R., Leonelli, L., Sonbuchner, L.S., McDonald, C.H., Cook, R.G., Dou, Y. *et al.* (2004) Human PAD4 regulates histone arginine methylation levels via demethylimination. *Science*, **306** (5694), 279–283.

93 Thompson, P.R. and Fast, W. (2006) Histone citrullination by protein arginine deiminase: is arginine methylation a green light or a roadblock? *ACS Chemical Biology*, **1** (7), 433–441.

94 Chang, B., Chen, Y., Zhao, Y. and Bruick, R.K. (2007) JMJD6 is a histone arginine demethylase. *Science*, **318** (5849), 444–447.

95 Lan, F., Nottke, A.C. and Shi, Y. (2008) Mechanisms involved in the regulation of histone lysine demethylases. *Current Opinion in Cell Biology*, **20** (3), 316–325.

96 Trewick, S.C., McLaughlin, P.J. and Allshire, R.C. (2005) Methylation: lost in hydroxylation? *EMBO Reports*, **6** (4), 315–320.

97 Tsukada, Y., Fang, J., Erdjument-Bromage, H., Warren, M.E., Borchers, C.H., Tempst, P. and Zhang, Y. (2006) Histone demethylation by a family of JmjC domain-containing proteins. *Nature*, **439** (7078), 811–816.

98 Chen, Y., Yang, Y., Wang, F., Wan, K., Yamane, K., Zhang, Y. and Lei, M. (2006) Crystal structure of human histone lysine-specific demethylase 1 (LSD1). *Proceedings of the National Academy of Sciences of the United States of America*, **103** (38), 13956–13961.

99 Stavropoulos, P., Blobel, G. and Hoelz, A. (2006) Crystal structure and mechanism of human lysine-specific demethylase-1. *Nature Structural & Molecular Biology*, **13** (7), 626–632.

100 Mimasu, S., Sengoku, T., Fukuzawa, S., Umehara, T. and Yokoyama, S. (2008) Crystal structure of histone demethylase LSD1 and tranylcypromine at 2.25 A. *Biochemical and Biophysical Research Communications*, **366** (1), 15–22.

101 Lee, M.G., Wynder, C., Cooch, N. and Shiekhattar, R. (2005) An essential role for CoREST in nucleosomal histone 3 lysine 4 demethylation. *Nature*, **437** (7057), 432–435.

102 Shi, Y.J., Matson, C., Lan, F., Iwase, S., Baba, T. and Shi, Y. (2005) Regulation of LSD1 histone demethylase activity by its associated factors. *Molecular Cell*, **19** (6), 857–864.

103 Yang, M., Gocke, C.B., Luo, X., Borek, D., Tomchick, D.R., Machius, M., Otwinowski, Z. and Yu, H. (2006) Structural basis for CoREST-dependent demethylation of nucleosomes by the human LSD1 histone demethylase. *Molecular Cell*, **23** (3), 377–387.

104 Forneris, F., Binda, C., Adamo, A., Battaglioli, E. and Mattevi, A. (2007) Structural basis of LSD1-CoREST selectivity in histone H3 recognition. *The Journal of Biological Chemistry*, **282** (28), 20070–20074.

105 Yang, M., Culhane, J.C., Szewczuk, L.M., Gocke, C.B., Brautigam, C.A., Tomchick, D.R., Machius, M., Cole, P.A. and Yu, H. (2007) Structural basis of histone demethylation by LSD1 revealed by suicide inactivation. *Nature Structural & Molecular Biology*, **14** (6), 535–539.

106 Yang, M., Culhane, J.C., Szewczuk, L.M., Jalili, P., Ball, H.L., Machius, M., Cole, P.A. and Yu, H. (2007) Structural basis for the inhibition of the LSD1 histone demethylase by the antidepressant trans-2-phenylcyclopropylamine. *Biochemistry*, **46** (27), 8058–8065.

107 Chen, Z., Zang, J., Whetstine, J., Hong, X., Davrazou, F., Kutateladze, T.G., Simpson, M., Mao, Q., Pan, C.H., Dai, S. *et al.* (2006) Structural insights into histone demethylation by JMJD2 family members. *Cell*, **125** (4), 691–702.

108 Chen, Z., Zang, J., Kappler, J., Hong, X., Crawford, F., Wang, Q., Lan, F., Jiang, C., Whetstine, J., Dai, S. *et al.* (2007) Structural basis of the recognition of a methylated histone tail by JMJD2A. *Proceedings of the National Academy of Sciences of the United States of America*, **104** (26), 10818–10823.

109 Ng, S.S., Kavanagh, K.L., McDonough, M.A., Butler, D., Pilka, E.S., Lienard, B.M., Bray, J.E., Savitsky, P., Gileadi, O., von Delft, F. *et al.* (2007) Crystal structures of histone demethylase JMJD2A reveal basis for substrate specificity. *Nature*, **448** (7149), 87–91.

110 Cuthbert, G.L., Daujat, S., Snowden, A.W., Erdjument-Bromage, H., Hagiwara, T., Yamada, M., Schneider, R., Gregory, P.D., Tempst, P., Bannister, A.J. *et al.* (2004) Histone deimination antagonizes arginine methylation. *Cell*, **118** (5), 545–553.

111 Arita, K., Hashimoto, H., Shimizu, T., Nakashima, K., Yamada, M. and Sato, M. (2004) Structural basis for Ca(2+)-induced activation of human PAD4. *Nature Structural & Molecular Biology*, **11** (8), 777–783.

112 Arita, K., Shimizu, T., Hashimoto, H., Hidaka, Y., Yamada, M. and Sato, M. (2006) Structural basis for histone N-terminal recognition by human peptidylarginine deiminase 4. *Proceedings of the National Academy of Sciences of the United States of America*, **103** (14), 5291–5296.

113 Goll, M.G. and Bestor, T.H. (2005) Eukaryotic cytosine methyltransferases. *Annual Review of Biochemistry*, **74**, 481–514.

114 Cheng, X. and Blumenthal, R.M. (2008) Mammalian DNA methyltransferases: a structural perspective. *Structure (London, England: 1993)*, **16** (3), 341–350.

115 Jia, D., Jurkowska, R.Z., Zhang, X., Jeltsch, A. and Cheng, X. (2007) Structure of Dnmt3a bound to Dnmt3L suggests a model for de novo DNA methylation. *Nature*, **449** (7159), 248–251.

116 Ooi, S.K., Qiu, C., Bernstein, E., Li, K., Jia, D., Yang, Z., Erdjument-Bromage, H., Tempst, P., Lin, S.P., Allis, C.D. *et al.* (2007) DNMT3L connects unmethylated lysine 4 of histone H3 to de novo methylation of DNA. *Nature*, **448** (7154), 714–717.

117 Klimasauskas, S., Kumar, S., Roberts, R.J. and Cheng, X. (1994) HhaI methyltransferase flips its target base out of the DNA helix. *Cell*, **76** (2), 357–369.

118 Reinisch, K.M., Chen, L., Verdine, G.L. and Lipscomb, W.N. (1995) The crystal structure of HaeIII methyltransferase convalently complexed to DNA: an extrahelical cytosine and rearranged base pairing. *Cell*, **82** (1), 143–153.

119 O'Gara, M., Klimasauskas, S., Roberts, R.J. and Cheng, X. (1996) Enzymatic

C5-cytosine methylation of DNA: mechanistic implications of new crystal structures for HhaL methyltransferase-DNA-AdoHcy complexes. *Journal of Molecular Biology*, **261** (5), 634–645.

120 Metivier, R., Gallais, R., Tiffoche, C., Le Peron, C., Jurkowska, R.Z., Carmouche, R.P., Ibberson, D., Barath, P., Demay, F., Reid, G. *et al.* (2008) Cyclical DNA methylation of a transcriptionally active promoter. *Nature*, **452** (7183), 45–50.

121 Kangaspeska, S., Stride, B., Metivier, R., Polycarpou-Schwarz, M., Ibberson, D., Carmouche, R.P., Benes, V., Gannon, F. and Reid, G. (2008) Transient cyclical methylation of promoter DNA. *Nature*, **452** (7183), 112–115.

122 Mujtaba, S., Zeng, L. and Zhou, M.M. (2007) Structure and acetyl-lysine recognition of the bromodomain. *Oncogene*, **26** (37), 5521–5527.

123 Perrakis, A. and Romier, C. (2008) Assembly of protein complexes by coexpression in prokaryotic and eukaryotic hosts: an overview. *Methods in Molecular Biology (Clifton, NJ)*, **426**, 247–256.

124 Rigaut, G., Shevchenko, A., Rutz, B., Wilm, M., Mann, M. and Seraphin, B. (1999) A generic protein purification method for protein complex characterization and proteome exploration. *Nature Biotechnology*, **17** (10), 1030–1032.

3 Computer- and Structure-Based Lead Identification for Epigenetic Targets

Ralf Heinke, Urszula Uciechowska, and Wolfgang Sippl

3.1 Introduction

The two major biochemical pathways of epigenetic regulation are DNA methylation and posttranslational modifications of amino acids in histone proteins. The modifications interact with each other and constitute a particular pattern of alterations in the chromatin structure, the so-called histone code [1]. The posttranslational modifications of histones have been shown to participate in a wide array of cellular processes, including regulation of gene transcription, gene repression and mitosis. The regulation of these covalent modifications and the implications of this regulation are currently of great interest in the scientific community [2]. Although histone proteins are under the control of various posttranslational modifications, such as acetylation, methylation, phosphorylation, ubiquitinlyation or glycosylation, the focus of most studies has been mainly on lysine acetylation/deacetylation and methylation/demethylation. Over the past decade, many of the enzymes that regulate these histone modifications have been identified and characterized on a molecular level. A large effort has been accompanied by a wealth of three-dimensional (3D) structures on epigenetic targets in an attempt to understand on an atomistic level epigenetic targets and regulation. (see Chapter 2 in this book). From the early discovery of histone deacetylase inhibitors, such as trichostatin A, to the more recent discovery of novel histone modifying enzyme inhibitors, structure- and computer-based approaches were applied to analyze target-ligand interaction and to rationalize the development of small molecule modulators [3]. This chapter summarizes the progress on small molecule inhibitors identified by structure- and computer-based approaches that can modulate the activity of histone deacetylases, histone acetyltransferases, histone methyltransferases and histone demethylases.

Epigenetic Targets in Drug Discovery. Edited by Wolfgang Sippl and Manfred Jung

ISBN: 978-3-527-32355-5

3.2 Computer-Based Methods in Drug Discovery

It has become common sense in drug discovery to use computer-based *in silico* design techniques to identify and optimize novel molecules with a desired biological activity [4]. As a practical matter, computer-based methods are frequently split into disciplines that focus on either structure-based or ligand-based approaches. When the 3D structure of a target protein is known, then it is possible to apply structure-based methods. New candidate molecules may be docked into a particular binding pocket in order to study whether they can interact with the protein in an optimal way. In an ideal situation, the target protein has already been crystallized in complex with a first lead structure. However, in particular for novel targets, structural information is frequently not available at the time of the first experiments (e.g. high-throughput screening). When no 3D structure is available, but a sufficient number of active analogs have already been synthesized, then pharmacophore-based methods can be applied to identify novel molecules that fit a particular pharmacophore model [5, 6]. It may seem straightforward to develop new molecules for known proteins by applying structure-based approaches, but there are significant problems invoked. Protein flexibility, multiple ligand binding modes, solvation and entropic effects are some of the problems that must be solved to end up with reliable models. There are also studies available that demonstrate the efficiency of ligand- and structure-based approaches in direct comparison [6], as well as synergies obtained by using both approaches in combination [7]. As the costs for computational power keep dropping and parallel computing are now available, *in silico* modeling techniques are no longer a limiting problem to analyze large databases comprising millions of compounds [4]. In general, *in silico* methods gained influence on the validation of targets, hit finding, hit to lead, expansion, lead optimization and also the prediction of suitable ADMET and off-target activity profiles [8].

3.2.1 Pharmacophore-Based Methods

The classic definition of a pharmacophore [9], the spatial arrangement of functional groups in a molecule necessary to mediate a biological effect, is based on a 3D point of view of molecules. It reflects the way medicinal chemists characterize the interaction pattern of molecules for a given target protein. However, depending on the different research areas, scientists have different views. Computational chemists often use the term pharmacophore in a more abstract way. Influenced by the structural representation of molecules, a set of topological connections is used to define the properties and dimension of a molecule in 2D. Here, the spatial and topological distribution of pharmacophoric features is converted to a lower dimensional representation, for example vectors. Such vectors, which represent pharmacophore descriptors, are referred to as "fingerprints," "keys," "bitstrings" or "correlation vectors," depending on the type of information stored. The pharmacophore descriptors or fingerprints can be regarded as a transformed molecular representation instead of an explicit

3D structure [10]. Both fingerprint and pharmacophore models are often used to rapidly screen large compound collections to identify novel potential hits [11].

3.2.2
3D Quantitative Structure–Activity Relationship

Three-dimensional quantitative structure–activity relationship (3D-QSAR) techniques are the most prominent computational means to support chemistry within indirect drug design projects. The primary aim of these techniques is to establish a correlation of biological activities of a series of structurally and biologically characterized compounds with the spatial fingerprints of numerous field properties of each molecule, such as steric demand, lipophilicity and electrostatic interactions. Typically, a 3D-QSAR study allows identifying a correlation between molecular structure and biological effect and provides guidelines for the design of next-generation compounds with enhanced biological activity. The most frequently applied methods include comparative molecular field analysis (CoMFA) [12], comparative molecular similarity indices analysis (CoMSIA) [13] and the GRID/GOLPE program (generating *o*ptimal *l*inear *PLS e*stimations) [14]. Several reviews have been published in the past few years focusing on the basic theory, the pitfalls and the application of 3D-QSAR approaches [15–18]. Apart from the commercial distribution, a major factor causing the ongoing enthusiasm for CoMFA-related approaches comes from the proven ability of several of these methods to correctly estimate the biological activity of novel compounds [15].

3.2.3
Ligand Docking

The increase of available structural data for protein–ligand complexes has accelerated the development of structure-based methods. Today, protein–ligand docking is considered as the most important tool for structure-based drug design. The docking process can be divided into two major parts: (1) the correct placement of a molecule in a protein binding pocket and (2) the prediction of ligand affinities by a so-called scoring function [6]. Considering the complexity of the underlying thermodynamics of the ligand binding process, this evidently is a challenging task. After more than 20 years of development, a large number of docking programs and even more scoring functions are available. In contrast to pharmacophore screening approaches, the performance of docking methods is a trade-off between computational demand and accuracy. A major problem of current docking programs is that they do not take into account protein flexibility or do not consider protein/ligand desolvation processes. Only very recently, docking programs were developed (e.g. AutoDock4 [19], GOLD4 [20], Glide [21], FlexE [22]) which consider protein flexibility to some extent. Another problem which often occurs in ligand docking is the correct placement of water molecules within the binding site, which represent putative ligand binding partners. Structure-based approaches are able to provide important information about the interaction between a ligand and a macromolecule, but the accurate prediction of the binding affinity is still an unsolved problem [23]. A detailed discussion about the limitations of docking and scoring programs can be found in recently published reviews [23, 24].

3.2.4
Virtual Screening

High-throughput screening of chemical libraries is a well established method for finding new lead structures in early drug discovery. However, the increasing number of purchasable compounds makes it necessary to have fast and reliable pre-filtering methods to reduce the number of compounds selected for experimental testing. In contrast to high-throughput screening, virtual screening (VS) compounds are selected on the basis of computer-based predictions. In this way, VS approaches try to select the most promising compounds from an electronic database for biological testing. VS can be carried out by applying different kind of approaches: (1) by searching databases for molecules with chemical similarity to a set of known actives [11], (2) by identifying compounds which match a given pharmacophore [4] or (3) by fitting molecules into the 3D structure of a macromolecular target [25]. In addition, pre-screening filters are usually applied that filter a compound library before docking towards compounds with favorable pharmacokinetics, optimum oral bioavailability, compatibility with some types of metabolisms and consequently low toxicity. The secret to success in VS lies in the choice of an appropriate combination of methods [23].

To evaluate the performance of a given VS technique, validation studies are usually carried out. For this purpose, known binders are pooled with a set of randomly selected compounds to assess how well the known binders "enrich" during the course of the screening process. Such considerations are relevant for the development of new methods; however, in actual drug discovery projects, at the end of the day, a newly discovered chemotype or a druglike lead structure represents the ultimate goal. Impressive enrichment rates of known actives will not be convincing [23]. Since the early VS attempts, a plethora of application studies has been performed and the list of success stories is steadily growing. Despite the fact that VS is still a developing discipline, it has been reviewed frequently [4, 8, 23–26], most recently in a comprehensive overview by Klebe [23].

3.2.5
Binding Free Energy Calculations

Accurate prediction of binding affinities for a diverse set of ligands using scoring functions turns out to be genuinely difficult [25]. In general, this is a problem of subtraction of large numbers, inaccurately calculated, to arrive at a small number. The large numbers are the protein-ligand interaction energy on one hand and the cost of bringing protein and ligand out of solvent and into a complex on the other hand. The result of this subtraction is the free energy of binding, the small number we want to know. As long as full protein–ligand flexibility and the complexity of protein–ligand–water interaction is not covered by docking and scoring, it cannot be expected to end up with accurate affinity prediction. Of course, more accurate methods may be considered. Among the most accurate today are thermodynamic integration/free energy calculation methods, which can sometimes calculate the differences in affinities between related molecules within 1 kcal/mol [27]. The problem with these methods is that they demand so much computation time as to be infeasible for a large compound selection usually studied in VS. Recent reports suggest that progress is being made in calculating absolute binding affinities, but these methods, too, remain too slow for docking screens, though they may be useful in rescoring docking hit lists [28, 29].

3.3
DNA Methyltransferases

Only a few studies have been published so far where rational approaches have been used to identify selective inhibitors of DNA methyltransferases (DNMTs). One reason might have been the missing crystal structures of therapeutically relevant DNMTs, such as DNMT1. Due to the lack of an experimental 3D structure of DNMT1, Lyko *et al.* generated a homology model for the catalytic domain based on the crystal structures of DNMT2 and bacterial homologs [30]. While this model demonstrated a significant conservation of the catalytic site – due to the high sequence identity of 50% between the related enzymes – it also revealed a number of unique structural features: His1459 of DNMT1 is substituted with alanine at the corresponding positions in the bacterial methyltransferases. In addition, the side-chains of Arg1310 and Arg1312 have different conformations compared to the corresponding side chains in the two bacterial methylases. The authors stated that these differences influence the binding of the ribose ring in the cytosine ligand by creating a tighter cavity.

To identify small molecule DNMT inhibitors Siedlecki *et al.* virtually screened the NCI Diversity Set [31]. The Diversity Set consists of 1990 compounds that are representative of the chemical diversity of more than 140 000 compounds. To refine the database for docking calculations, unwanted compounds not suitable for the DNMT1 active site (considering size, hydrophobicity, uncommon atom types) were removed. To test whether the applied scoring function was suitable for the DNMT binding pocket, known binders were used first as a training set. The DOCK5 [32] program was able to correctly predict the bioactive conformation of the training set ligands. The validated protocol was then applied to screen the NCI Diversity Set. The visual analysis of the docking and scoring data resulted in seven identified virtual hits. Two of them were experimentally tested in a cell-free *in vitro* assay and were found to be active in the range between 10 and 100 μM. The most interesting and most active compound is the tryptophan derivative RG108 (NSC401077; Figure 3.1). In the same study, NSC303530 was also identified as a somewhat weaker inhibitor. Analogs of R108 that do not contain the carboxylic acid group were found to be inactive.

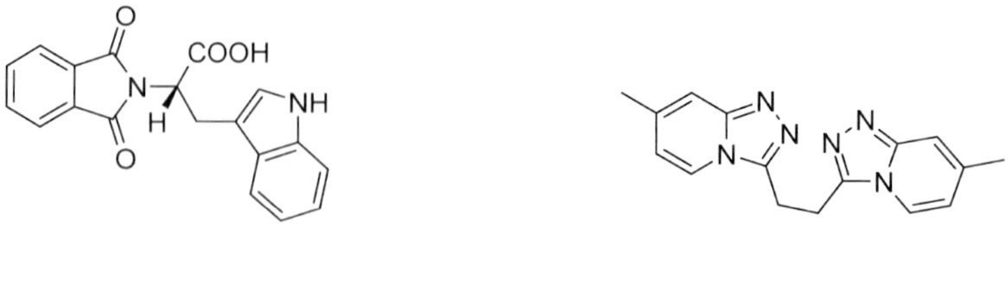

RG108 (NSC401077)   NSC303530

Figure 3.1 Molecular structures of two DNMT inhibitors identified by virtual screening of the NCI diversity set [31].

3.4
Histone Deacetylases

3.4.1
Classic HDACs

So far 18 different members of HDACs have been discovered in humans and classified into four classes based on their homology to yeast histone deacetylases [33]. Class I includes four different subtypes (HDAC1, 2, 3, 8), class II contains six subtypes which are divided into two subclasses: class IIa with subtypes HDAC4, 5, 7, 9 and class IIb with HDAC6, 10. Class I and class II HDAC share significant structural homology, especially within the highly conserved catalytic domains. HDACs 6 and 10 are unique as they have two catalytic domains. HDAC11 is referred to as class IV. While the activity of class I, II and IV HDACs depends on a zinc based catalysis mechanism, the class III enzymes, also called sirtuins, require nicotinamide adenine dinucleotide as a cofactor for their catalysis.

Cocrystal structures of HDACs in complex with hydroxamic acid containing ligands have been useful in dissecting the molecular details of HDAC inhibition [34]. The first of these structures was obtained with HDAC-like protein (HDLP) complexed with two different inhibitors [3]. Later, crystal structures of human HDAC4, HDAC7 and HDAC8, as well as bacterial FB188 HDAH have been resolved (see Chapter 2 in this book for more details). Unfortunately, for two of the most promising HDAC subtypes for drug discovery, HDAC1 and HDAC6, no structural data are available at the moment. The architecture of the solved HDACs is very similar, with the residues in the active site being conserved between bacterial and human HDACs. However, the organization of the loop and distal helices is different in the known HDAC structures, for example HDAC8 shows a more open and accessible substrate binding channel. The deacetylase active site with the zinc ion is located at the end of an approximately 12 Å tunnel. The zinc ion is penta-coordinated by two aspartic acids and one histidine. The remainder of the substrate channel is made up of lipophilic amino acids which are highly conserved across the isoforms. Especially, two aromatic side-chains which restrict the width of the tunnel can be found at the same position in the different HDAC structures. At the top of the binding cavity is a rim leading to the surface, which is formed by several loop regions that differ between subtypes.

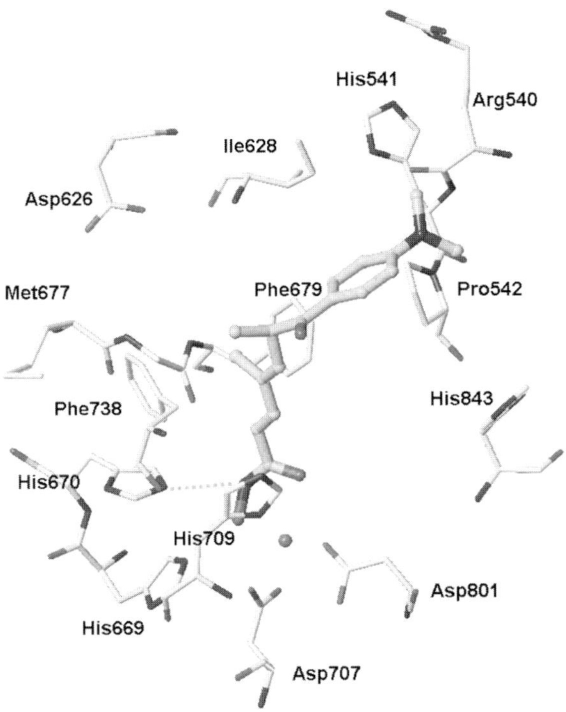

Figure 3.2 X-ray structure of HDAC7 (2PQP.pdb) in complex with the inhibitor TSA (shown in ball and stick mode). Only the residues in the binding pocket are shown. Hydrogen bonds are displayed as dashed lines.

As an example, the binding mode of the cocrystallized inhibitor trichostatin A (TSA) at HDAC7 is shown in Figure 3.2.

In the crystal structures, the inhibitors coordinate to the active site zinc and make a series of hydrogen bonds via their hydroxamic acid moiety. The hydroxamic acids are linked by a flexible spacer with bulky cap groups. The aromatic or aliphatic spacer participates in van der Waals interactions throughout the long channel, whereas the terminal part of the inhibitor interacts with residues at the rim of HDAC. In general, the binding mode of the cocrystallized inhibitors TSA and SAHA is conserved among the different species and subtypes [35].

3.4.1.1 **Docking Studies Using X-Ray Structures and Homology Models**

Ligand-bound structures of the target protein provide a suitable starting point for structure-based drug design. Since the first of the solved structures was that of HDLP, molecular modeling studies started with the analysis of the inhibitor binding mode for this bacterial enzyme. A variety of studies were reported in the meantime where structure-based optimization of HDAC inhibitors was successfully guided by docking the compounds into the HDLP active site [36–44] (see also Chapter 9 in this book). In the case of HDAC-1 and HDAC-6 a crystal structure of the enzyme is yet to be elucidated and, in its absence, homology models of HDAC-1 and HDAC-6 complexed with hydroxamate-based inhibitors were generated by several groups [45–56]. The refined models were generally checked for structural integrity using molecular dynamics simulations and various protein structure checking tools. The predictive ability of the models was evaluated through docking studies of known hydroxamate- or benzamide-based HDAC inhibitors. For constructing the homology models the available crystal structures of HDLP and HDAC8 were considered in the case of HDAC1. The models show a high degree of similarity compared to the HDAC8 crystal structure. The two conserved aromatic amino acids (Phe150 and Phe205 in the case of HDAC1) face each other and form the most slender part of the substrate channel. The channel exit is composed of nonstructured loop regions. Molecular dynamics simulations indicate a high flexibility of this region, which makes structure-based design a challenging task [45, 48, 49]. For HDAC6, which has two catalytic domains, so far only two 3D models have been reported. Whereas one was generated on the basis of the bacterial FB188 HDAH (38% sequence identity) [57], a further model was derived using the recently published human HDAC7 crystal structure in complex with SAHA and TSA (49% sequence identity) [53]. Both HDAC6 models were generated for the catalytic domain located at the C-terminal region and have been used to explain structure–activity relationships for a series of HDAC6-selective inhibitors. In the study by Schäfer *et al.* [53, 58] the generated HDAC6 model was used to dock a series of biaryl- and pyridylalanine-containing hydroxamate inhibitors. The HDAC6 structure showed a clearly defined hydrophobic binding cavity formed by several aromatic and hydrophobic residues (His499, His560, Phe566, Ile569) which accommodated the hydrophobic cap group of the inhibitors. As an example, the binding mode of the HDAC6-selective phenylalanine-containing hydroxamate inhibitor **5a** is show in Figures 3.3 and 3.4.

3.4.1.2 3D-QSAR Studies

The published QSAR [59–61] and 3D-QSAR [62–65] models for HDAC inhibitors were used to explain the differences in activity of hydroxamate-based compounds. All the reported models, which showed moderate to good internal predictivity, were mainly used in a retrospectively way to explain the biological activities of HDAC inhibitors. Generally, the 3D-QSAR models were compared with ligand docking results to get insight into the structural requirements for anti-HDAC activity.

3.4.1.3 Virtual Screening Studies

Only a few virtual screening studies focusing on HDACs have been published so far. The rationale for that might be the as yet unsolved crystal structure of the therapeutically interesting subtypes HDAC1 and HDAC6 and the limited number of commercially available hydroxamates. At Argenta, a virtual screening approach was initiated based on the published crystal structure (PDB code: 1C3R) of the HDAC-like protein (HDLP) [66]. A virtual library of 644 hydroxamic acids was generated from a database of available carboxylic acids. The designed compounds were docked and scored using the FlexX program [22]. Based on the virtual screening results, 75 compounds were selected and tested in an HDAC (subtype) enzyme assay. ADS100380 (Figure 3.4) was

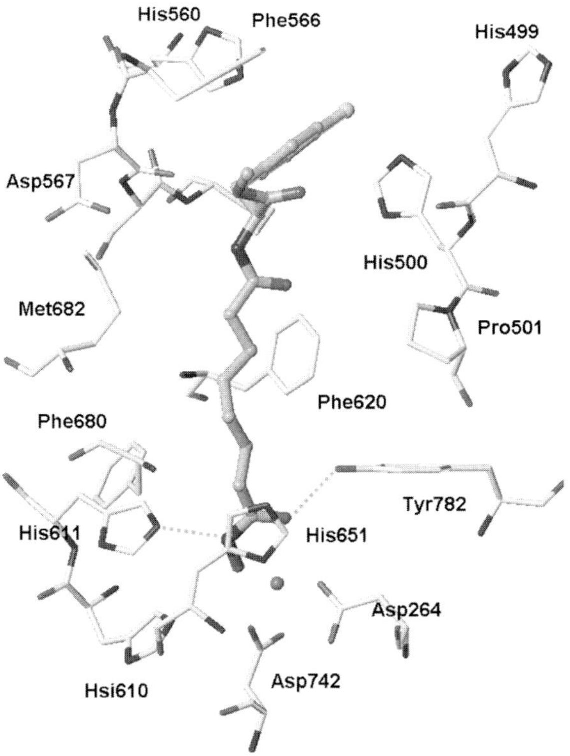

Figure 3.3 Interaction mode of the phenylalanine-containing hydroxamate HDAC inhibitor **5a** [53] at HDAC6. The binding mode was derived by docking the inhibitor into a HDAC6 homology model.

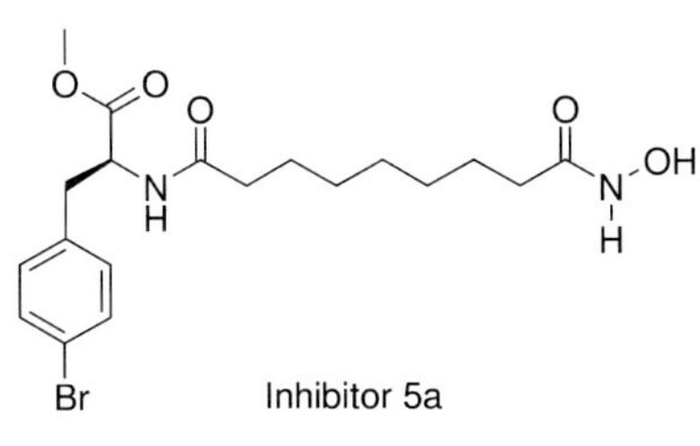

Inhibitor 5a

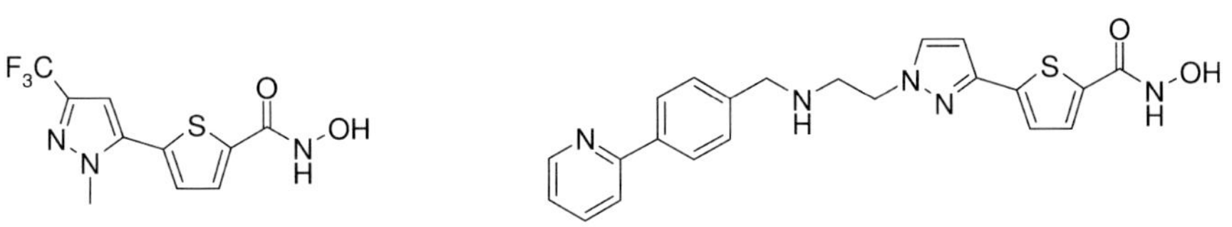

ADS100380 Inhibitor 6p

Figure 3.4 Molecular structures of HDAC inhibitors mentioned in the text.

identified as a sub-micromolar ($IC_{50} = 0.75\,\mu M$) HDAC inhibitor. As expected, the corresponding carboxylic acid of ADS100380 was inactive. The docking study indicated that the catalytic zinc ion to which the hydroxamic acid group of ADS100380 binds is located at the bottom of a tube-shaped pocket. Thus, optimization of ADS100380 was designed to make additional interactions at the entrance to the HDAC active site by tethering hydrophobic aromatic groups to the pyrazole nitrogen. Several nanomolar HDAC inhibitors were obtained by the structure-guided optimization process (e.g. inhibitor **6p** in Figure 3.4).

To test the performance of a ligand-based VS Jagarlapudi *et al.* used a total of 20 well defined HDAC inhibitors [67]. On the basis of the known inhibitors the authors generated a pharmacophore model using the Catalyst software. The derived HypoGen pharmacophore model consists of four pharmacophore features: one hydrogen bond acceptor, one hydrophobic aliphatic and two ring aromatic centers. This model was validated against 378 known HDAC inhibitors from literature with a correlation of 0.897 as well as a significant enrichment in VS. The validated model was further used to retrieve molecules from the NCI database (238 819 compounds). The pharmacophore screening retrieved 4638 molecules while 297 molecules were indicated as "highly active." Unfortunately, no experimental validation of the identified compounds was carried out thus making it impossible to judge whether the approach has some relevance for real life studies.

Another retrospective analysis of already known HDAC inhibitors was carried out by You *et al.* [68]. They generated a 3D chemical-feature-based pharmacophore model and compared the ligand-based model with the structural–functional requirements for the binding of the HDAC inhibitors. Using this model, the interactions between the benzamide MS-275 and HDAC were explored. The result showed that the type and spatial location of chemical features encoded in the pharmacophore are in full agreement with the enzyme–inhibitor interaction pattern identified from molecular docking. However, also in this study no experimental validation of the modeling results was provided.

3.4.2 Sirtuins

The class III deacetylases, named sirtuins, are structurally and functionally different from other HDACs. In contrast to the zinc-dependent deacetylation of classic HDACs, sirtuins depend on NAD^+ to carry out catalytic reactions. A variety of sirtuin crystal structures have been published over the past few years. The structures of human Sirt2 and Sirt5 as well as several bacterial Sir2 proteins could be derived, whereas no 3D structure is available for Sirt1 and the other subtypes [69]. All solved sirtuin structures contain a conserved 270-amino-acid catalytic domain with variable N- and C-termini. The structure of the catalytic domain consists of a large classic Rossmann fold and a small zinc binding domain. The interface between the large and the small subdomain is commonly subdivided into A, B and C pockets. This division is based on the interaction of adenine (A), ribose (B) and nicotinamide (C) which are parts of the NAD^+ cofactor. (Figure 3.5) Whereas the interaction of adenine and

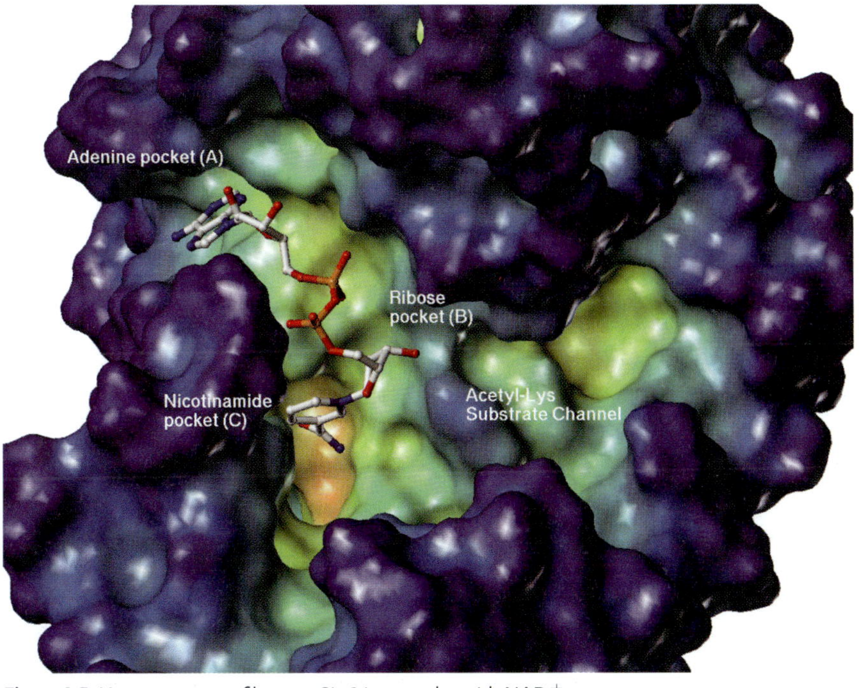

Figure 3.5 X-ray structure of human Sirt2 in complex with NAD$^+$ (predicted by docking). The molecular surface of the protein is colored according to the cavity depth.

ribose is similar in all available sirtuin X-ray structures, the interaction of the nicotinamide part is less clearly defined. Several, so-called productive and nonproductive conformations of nicotinamide have been observed in the crystal structures, reflecting the high flexibility of this part of the cofactor. In the X-ray structure of a Sirt2 homolog from Archeabacteria it was shown that the acetylated peptide binds in a cleft between the two domains [70]. The acetyl-lysine residue inserts into a conserved hydrophobic pocket, where NAD$^+$ binds nearby (Figure 3.5). In case of the human Sirt2 X-ray structure no structural information about the NAD$^+$ or substrate binding is available. However, due to the homology with bacterial sirtuins, docking studies showed that NAD$^+$ interacts in a comparable way with human and bacterial enzyme [71].

Several inhibitors are available for Sirt2 that have been discovered by virtual screening approaches [72–74]. Based on docking studies that were carried out for human Sirt2 and competition experiments with NAD$^+$, it was found that adenosine mimetics (e.g. the kinase inhibitor Ro-318220) are potent Sirt2 inhibitors which interact with the adenine subpocket [73]. The planar ring systems of the docked maleimides fit perfectly in the adenine-binding pocket and make hydrogen bonds bond with Cys324 and Asp325. The docking of the most potent inhibitor Ro-318220 revealed a second putative binding site for the polar amidine group near Ile93 and Asp95 (Figures 3.6 and 3.7).

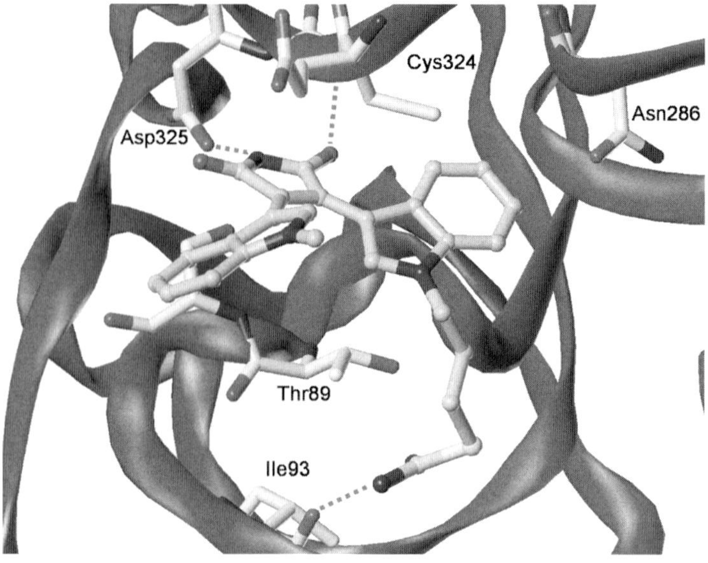

Figure 3.6 Interaction of the inhibitor Ro-318220 (gray carbon atoms) at the adenosine binding site of Sirt2 as predicted by docking.

Tervo *et al.* carried out a receptor-based VS on the screening collection from Maybridge, comprising about 60 000 compounds [74]. Using the UNITYsoftware [75] a simple pharmacophore query was generated first to select potential Sirt2 hits. The database searching returned 66 candidate compounds, of which 44 compounds passed an *in silico* intestinal absorption model generated with the VOLSURF program [76]. The retrieved hits were subsequently docked in the Sirt2 binding pocket using the GOLD program. The location of the docking poses at the active site, as well as their ability to match the requirements of the search queries, was visually analyzed. On the basis of the visual inspection 15 compounds were selected for test their ability to inhibit Sirt2 *in vitro*. Two out of 15 experimentally tested compounds showed a moderate *in vitro* inhibitory activity toward Sirt2 (JFD00244, $IC_{50} = 57\,\mu M$; CD04097, $IC_{50} = 74\,\mu M$; Figure 3.7). The docking study which was carried out with the human Sirt2 crystal structure revealed that the active inhibitors interact mainly with Asp95, Gln167, Asn168 and with Ile169, mostly by forming hydrogen bonds to the backbone atoms. On the basis of the docking study, the authors suggested that this region, which is also the postulated binding site for nicotinamide, is also important for the inhibitor binding. This observation is also supported by the finding that the docked inactive compounds do not show hydrogen bonds to these amino acid residues. Using the same approach Poso *et al.* performed further VS on other compound libraries [77–79]. Several moderately active inhibitors could be identified from the Leadquest and Maybridge compound collections.

A recent effort to identify a Sirt2 inhibitors culminated in the report of the vinylnitrile AGK2 (Figure 3.7). AKG2 and chemically similar analogs were identified

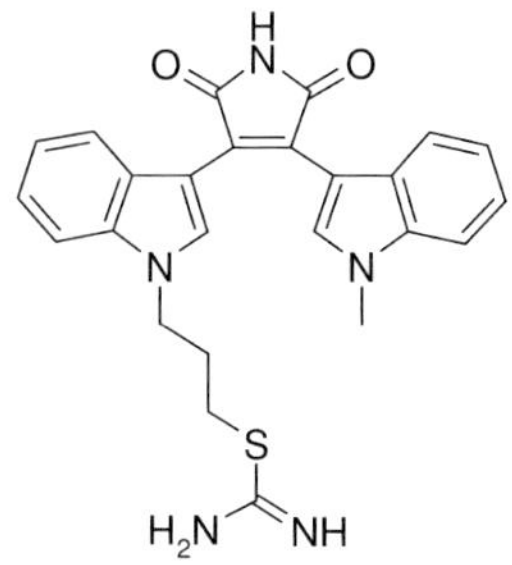

Ro-318220

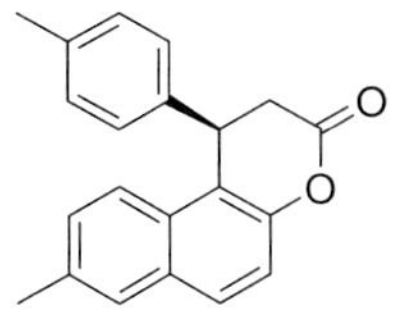

β-Phenylspitomicin *(R)*-8c

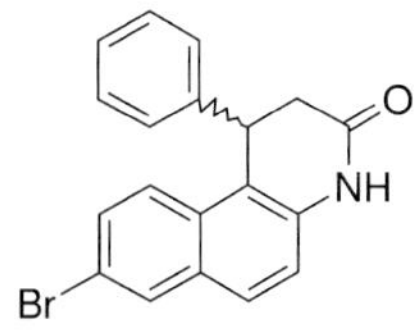

Lactam 12

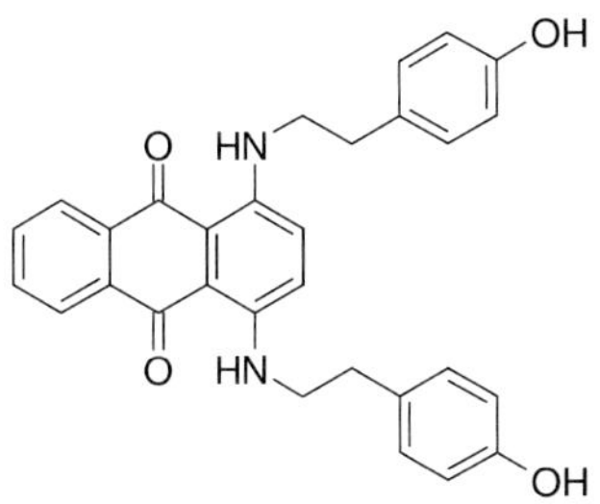

JFD00244

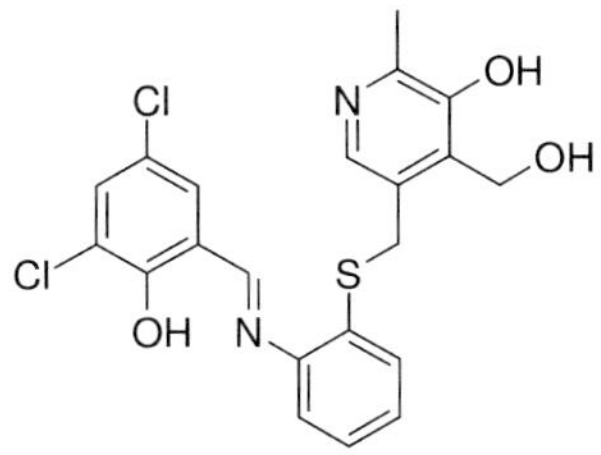

CD04097

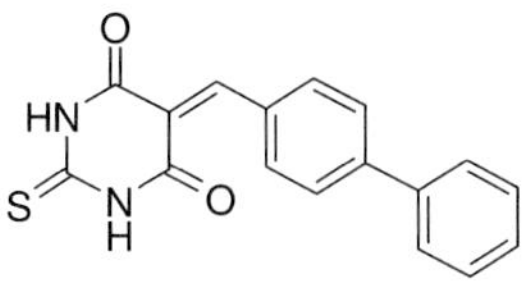

Thiobarbiturate 25

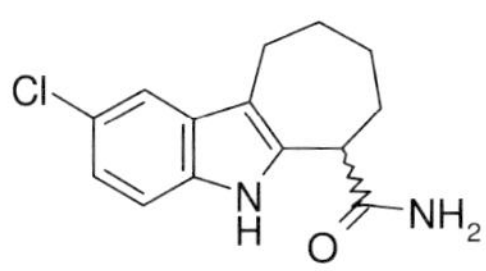

Indole 35

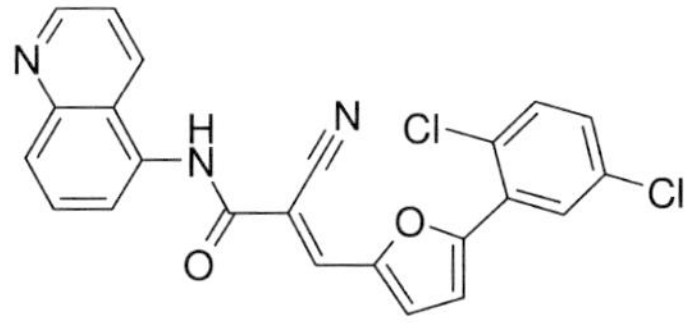

AKG2

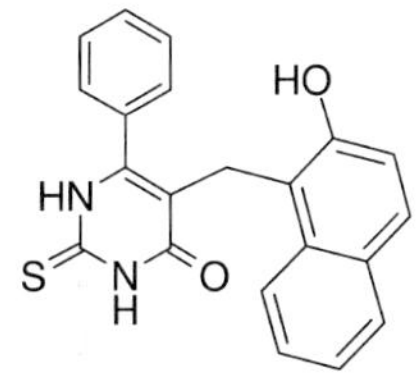

Cambinol

Figure 3.7 Molecular structures of sirtuin inhibitors mentioned in the text.

in a focused library screening. To elucidate the structural mechanism of Sirt2 inhibition by AGK2 Outeiro *et al.* [80] developed 3D models of human Sirt2 in several different conformations by combining available human and yeast crystal structures. The high flexibility of the active site loop made this strategy necessary. The different Sirt2 conformations were subsequently used for docking the identified inhibitors using the ICM program [81]. Comparative analysis of the low-energy ligand conformations confirmed that the preferred site for ligand binding is pocket C, where the nicotinamide part of NAD^+ interacts. A hydrogen-bonding pattern for AKG2 was observed which is similar to that of other Sirt2 inhibitors. AGK2 inhibits Sirt2 with an IC_{50} value of 3.5 μM and shows more than 10-fold selectivity versus Sirt1 and Sirt3. In further biological experiments AGK2 displayed the ability to block α-synuclein-mediated toxicity in a Parkinson's disease model, possibly by modulating tubulin acetylation.

Neugebauer *et al.* used docking simulations to analyze the binding of several Sirt2 inhibitors and to rationalize the structure–activity relationships of a series of arylsplitomicins (Figure 3.7) [82]. Docking studies using the human Sirt2 X-ray structure showed that the Sirt2 inhibitor cambinol (Figure 3.8a) interacts with the

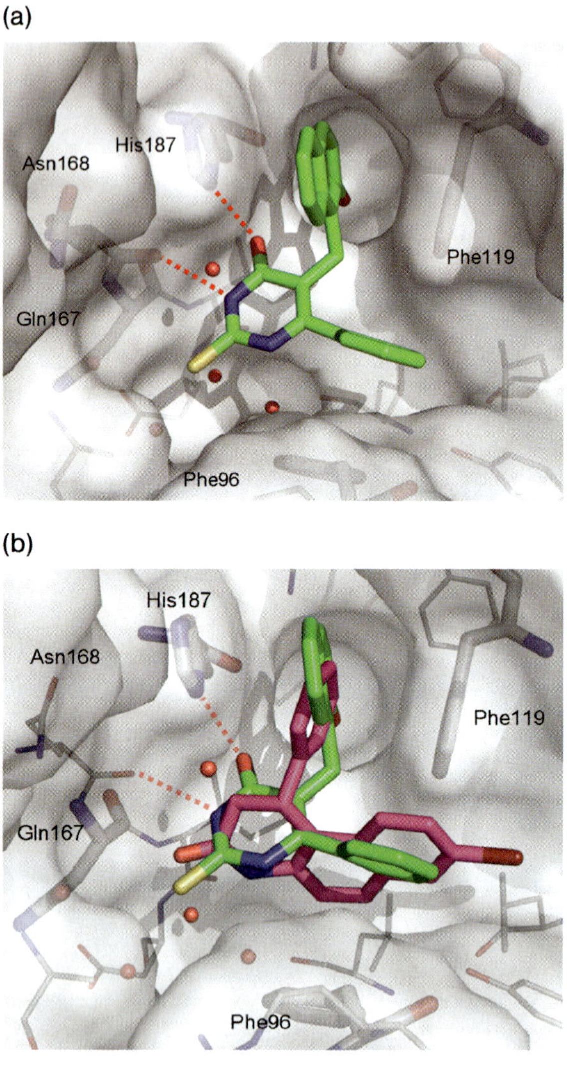

Figure 3.8 (a) Binding mode of cambinol (green carbons) at the Sirt2 binding pocket. Hydrogen bonds are shown as dashed lines. (b) Binding mode of the lactam-based inhibitor **12** (magenta) and cambinol (green) at the Sirt2 binding pocket. Hydrogen bonds are shown as dashed lines.

nicotinamide subpocket (C). Several conserved water molecules are observed in the nicotinamide subpocket of human and bacterial X-ray structures. The polar moieties of cambinol and the indole **35** [83] (Figure 3.7) were found to interact with the polar residues Gln167, Asn168 and the water molecules of the nicotinamide subpocket (Figure 3.8a). Also the docked β-phenylsplitomicin showed the same binding mode, including a hydrogen bond to the water molecule bonded to Gln167. The β-phenyl substituent of the (*R*)-isomer fits into a hydrophobic channel and is sandwiched between Phe119 and His187. By synthesizing and assaying the pure enantiomers of a β-phenylsplitomicin rac-**8c** (Figure 3.7) the postulated binding mode could be validated. As predicted by the docking study only the (*R*)-isomer is a potent Sirt2 inhibitor with an IC_{50} value of 1.0 μM whereas the (*S*)-isomer is weakly active.

One of the limitations of splitomicins has been found the instability of the lactone ring, which led to a short half-life particularly at physiological pH [84]. Therefore, VS was used to discover novel more drug-like chemotypes. Similarity-based searching of commercial databases and subsequent docking the hits into the Sirt2 binding site yielded two novel classes of sirtuin inhibitors. In the first series of inhibitors the lactone of β-phenylsplitomicin is replaced with the lactam ring, resulting in equally active inhibitors. The predicted binding mode of the lactam-based inhibitor **12** is shown in Figure 3.8B. Provided that the lactams retain the *in vivo* activity, their stability makes them more suitable for further development as sirtuin inhibitors.

The second series of inhibitors are based on a common thiobarbiturate structure, which shows similarity to the cambinol structure [85]. A set of seven active Sirt1 and Sirt2 inhibitors could be identified and the binding mode was predicted using the GOLD docking program. To rationalize the experimental results, binding free energy calculations were carried out by molecular mechanics Poisson–Boltzmann/surface area (MM-PBSA) calculations [86]. A significant correlation was observed between calculated binding free energies and measured Sirt2 inhibitory activities. Thus, the prediction model could be used to estimate the inhibitory activity of novel candidate drugs. The analyses suggested a molecular basis for the interaction of the identified thiobarbiturate derivatives with human Sirt2. The interaction of the most potent thiobarbiturate **25** ($IC_{50} = 8.7$ μM) with human Sirt2 is shown as an example in Figure 3.9. A common feature of the active inhibitors is the interaction (hydrogen bond) of one thiobarbiturate NH-group with the backbone carbonyl of Gln167 and the hydrogen bond between the barbiturate CO-group and His187. The bulky naphthyl or biaryl substituent is facing in the acetyl-lysine substrate channel and makes van der Waals interactions with the aromatic ring system of Phe119 and His187.

Suramin (Figure 3.10), a symmetric polyanionic naphthylurea derivative, is originally used for the treatment of trypanosomiasis. Additionally, it shows a wide range of biological activities such as antiproliferative and antiviral activity. The observation that suramin inhibited Sirt1 [87] inspired Trapp *et al.* [71] to test a diverse set of suramin analogs to carry out structure–activity studies and to investigate the structural requirements for the binding of suramin derivatives by molecular docking. Suramin exhibited an IC_{50} value of 297 nM against Sirt1 and 1150 nM

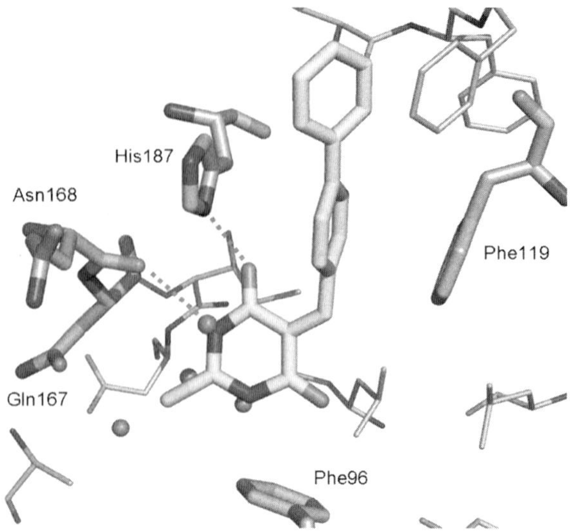

Figure 3.9 Interaction of the thiobarbiturate **25** (white carbons) with the Sirt2 binding site. Hydrogen bonds are shown as dashed lines.

against Sirt2. Whereas variations on the benzoyl portion of suramin only led to a slight increase of the inhibitory potency, variation of the suramin core structure afforded the small urea compound NF675 (Figure 3.10) that showed an IC_{50} value of 93 nM for Sirt2. The putative binding site of suramin derivatives was examined using the recently published X-ray structure of suramin cocrystallized with human Sirt5 [69] and a Sirt2 model that was generated on the available X-ray data for this subtype. Consideration of the binding mode of suramin with Sirt5 and subsequent docking studies suggested that the binding site for suramins is localized between the nicotinamide binding pocket and the peptide substrate binding region, thus inhibiting the deacetylation step. This finding was in agreement with the results obtained by competition analyses in which suramin inhibited sirtuins in a noncompetitive manner regarding both NAD^+ and peptide substrate. Despite their so far unmatched inhibitory potency, the application of suramins within cellular studies or even therapeutic approaches is problematic due to their high polarity. However, suramin derivatives may be useful tools for the investigation of polar motifs in new sirtuin inhibitors that address the same binding pocket.

The available structural information on human sirtuins and the derived docking results suggest that inhibitors can interact with different binding pockets. Whereas for adenosine analogs an interaction was predicted for the adenine pocket and verified by competition experiments, for a variety of inhibitors (e.g. AKG2, β-phenylsplitomicins, cambinol, thiobarbiturates and the indole **35**) bearing polar moieties the interaction with the nicotinamide or the substrate pocket is postulated. Crystal structures of human sirtuins together with inhibitors from the different structural classes will be helpful for structure-based optimization.

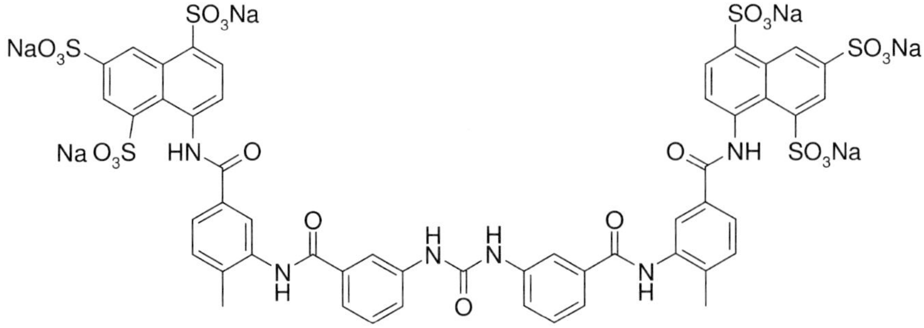

Suramin

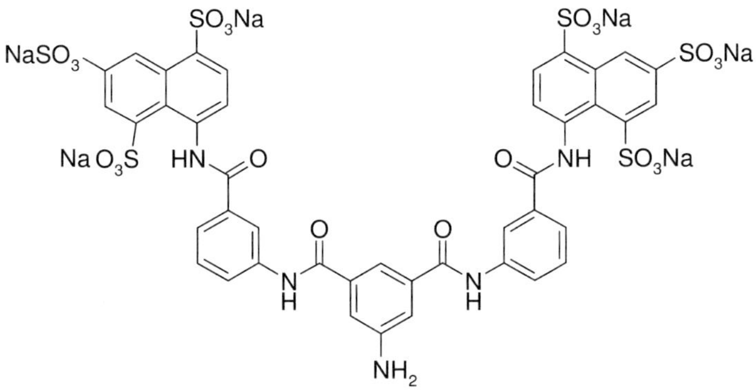

NF675

Figure 3.10 Molecular structure of the sirtuin inhibitors suramin and NF675.

Since no crystal structure has been reported so far for Sirt1, Poso *et al.* generated a homology model for the domain area at residues 244 to 498 of the full-length Sirt1 [88]. The authors proposed the binding-mode of recently reported set of indole-based Sirt1 inhibitors [3]. The interaction site and the ligand conformation were predicted by the use of molecular docking techniques. To distinguish between active and inactive compounds, a structure-based pharmacophore model was constructed. The validated pharmacophore was suggested as a filter for further database screening. However, an experimental validation of the described approach has not been reported so far.

3.5 Histone Acetyltransferases

Histone acetyltransferase (HAT) enzymes are divided into several families based on conserved sequence motifs. The two major families are named GNAT (Gcn5-related

N-acetyltransferases) and MYST (MOZ, Ybf2/Sas3, Sas2, Tip60; for details see Chapter 2 in this book). Numerous structural studies were carried out on HATs in the past decade that lead to a wealth of structural data on the GNAT, MYST and p300/CBP families [89–91]. Despite the large number of available crystal structures derived for HATs, HAT-cofactor and HAT-substrate complexes, no study was reported so far which used 3D structural information for virtual screening or molecular design of HAT inhibitors. The few available HAT inhibitors were mostly identified by random screening campaigns or empirical findings (see Chapter 11 in this book for more details).

3.6
Histone Methyltransferases

During the past several years, a variety of crystal structures of histone lysine and arginine methyltransferase in complex with the cofactor analog SAH and/or in complex with peptide substrates have been reported [92]. However, no 3D structure of a complex between a histone methyltransferase (HMT) and an inhibitor has been reported so far. Due to the lack of experimental structures, a variety of molecular modeling and docking studies has been carried out for HMTs in order to understand the structural requirements for inhibitor binding.

The first crystal structure for a PRMT enzyme was reported in 2000 for rat PRMT3 in complex with the cofactor analogue SAH [93]. The results revealed a two-domain structure – a SAM binding domain and a barrel-like domain – with the active site pocket located between the two domains. The rat PRMT1 crystal structure in complex with SAH and a substrate peptide were published in 2003 and allowed for the first time the analysis of the enzyme–substrate interaction [94]. Mutagenesis studies on rat PRMT1 confirmed that two active site glutamate residues (Glu144 and Glu153) are essential for enzymatic activity and that dimerization of PRMT1 is essential for cofactor binding. The crystal structures of rat PRMT1 were obtained at a nonphysiological pH value (pH 4.7; maximum enzymatic activity at pH 8.5), resulting in a conformational change of one of the active site glutamates (Glu153) and a disordered helix αX which is part of the substrate binding pocket.

The available rat PRMT1 and PRMT3 crystal structures have been used to provide a structural explanation for the inhibitory activity of a set of synthesized analogues of AMI-1 (Figure 3.11). Docking of inhibitors such as **4b** (Figure 3.11) into PRMT1 and the *Aspergillus* homologue RmtA revealed a potential interaction with the arginine substrate and the cofactor binding pocket. In contrast, related analogs could be docked either in the SAM or substrate binding site. However, no experimental confirmation by competition experiments has been reported to support the postulated binding mode [95]. The reported series of dye-related small molecules was further used to establish a receptor-based 3D-QSAR model for nine selected inhibitors from the study. The 3D-QSAR model which was generated using the GRID/GOLPE [14] approach showed good internal predictivity ($q^2 = 0.93$). However, due to the limited number of molecules in the 3D-QSAR analysis, the model is of limited validity.

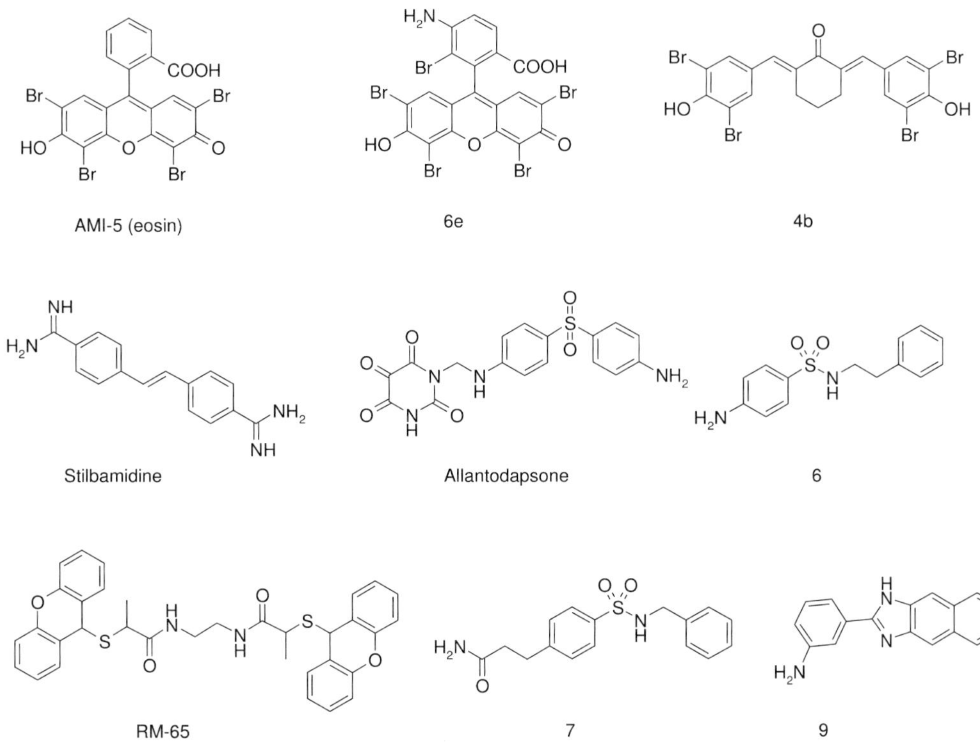

Figure 3.11 Molecular structures of PRMT inhibitors mentioned in the text.

In a further study Mai *et al.* [96] chose the AMI-5 (eosin; Figure 3.11) chemical structure as a template to design a new series of simplified analogs, starting from a pharmacophore hypothesis. In this hypothesis, the presence of two o-bromo- or o,o-dibromophenol moieties inserted into hydrophobic moieties were identified as crucial for having antimethyltransferase activity. They prepared a series of substituted 1,5-diphenyl-1,4-pentadien-3-ones (e.g. compound **4b**; Figure 3.11) and docked them into the generated model structures of human PRMT1, CARM1 and into the SET7 crystal structure. The analysis of the AutoDock-proposed binding modes revealed that the compounds are able to bind in the SAM or in the Arg/Lys substrate binding sites. The most active compounds could be docked in the SAM binding pocket of the two PRMTs (PRMT1 and CARM1), whereas for SET7 most of the developed compounds occupied both the lysine and SAM binding site.

Applying a combination of structure-based virtual screening and biochemical characterization, two drug-like substrate competitive PRMT1 inhibitors (allantodapsone, stilbamidine; Figure 3.11) were reported recently [97]. Based on a generated homology model of human PRMT1 and subsequent docking into the substrate binding site, key interactions between the identified inhibitors and PRMT1 could be derived. A common feature of the actively tested inhibitors is the hydrogen bonding of a basic or polar group with the active site Glu152 (which corresponds to Glu144 in rat PRMT1). A basic or polar moiety of the inhibitors mimics the guanidine group of the arginine side-chain of the substrate peptide. In addition, the inhibitors show van der Waals interactions with several aromatic residues of the binding pocket (Tyr47, Tyr156, Trp302; Figures 3.12a and 3.12b). The proposed binding mode could be confirmed by competition expriment using a synthetic histone substrate.

Based on the identified PRMT1 inhibitors stilbamidine and allantodapsone, Heinke *et al.* [98] expanded their virtual and biological screening for novel inhibitors. Structure-based VS of the Chembridge database comprising 328 000 molecules was performed using a combination of ligand- and target-based in silico screening. To focus on lead-like PRMT inhibitors, the authors filtered the Chembridge database for molecules with a molecular weight below 400, a topological polar surface area (TPSA) below 150 Å^2 and at least one nitrogen atom. This resulted in 189 000 molecules which were virtually screened using a structure-based pharmacophore model. The model was generated with the LigandScout program on the basis of the PRMT1-allantodapsone interaction model. The pharmacophore-based screening resulted in 6232 compounds (3.3%) which passed the LigandScout pharmacophore. The 6232 compounds were docked subsequently into the substrate binding pocket of PRMT1. Due to the fact that docking scores are not good discriminators between true actives and false positives, the authors focused not only on the derived Gold-scores but used additional filters for selecting potential candidates for the biological testing (i.e. compounds were automatically selected which showed a binding mode similar to the known PRMT1 inhibitors). Among the top-ranked 100 docking poses which fulfilled the distance constraints, nine compounds from clusters of similar molecules were selected and experimentally tested using human PRMT1 and an antibody-based assay with a time-resolved fluorescence readout. Among several aromatic amines (inhibitors **6** and **9**; Figure 3.11), an aliphatic amine and an amide (inhibitor **7**) were also found to be active in the micromolar range.

A further fragment-based virtual screening identified α-methylthioglycolic amides as new lead PRMT inhibitors [99]. Similarity-based searching for analogs resulted in RM-65 (Figure 3.11), which was identified as bisubstrate PRMT1 inhibitor. Docking of RM-65 showed that the compound blocks the cofactor and the substrate channel, showing mainly favorable van der Waals interaction with aromatic residues (Tyr43, Tyr47, Met56, Val108, Tyr156, Tyr160) of the SAM and Arg-binding pocket [101].

Jenuwein *et al.* applied both VS and HTS to screen the Boehringer Ingelheim chemical compound library for inhibitors of the lysine methyltransferase G9a. Cheminformatic tools were used to identify molecules that would have an increased probability to function as potential G9a inhibitors. A similarity searching approach was carried out using nine known inhibitors of Arg- and Lys-methyltransferases (AMI compounds 1–9) [100]. The similarity was calculated on the basis of ligand/protein-based fingerprints/site-points [101]. The approach was used both for a ligand-based and protein-based VS. For the protein-based screening a homology model was developed, based on the crystal structure of DIM-5 (1PEG.pdb) [102], a lysine methyltransferase with 30% identity in the SET domain to G9a. Each method scored the compounds in the screening collection. Additional compounds were randomly selected, and a total of 125 000 substances were subsequently evaluated

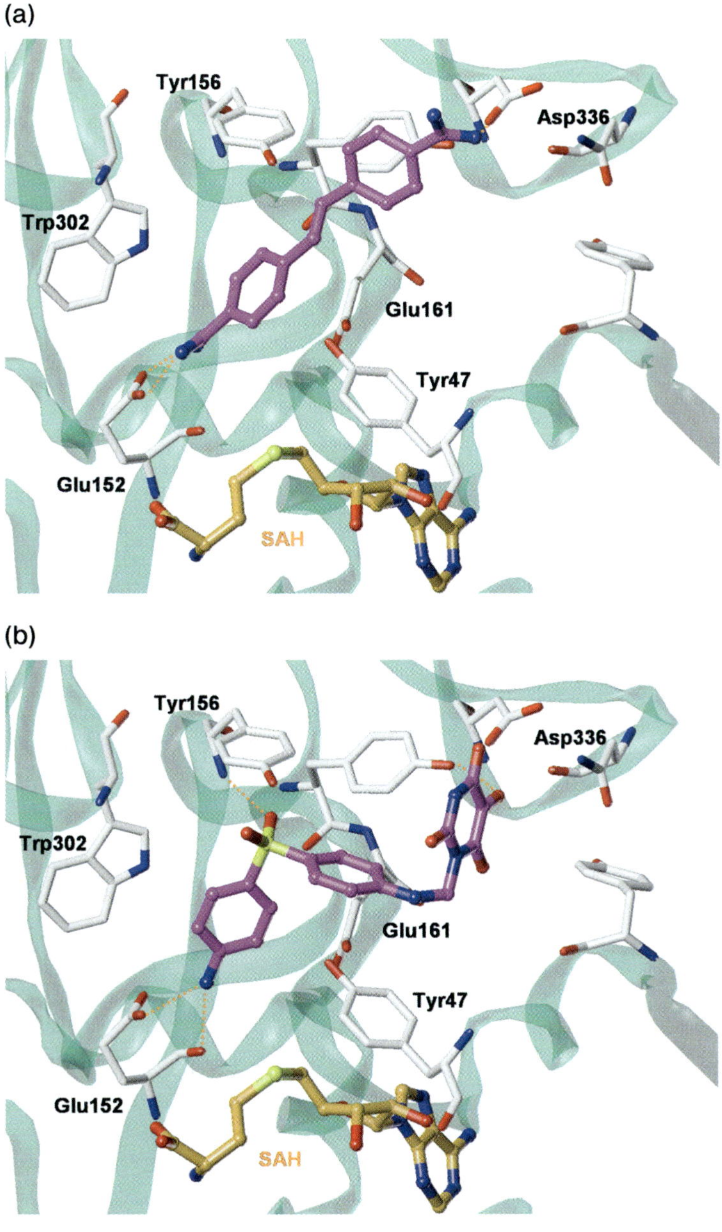

Figure 3.12 (a) Predicted binding mode of stilbamidine (colored magenta) at the substrate binding pocket of PRMT1. The cofactor analog SAH is shown in orange at the bottom of the figure. Hydrogen bonds are shown as dashed lines. Only residues of the binding site are displayed. (b) Predicted binding mode of allantodapsone (colored magenta) at the substrate binding pocket of PRMT1. The cofactor analog SAH is shown in orange at the bottom of the figure. Hydrogen bonds are shown as dashed lines. Only residues of the binding site are displayed.

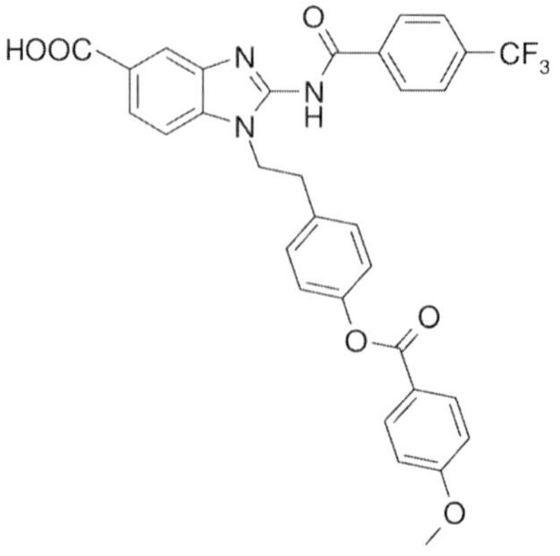

Bix-01338 (5 μM, G9a; 6 μM, PRMT1)

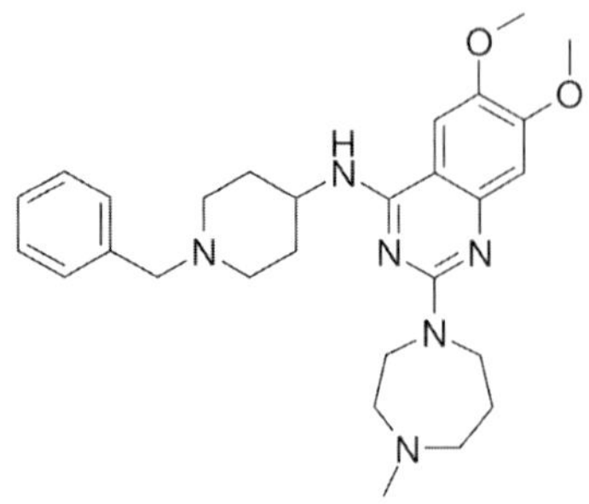

Bix-01294 (3 μM, G9a)

Figure 3.13 Molecular structures of G9a inhibitors mentioned in the text.

in HTS. The experimental in vitro testing on G9a revealed seven hits with activities in the low micromolar range. Beside the unselective inhibitor acylbenzimidazole BIX-01338, one selective inhibitor was identified (BIX-01294; Figure 3.13). BIX-01294 inhibited G9a at an IC_{50} of 2.7 μM and showed no activity against SUV39H1 or PRMT1. Cell lines treated with BIX-01294 showed a reduction in histone H3 lysine 9 dimethylation; the mono- or trimethyl stages appeared unaffected. In addition the mode of action for two inhibitors was examined by measuring the dependence of the reaction kinetics on the concentration of the cofactor SAM. Whereas the unselective inhibitor BIX-01338 displayed competitive inhibition with SAM, BIX-01294 inhibited G9a in an uncompetitive manner with SAM, suggesting that it can only bind the enzyme–cofactor complex, but not the free enzyme.

3.7
Histone Demethylases

The first histone demethylases (HDMs) were identified only recently. In 2004, Shi and co-workers discovered the first demethylase specifically demethylating histone H3 at lysine 4 and named it lysine-specific demethylase-1 (LSD1) [103]. LSD1 shows a high sequence homology with FAD-dependent amine oxidases. Two years later, another family of histone demethylases was identified and termed JmjC protein [104]. These demethylases use Fe(II) and α-ketoglutarate in an oxygenation reaction to remove the methyl groups from lysine residues. Since the expression levels of several of these demethylases are increased in primary tumors, HDMs are considered as potential drug targets [105]. Therefore it is not surprising that a huge effort is now being made to explore the structural requirements of modulating these targets and to identify small molecule inhibitors. A variety of crystal structures have been solved in the past four years, which helped in understanding the binding of substrates and first available unselective inhibitors (for more details see Chapter 13 of this book). It is likely that the available 3D structures of HDMs will soon result in the structure-guided design of druglike and selective inhibitors [106].

3.8 Summary

Despite many technical challenges, structure-based virtual screening has an important role in drug discovery. As a steadily growing number of epigenetic targets are characterized biologically and also structurally, structure-based methods are more and more applied to design specific inhibitors to elucidate their therapeutic potential. Ligand docking and scoring technologies have steadily improved and the importance of the adequate validation of pragmatic virtual screening protocols is now well recognized. While both ligand- and receptor-based approaches already have demonstrated their worth in identification of novel lead compounds for epigenetic targets, there is still the challenge to improve the predictive accuracy of scoring functions, particularly to enable scoring-based methods to have a greater impact in guiding lead optimization.

Acknowledgement

We thank Barbara Elsner, Institute of Pharmacy, Martin-Luther-University of Halle-Wittenberg, for technical assistance.

References

1 Wolffe, A.P. and Matzke, M.A. (1999) Epigenetics: regulation through repression. *Science*, **286**, 481–486.

2 Kouzarides, T. (2007) Chromatin modifications and their function. *Cell*, **128**, 693–705.

3 Finnin, M.S., Donigian, J.R., Cohen, A., Richon, V.M., Rifkind, R.A., Marks, P.A. *et al.* (1999) Structures of a histone deacetylase homologue bound to the TSA and SAHA inhibitors. *Nature*, **401**, 188–193.

4 Kirchmair, J., Distinto, S., Schuster, D., Spitzer, G., Langer, T. and Wolber, G. (2008) Enhancing drug discovery through *in silico* screening: strategies to increase true positives retrieval rates. *Current Medicinal Chemistry*, **15**, 2040–2053.

5 Hawkins, P.C.D., Skillman, A.G. and Nicholls, A. (2007) Comparison of shape-matching and docking as virtual screening tools. *Journal of Medicinal Chemistry*, **50**, 74–82.

6 Evers, A., Hessler, G., Matter, H. and Klabunde, T. (2005) Virtual screening of biogenic amine-binding G-protein coupled receptors: comparative evaluation of protein- and ligand-based virtual screening protocols. *Journal of Medicinal Chemistry*, **48**, 5448–5465.

7 Kirchmair, J., Laggner, C., Wolber, G. and Langer, T. (2005) Comparative analysis of

protein-bound ligand conformations with respect to catalyst's conformational space subsampling algorithms. *Journal of Chemical Information and Modeling*, **45**, 422–430.

8 Stahl, M., Guba, W. and Kansy, M. (2006) Integrating molecular design resources within modern drug discovery research: the Roche experience. *Drug Discovery Today*, **11**, 326–333.

9 Wermuth, C.G., Ganellin, C.R., Lindberg, P. and Mitschler, L.A. (1998) Glossary of terms used in medicinal chemistry (IUPAC Recommendations 1997). *Annual Reports in Medicinal Chemistry*, **33**, 385–395.

10 Ahlstrom, M.M., Ridderstrom, M., Luthman, K. and Zamora, I. (2005) Virtual screening and scaffold hopping based on GRID molecular interaction fields. *Journal of Chemical Information and Modeling*, **45**, 1313–1323.

11 Stahura, F.L. and Bajorath, J. (2005) New methodologies for ligand-based virtual screening. *Current Pharmaceutical Design*, **11**, 1189–1192.

12 Cramer, R.D. III, Patterson, D.E. and Bunce, J.D. (1988) Comparative molecular field analysis (CoMFA) 1. Effect of shape on binding of steroids to carrier proteins. *Journal of the American Chemical Society*, **110**, 5959–5967.

13 Klebe, G. and Abraham, U. (1993) On the prediction of binding properties of drug molecules by comparative molecular field analysis. *Journal of Medicinal Chemistry*, **36**, 70–80.

14 Baroni, M., Constantino, G., Cruciani, G., Riganelli, D., Valigli, R. and Clementi, S. (1993) Generating optimal linear pls estimations (GOLPE): An advanced chemometric tool for handling 3D-QSAR problems. *Quantitative Structure-Activity Relationships*, **12**, 9–20.

15 Sippl, W. (2006) in *Methods and Principles in Medicinal Chemistry – Pharmacophore Generation and Concepts* (eds T. Langer and R. Hofmann) (series eds H. Kubinyi, G. Folkers and R. Mannhold), VCH Publisher, New York.

16 Cruciani, G. (ed.) (2006) *Methods and Principles in Medicinal Chemistry – Molecular Interaction Fields* (series eds H. Kubinyi, G. Folkers and R. Mannhold), VCH Publisher, New York.

17 Akamatsu, M. (2002) Current state and perspectives of 3D QSAR. *Current Topics in Medicinal Chemistry*, **2**, 1381–1394.

18 Doweyko, A.M. (2004) 3D QSAR illusions. *Journal of Computer-Aided Molecular Design*, **18**, 587–596.

19 Osterberg, F., Morris, G.M., Sanner, M.F., Olson, A.J. and Goodsell, D.S. (2002) Automated docking to multiple target structures: incorporation of protein mobility and structural water heterogeneity in AutoDock. *Proteins*, **46**, 34–40.

20 Gold, Cambridge Crystallographic Data Centre, Cambridge, UK, http://www.ccdc.cam.ac.uk.

21 Glide, Schrödinger, Portland, OR, http://www.schroedinger.com.

22 FlexE, BiosolveIT, St. Augustin, Germany, http://www.biolsolveit.de.

23 Klebe, G. (2006) Virtual ligand screening. *Drug Discovery Today*, **11**, 580–594.

24 Tame, J.R. (2005) Scoring functions-the first 100 years. *Journal of Computer-Aided Molecular Design*, **17**, 445–451.

25 Leach, A.R., Shoichet, B.K. and Peishoff, C.E. (2006) Prediction of protein-ligand interactions. Docking and scoring: successes and gaps. *Journal of Medicinal Chemistry*, **49**, 5852–5855.

26 Kitchen, D.B., Decornez, H., Furr, J.R. and Bajorth, J. (2004) Docking and scoring in virtual screening for drug discovery: Methods and applications. *Nature Reviews. Drug Discovery*, **3**, 935–949.

27 Pearlman, D.A. (2005) Evaluating the molecular mechanics Poisson-Boltzmann surface area free energy method using a congeneric series of ligands to p38 MAP kinase. *Journal of Medicinal Chemistry*, **48**, 7796–7807.

28 Chang, C.E. and Gilson, M.K. (2004) Free energy, entropy, and induced fit in host-guest recognition: calculations with the second-generation mining minima

algorithm. *Journal of the American Chemical Society*, **126**, 13156–13164.

29 Deng, Y. and Roux, B. (2006) Calculation of standard binding free energies: Aromatic molecules in the T4 lysozyme L99A mutant. *Journal of Chemical Theory and Computation*, **2**, 1255–1273.

30 Siedlecki, P., Boy, R.G., Comagic, S., Schirrmacher, R., Wiessler, M., Zielenkiewicz, P., Suhai, S. and Lyko, F. (2003) Establishment and functional validation of a structural homology model for human DNA methyltransferase 1. *Biochemical and Biophysical Research Communications*, **306**, 558–563.

31 Siedlecki, P., Boy, R.G., Musch, T., Brueckner, B., Suhai, S., Lyko, F. and Zielenkiewicz, P. (2006) Discovery of two novel, small-molecule inhibitors of DNA methylation. *Journal of Medicinal Chemistry*, **49**, 678–683.

32 Moustakas, D.T., Lang, P.T., Pegg, S., Pettersen, E., Kuntz, I.D. *et al.* (2006) Development and validation of a modular, extensible docking program: DOCK 5. *Journal of Computer-Aided Molecular Design*, **20**, 601–619.

33 de Ruijter, A.J., van Gennip, A.H., Caron, H.N., Kemp, S. and van Kuilenburg, A.B. (2003) Histone deacetylases (HDACs): characterization of the classical HDAC family. *The Biochemical Journal*, **370**, 737–749.

34 Hodawadekar, S.C. and Marmorstein, R. (2007) Chemistry of acetyl transfer by histone modifying enzymes: structure, mechanism and implications for effector design. *Oncogene*, **26**, 5528–5540.

35 Zhang, Y., Fang, H., Jiao, J. and Xu, W. (2008) The structure and function of histone deacetylases: The target for anti-cancer therapy. *Current Medicinal Chemistry*, **15**, 2840–2849.

36 Massa, S., Mai, A., Sbardella, G., Esposito, M., Ragno, R., Loidl, P. *et al.* (2001) G. 3-(4-Aroyl-1*H*-pyrrol-2-yl)-*N*-hydroxy-2-propenamides, a new class of synthetic histone deacetylase inhibitors. *Journal of Medicinal Chemistry*, **44**, 2069–2072.

37 Van Ommeslaeghe, K., Elaut, G., Brecx, V., Papeleu, P., Iterbeke, K., Geerlings, P. *et al.* (2003) Amide analogues of TSA: Synthesis, binding mode analysis and HDAC inhibition. *Bioorganic & Medicinal Chemistry Letters*, **13**, 1861–1864.

38 Wang, D.F., Wiest, O., Helquist, P., Lan-Hargest, H.Y. and Wiech, N.L. (2004) On the function of the 14 A long internal cavity of histone deacetylase-like protein: implications for the design of histone deacetylase inhibitors. *Journal of Medicinal Chemistry*, **47**, 3409–3417.

39 Lu, Q., Wang, D.S., Chen, C.S., Hu, Y.D. and Chen, C.S. (2005) Structure-based optimization of phenylbutyrate-derived histone deacetylase inhibitors. *Journal of Medicinal Chemistry*, **48**, 5530–5535.

40 Rodriquez, M., Terracciano, S., Cini, E., Settembrini, G., Bruno, I., Bifulco, G. *et al.* (2006) Total synthesis, NMR solution structure, and binding model of the potent histone deacetylase inhibitor FR235222. *Angewandte Chemie-International Edition*, **45**, 423–427.

41 Maulucci, N., Chini, M.G., Di Micco, S., Izzo, I., Cafaro, E., Russo, A. *et al.* (2007) Molecular insights into azumamide E histone deacetylases inhibitory activity. *Journal of the American Chemical Society*, **129**, 3007–3012.

42 Liu, T., Kapustin, G. and Etzkorn, F.A. (2007) Design and synthesis of a potent histone deacetylase inhibitor. *Journal of Medicinal Chemistry*, **50**, 2003–2006.

43 Micco, D.S., Terracciano, S., Bruno, I., Rodriquez, M., Riccio, R., Taddei, M. *et al.* (2008) Molecular modeling studies toward the structural optimization of new cyclopeptide-based HDAC inhibitors modeled on the natural product FR235222. *Bioorganic and Medicinal Chemistry*, **16**, 8635–8642.

44 Chen, P.C., Patil, V., Guerrant, W., Green, P. and Oyelere, A.K. (2008) Synthesis and structure–activity relationship of histone deacetylase (HDAC) inhibitors with triazole-linked cap group. *Bioorganic and Medicinal Chemistry*, **16**, 4839–4853.

45 Lavoie, R., Bouchain, G., Frechette, S., Woo, S.H., Khalil, E.A., Leit, S. *et al.* (2001) Design and synthesis of a novel class of histone deacetylase inhibitors. *Bioorganic & Medicinal Chemistry Letters*, **11**, 2847–2850.

46 Remiszewski, S.W., Sambucetti, L.C., Atadja, P., Bair, K.W., Cornell, W.D., Green, M.A. *et al.* (2002) Inhibitors of human histone deacetylase: Synthesis and enzyme and cellular activity of straight chain hydroxamates. *Journal of Medicinal Chemistry*, **45**, 753–757.

47 Mai, A., Massa, S., Ragno, R., Cerbara, I., Jesacher, F., Loidl, P. and Brosch, G. (2003) 3-(4-Aroyl-1-methyl-1H-2-pyrrolyl)-N-hydroxy-2-alkylamides as a new class of synthetic histone deacetylase inhibitors. 1. Design, synthesis, biological evaluation, and binding mode studies performed through three different docking procedures. *Journal of Medicinal Chemistry*, **46**, 512–524.

48 Park, H. and Lee, S. (2004) Homology modeling, force field design, and free energy simulation studies to optimize the activities of histone deacetylase inhibitors. *Journal of Computer-Aided Molecular Design*, **16**, 375–388.

49 Wang, D.-F., Helquist, P., Wiech, N.L. and Wiest, O. (2005) Toward selective histone deacetylase inhibitor design: homology modeling, docking studies, and molecular dynamics simulations of human class I histone deacetylases. *Journal of Medicinal Chemistry*, **48**, 6936–6947.

50 Kim, H.M., Hong, S.H., Kim, M.S., Lee, C.W., Kang, J.S., Lee, K. *et al.* (2007) Modification of cap group in d-lactam-based histone deacetylase (HDAC) inhibitors. *Bioorganic & Medicinal Chemistry Letters*, **17**, 6234–6237.

51 Witter, D.J., Harrington, P., Wilson, K.J., Chenard, M., Fleming, J.C., Haines, H. *et al.* (2008) Optimization of biaryl selective HDAC1&2 inhibitors. *Bioorganic & Medicinal Chemistry Letters*, **18**, 726–731.

52 Moradei, O.M., Mallais, T.C., Frechette, S., Paquin, I., Tessier, P.E., Leit, S.M. *et al.* (2007) Novel aminophenyl benzamide-type histone deacetylase inhibitors with enhanced potency and selectivity. *Journal of Medicinal Chemistry*, **50**, 5543–5546.

53 Schäfer, S., Saunders, L., Eliseeva, E.A. Jung, M., Schwienhorst, A., Dickmanns, A. *et al.* (2008) Phenylalanine-containing hydroxamic acids as selective inhibitors of class IIb histone deacetylases (HDACs). *Bioorganic and Medicinal Chemistry*, **16**, 2011–2033.

54 Yan, C., Xiu, Z., Li, X., Li, S., Hao, C. and Teng, H. (2008) Comparative molecular dynamics simulations of histone deacetylase-like protein: Binding modes and free energy analysis to hydroxamic acid inhibitors. *Proteins*, **73**, 134–149.

55 Mukherjee, P., Pradhan, A., Shah, F., Tekwanib, B.L. and Averya, M.A. (2008) Structural insights into the Plasmodium falciparum histone deacetylase 1 (PfHDAC-1): A novel target for the development of antimalarial therapy. *Bioorganic and Medicinal Chemistry*, **16**, 5254–5265.

56 Weerasinghe, S.V.W., Estiu, G., Wiest, O. and Pflum, M.K.H. (2008) Residues in the 11 Å channel of histone deacetylase 1 promote catalytic activity: implications for designing isoform-selective histone deacetylase inhibitors. *Journal of Medicinal Chemistry*, **51**, 5542–5551.

57 Estiu, G., Greenberg, E., Harrison, C.B., Kwiatkowski, N.P., Mazitschek, R., Bradner, J.E. *et al.* (2008) Structural origin of selectivity in class II-selective histone deacetylase inhibitors. *Journal of Medicinal Chemistry*, **51**, 2898–2906.

58 Schäfer, S., Saunders, L., Schlimme, S., Valkov, V., Wagner, J., Kratz, F. *et al.* (2009) Pyridylalanine-containing hydroxamic acids as selective HDAC6 inhibitors. *ChemMedChem*, **4**, 283–290.

59 Wang, D.F., Wiest, O., Helquist, P., Lan-Hargest, H.Y. and Wiech, N.L. (2004) QSAR studies of PC-3 cell line inhibition activity of TSA and SAHA-like hydroxamic acids. *Bioorganic & Medicinal Chemistry Letters*, **14**, 707–711.

60 Xie, A., Liao, C., Li, Z., Ning, Z., Hu, W., Lu, X., Shi, L. and Zhou, J. (2004) Quantitative structure-activity relationship study of histone deacetylase inhibitors. *Current Medicinal Chemistry Anticancer Agents*, **4**, 273–299.

61 Eikel, D., Lampen, A. and Nau, H. (2006) Teratogenic effects mediated by inhibition of histone deacetylases: evidence from quantitative structure activity relationships of 20 valproic acid derivatives. *Chemical Research in Toxicology*, **19**, 272–278.

62 Guo, Y., Xiao, J., Guo, Z., Chu, F., Cheng, Y. and Wu, S. (2005) Exploration of a binding mode of indole amide analogues as potent histone deacetylase inhibitors and 3D-QSAR analyses. *Bioorganic and Medicinal Chemistry*, **13**, 5424–5434.

63 Juvale, D.C., Kulkarni, V.V., Deokar, H.S., Wagh, N.K., Padhye, S.B. and Kulkarni, V.M. (2006) 3D-QSAR of histone deacetylase inhibitors: hydroxamate analogues. *Organic and Biomolecular Chemistry*, **4**, 2858–2868.

64 Ragno, R., Simeoni, S., Valente, S., Massa, S. and Mai, A. (2006) 3-D QSAR studies on histone deacetylase inhibitors. A GOLPE/GRID approach on different series of compounds. *Journal of Chemical Information and Modeling*, **46**, 1420–1430.

65 Ragno, R., Simeoni, S., Rotili, D., Caroli, A., Botta, G., Brosch, G., Massa, S. and Mai, A. (2008) Class II-selective histone deacetylase inhibitors. Part 2: alignment-independent GRIND 3-D QSAR, homology and docking studies. *European Journal of Medicinal Chemistry*, **43**, 621–632.

66 Price, S., Bordogna, W., Bull, R.J., Clark, D.E., Crackett, P.H., Dyke, H.J. *et al.* (2007) Identification and optimisation of a series of substituted 5-(1H-pyrazol-3-yl)-thiophene-2-hydroxamic acids as potent histone deacetylase (HDAC) inhibitors. *Bioorganic & Medicinal Chemistry Letters*, **17**, 370–375.

67 Vadivelan, S., Sinha, B.N., Rambabu, G., Boppana, K. and Jagarlapudi, S. (2008) Pharmacophore modeling and virtual screening studies to design some potential histone deacetylase inhibitors as new leads. *Journal of Molecular Graphics & Modelling*, **26**, 935–946.

68 Chen, Y., Jiang, Y.J., Zhou, J.W., Yu, Q.S. and You, Q.D. (2008) Identification of ligand features essential for HDACs inhibitors by pharmacophore modeling. *Journal of Molecular Graphics & Modelling*, **25**, 1160–1168.

69 Schuetz, A., Min, J., Antoshenko, T., Wang, C.L., Allali-Hassani, A., Dong, A. *et al.* (2007) Structural basis of inhibition of the human NAD+-dependent deacetylase SIRT5 by suramin. *Structure (London, England: 1993)*, **15**, 377–389.

70 Sanders, B.D., Zhao, K., Slama, J.T. and Marmorstein, R. (2007) Structural basis for nicotinamide inhibition and base exchange in Sir2 enzymes. *Molecular Cell*, **25**, 463–472.

71 Trapp, J., Meier, R., Hongwiset, D., Kassack, M.U., Sippl, W. and Jung, M. (2007) Structure-activity studies on suramin analogues as inhibitors of NAD(+)-dependent histone deacetylases (sirtuins). *ChemMedChem*, **2**, 1419–1431.

72 Neugebauer, R.C., Sippl, W. and Jung, M. (2008) Inhibitors of NAD+ dependent histone deacetylases (sirtuins). *Current Pharmaceutical Design*, **14**, 562–573.

73 Trapp, J., Jochum, A., Meier, R., Saunders, L., Marshall, B., Kunick, C. *et al.* (2006) Adenosine mimetics as inhibitors of NAD(+)-dependent histone deacetylases, from kinase to sirtuin inhibition. *Journal of Medicinal Chemistry*, **49**, 7307–7316.

74 Tervo, A.J., Kyrylenko, S., Niskanen, P., Salminen, A., Leppänen, J., Nyrönnen, T.H. *et al.* (2004) An in silico approach to discovering novel inhibitors of human

sirtuin type 2. *Journal of Medicinal Chemistry*, **47**, 6292–6298.

75 UNITY, Tripos Assoc., St. Louis, USA.

76 Crivori, P., Cruciani, G., Carrupt, P.A. and Testa, B. (2000) Predicting blood-brain barrier permeation from three-dimensional molecular structure. *Journal of Medicinal Chemistry*, **43**, 2204–2216.

77 Tervo, A.J., Suuronen, T., Kyrylenko, S., Kuusisto, E., Kiviranta, P.H., Salminnen, A. *et al.* (2006) Discovering inhibitors of human sirtuin type 2: novel structural scaffolds. *Journal of Medicinal Chemistry*, **49**, 7239–7241.

78 Kiviranta, P.H., Leppanen, J., Kyrylenko, S., Salo, H.S., Lahtela-Kakkonen, M., Tervo, A.J. *et al.* (2006) N, N′-bisbenzylidenebenzene-1,4-diamines and N,N′-bisbenzylidenenaphthalene-1,4-diamines as sirtuin type 2 (SIRT2) inhibitors. *Journal of Medicinal Chemistry*, **49**, 7907–7911.

79 Huhtiniemi, T., Suuronen, T., Rinne, V.M., Wittekindt, C., Lahtela-Kakkonen, M., Jarho, E. *et al.* (2008) Oxadiazole-carbonylaminothioureas as SIRT1 and SIRT2 inhibitors. *Journal of Medicinal Chemistry*, **51**, 4377–4380.

80 Outeiro, T.F., Kontopoulos, E., Altmann, S.M., Kufareva, I., Strathearn, K.E., Amore, A.M. *et al.* (2007) Sirtuin 2 inhibitors rescue alpha-synuclein-mediated toxicity in models of Parkinson's disease. *Science*, **317**, 516–519.

81 Abagyan, R., Totrov, M. and Kuznetsov, D. (1994) ICM – a new method for modeling and design: applications to docking and structure prediction. *Journal of Computational Chemistry*, **15**, 488–498.

82 Neugebauer, R.C., Uchiechowska, U., Meier, R., Hruby, H., Valkov, V., Verdin, E. *et al.* (2008) Stucture activity studies on splitomicin derivatives as sirtuin inhibitors and computational prediction of binding mode. *Journal of Medicinal Chemistry*, **51**, 1203–1213.

83 Napper, A.D., Hixon, J., McDonagh, T., Keavey, K., Pons, J.F., Barker, J. *et al.* (2005) Discovery of indoles as potent and selective inhibitors of the deacetylase SIRT1. *Journal of Medicinal Chemistry*, **48**, 8045–8054.

84 Posakony, J., Hirao, M., Stevens, S., Simon, J.A. and Bedalov, A. (2004) Inhibitors of Sir2: evaluation of splitomicin analogues. *Journal of Medicinal Chemistry*, **47**, 2635–2644.

85 Heltweg, B., Gatbonton, T., Schuler, A.D., Posakony, J., Li, H., Goehle, S. *et al.* (2006) Antitumor activity of a small-molecule inhibitor of human silent information regulator 2 enzymes. *Cancer Research*, **66**, 4368–4377.

86 Wang, J., Wolf, R.M., Caldwell, J.W., Kollman, P.A. and Case, D.A. (2004) Development and testing of a general amber force field. *Journal of Computational Chemistry*, **25**, 1157–1174.

87 Howitz, K.T., Bitterman, K.J., Cohen, H.Y., Lamming, D.W., Lavu, S., Wood, J.G. *et al.* (2003) Small molecule activators of sirtuin expan Saccharomyces cerevisiae lifespan. *Nature*, **425**, 191–196.

88 Huhtiniemi, T., Wittekindt, C., Laitinen, T., Leppänen, J., Salminen, A., Poso, A. *et al.* (2006) Comparative and pharmacophore model for deacetylase SIRT1. *Journal of Computer-Aided Molecular Design*, **20**, 589–599.

89 Lin, Y., Fletcher, C.M., Zhou, J., Allis, C.D. and Wagner, G. (1999) Solution structure of the catalytic domain of GCN5 histone acetyltransferase bound to coenzyme A. *Nature*, **400**, 86–89.

90 Trievel, R.C., Rojas, J.R., Sterner, D.E., Venkataramani, R.N., Wang, L., Zhou, J., Allis, C.D., Berger, S.L. and Marmorstein, R. (1999) Crystal structure and mechanism of histone acetylation of the yeast GCN5 transcriptional coactivator. *Proceedings of the National Academy of Sciences of the United States of America*, **96**, 8931–8936.

91 Liu, X., Wang, L., Zhao, K., Thompson, P.R., Hwang, Y., Marmorstein, R. and Cole, P.A. (2008) The structural basis of protein acetylation by the p300/CBP transcriptional coactivator. *Nature*, **451**, 846–850.

92 Bhaumik, S.R., Smith, E. and Shilatifard, A. (2007) Covalent modifications of histones during development and disease pathogenesis. *Nature Structural & Molecular Biology*, **14**, 1008–1016.

93 Zhang, X., Zhou, L. and Cheng, X. (2000) Crystal structure of the conserved core of protein arginine methyltransferase PRMT3. *The EMBO Journal*, **19**, 3509–3519.

94 Zhang, X. and Cheng, X. (2003) Structure of the predominant protein arginine methyltransferase PRMT1 and analysis of its binding to substrate peptides. *Structure (Camb)*, **11**, 509–520.

95 Ragno, R., Simeoni, S., Castellano, S., Vicidomini, C., Mai, A., Caroli, A. *et al.* (2007) Small molecule inhibitors of histone arginine methyltransferases: homology modeling, molecular docking, binding mode analysis, and biological evaluations. *Journal of Medicinal Chemistry*, **50**, 1241–1253.

96 Mai, A., Valente, S., Cheng, D., Perrone, A., Ragno, R., Simeoni, S. *et al.* (2007) Synthesis and biological validation of novel synthetic histone/protein methyltransferase inhibitors. *ChemMedChem*, **3**, 987–991.

97 Spannhoff, A., Heinke, R., Bauer, I., Trojer, P., Metzger, E., Gust, R. *et al.* (2007) Target-based approach to inhibitors of histone arginine methyltransferases. *Journal of Medicinal Chemistry*, **50**, 2319–2325.

98 Heinke, R., Spannhoff, A., Huda, E., Meier, R., Jung, M. and Sippl, W. (2009) Virtual screening and biological characterization of histone methyltransferase inhibitors PRMT1. *ChemMedChem*, **4**, 69–77.

99 Spannhoff, A., Machmur, R., Heinke, R., Trojer, P., Bauer, I., Brosch, G. *et al.* (2007) A novel arginine methyltransferase inhibitor with cellular activity. *Bioorganic & Medicinal Chemistry Letters*, **17**, 4150–4153.

100 Cheng, D., Yadav, N., King, R.W., Swanson, M.S., Weinstein, E.J. and Bedford, M.T. (2004) Small molecule regulators of protein arginine methyltransferases. *The Journal of Biological Chemistry*, **279**, 23892–23899.

101 Mason, J.S., Morize, I., Menard, P.R., Cheney, D.L., Hulme, C. and Labaudiniere, R.F. (1999) New 4-point pharmacophore method for molecular similarity and diversity applications: overview of the method and applications, including a novel approach to the design of combinatorial libraries containing privileged substructures. *Journal of Medicinal Chemistry*, **42**, 3251–3264.

102 Zhang, X., Yang, Z., Khan, S.I., Horton, J.R., Tamaru, H., Selker, E.U. *et al.* (2003) Structural basis for the product specificity of histone lysine methyltransferases. *Molecular Cell*, **12**, 177–185.

103 Shi, Y.J., Lan, F., Matson, C., Mulligan, P., Whetstine, J.R., Cole, P.A. *et al.* (2004) Histone demethylation mediated by the nuclear arnine oxidase homologue LSD1. *Cell*, **119**, 941–953.

104 Tsukada, Y., Fang, J., Erdjument-Bromage, H., Warren, M.E., Borchers, C.H., Tempst, P. *et al.* (2006) Histone demethylation by a family of JmjC domain-containing proteins. *Nature*, **439**, 811–816.

105 Wang, G.G., Allis, C.D. and Chi, P. (2007) Chromatin remodeling and cancer, Part I: Covalent histone modifications. *Trends in Molecular Medicine*, **13**, 363–372.

106 Rose, N.R., Ng, S.S., Mecinovi,ć J., Liénard, B.M., Bello, S.H., Sun, Z. *et al.* (2008) Inhibitor scaffolds for 2-oxoglutarate-dependent histone lysine demethylases. *Journal of Medicinal Chemistry*, **51**, 7053–7055.

4
Histone Modification Analysis Using Mass Spectrometry

Ana Villar-Garea and Axel Imhof

4.1
Introduction

The biological function of histones is strongly regulated through posttranslational modifications (PTMs). Different modifications affect each other and lead to an intricate network of interdependent modification patterns, which has been suggested to constitute a "histone code." Histones are very abundant, small basic proteins that package DNA in the eukaryotic nucleus to form chromatin. The four core histones are densely modified within their first 20–40 N-terminal amino acids, which are evolutionarily extremely well conserved despite having no structural function. The presumptive histone code consists of combinations of multiple PTMs of amino acids within these N-terminal tails. It has been suggested that cells use the modifications to encrypt various chromatin conformations and gene expression states. The analysis of modified histones can be used as a model to dissect complex modification patterns and to investigate their molecular functions. Here we review analytical methods that have been used to decipher complex histone modification patterns and we discuss the implication of these findings for chromatin structure and function.

Posttranslational modifications (PTMs) of proteins play a key role in regulating the biological function of many polypeptides. The spectrum of modifications ranges from the addition of relatively small groups such as methyl, acetyl and phosphate groups to the attachment of larger sugar moieties or the generation of isopeptidic bonds between the molecule of interest and the small peptides ubiquitin or SUMO [1]. In this review we focus on two of those modifications that are commonly found to regulate histone function: acetylation and methylation of lysine residues. Mass spectrometry provides key tools for the analysis of PTMs [2–5]. Every modification adds a distinct mass to the molecule studied and, thanks to the high resolution of modern mass spectrometers and the development of "soft" ionization techniques, the mapping of posttranslational modifications has been greatly facilitated during the past couple of years. The increased usage of these high-resolution methods not only

Epigenetic Targets in Drug Discovery. Edited by Wolfgang Sippl and Manfred Jung

ISBN: 978-3-527-32355-5

allowed a much faster detection of PTMs but also revealed a much higher abundance of PTMs on histone molecules than previously anticipated. However, in order to precisely map the residue that is modified, elaborate methods have been established to enrich peptides that carry particular modifications [6–9] and to study them by MS/MS or MS^n mass spectrometry. Frequently, histones carry several different modifications, which can be localized on a single peptide within a protease digest [10–13].

4.2
Histone Molecules

Histones are very basic proteins with an isoelectric point between 10.31 and 11.27 for human complement. They are present in virtually all eukaryotes (with the exception of dinoflagellates [14]) where they are associated with most of the nuclear DNA. The DNA is wrapped around an octamer formed by the four core histones H2A, H2B, H3 and H4 to build a nucleosome. This particle is the fundamental repeating unit of chromatin [15]. A string of nucleosomes can fold into a higher order structure, the exact molecular nature of which is still not fully understood but clearly has a strong influence on gene expression.

Since the crystal structures of the octamer and nucleosome have been solved at high resolution [16], we know that the C-terminal "globular" domains of the core histones form the proteinacaeous core of the nucleosome. The N-termini ("the tails") in contrast protrude into solution and do not adopt a defined structure, which could be resolved by X-ray crystallography. These N-terminal tails are extremely well conserved during evolution [15], suggesting an important role in nucleosome function. This notion is further supported by the fact that the histone tails are essential for viability in yeast [17]. The likely reason why these tails have been conserved during evolution is their intense posttranslational modification. The histone H3 tail for example is formed by about 38 amino acids, with 19 of them being potentially modified. This not only generates a very high density of PTMs on a short stretch of the protein but also produces a challenge for the analysis of the modification pattern within this stretch. In the following review, we briefly describe methods that allow a prefractionation of histone molecules or protease digestion products of histones.

4.3
Capillary Electrophoresis

A further improvement of the more traditional slab gel analysis is the use of high-performance capillary electrophoresis (HPCE), which combines the separation power of high-performance liquid chromatography (HPLC) with the selectivity and speed of conventional gel electrophoresis. However, as HPCE separations are often performed using fused silica capillaries the positively charged histone molecules interact with the negatively charged silanol groups of the capillary, leading to an extreme peak broadening and a low resolution. To circumvent this problem several additives such as hydroxypropyl methylcellulose have been added to the running buffer to suppress the interaction between histones and the inner surface of the capillary [18–20]. Although easy to handle and very reliable, the dynamic coating procedure does not allow online coupling to an ESI mass spectrometer. In order to allow a combination of CE and the high analytical power of mass spectrometry permanently coated capillaries are used to analyze core histone molecules using 0.1 M formic acid and a sheath liquid of methanol/water (80 : 20) to facilitate ionization [21].

4.4
Reversed Phase Chromatography

Another powerful method that is frequently used to separate core histones from each other as well as the peptides resulting from a tryptic digest is reversed phase chromatography [22]. As the histones contain a highly hydrophobic core they bind very efficiently to a C4 reversed phase column. These columns have an extremely high resolution and are able to differentiate between histone variants that differ in just a few amino acids, such as H3.1 and H3.3 [23, 24]. Besides the separation of intact histones, reversed phase columns are also frequently used to separate peptides generated by a protease digest of histone molecules to reduce the complexity of a peptide mixture and to facilitate the analysis of the individual peptides. Although LC separations are generally much more time-intensive that the CE separation discussed in the section above, it is by far the preferred pre-fractionation method for online couplings to mass spectrometers, as the coupling to a MS detector is much more reliable and reproducible. For example, the high resolution power of C18 reversed phase chromatography coupled to high resolution mass spectrometry allows the distinction of trimethylated and acetylated peptides not only based on their different mass but also based on the difference in retention time from a C-18 column (Figure 4.1).

4.5
Mass Spectrometry

Mass spectrometry provides a more direct and precise technique to study histone modifications. As with the other methods discussed above, mass spectrometry also has several pitfalls that should be taken into account when analyzing histone modifications. First of all histones and especially the core histones H3 and H4 are rich in lysine residues. Consequently, trypsin as an enzyme that is routinely used for the identification of proteins via peptide mass fingerprints cannot be used for regular "in gel" digestion of histones. Other enzymes that have a different specificity (such as Asp-N or Arg-C) are more frequently used in the analysis of histones [25]. A drawback

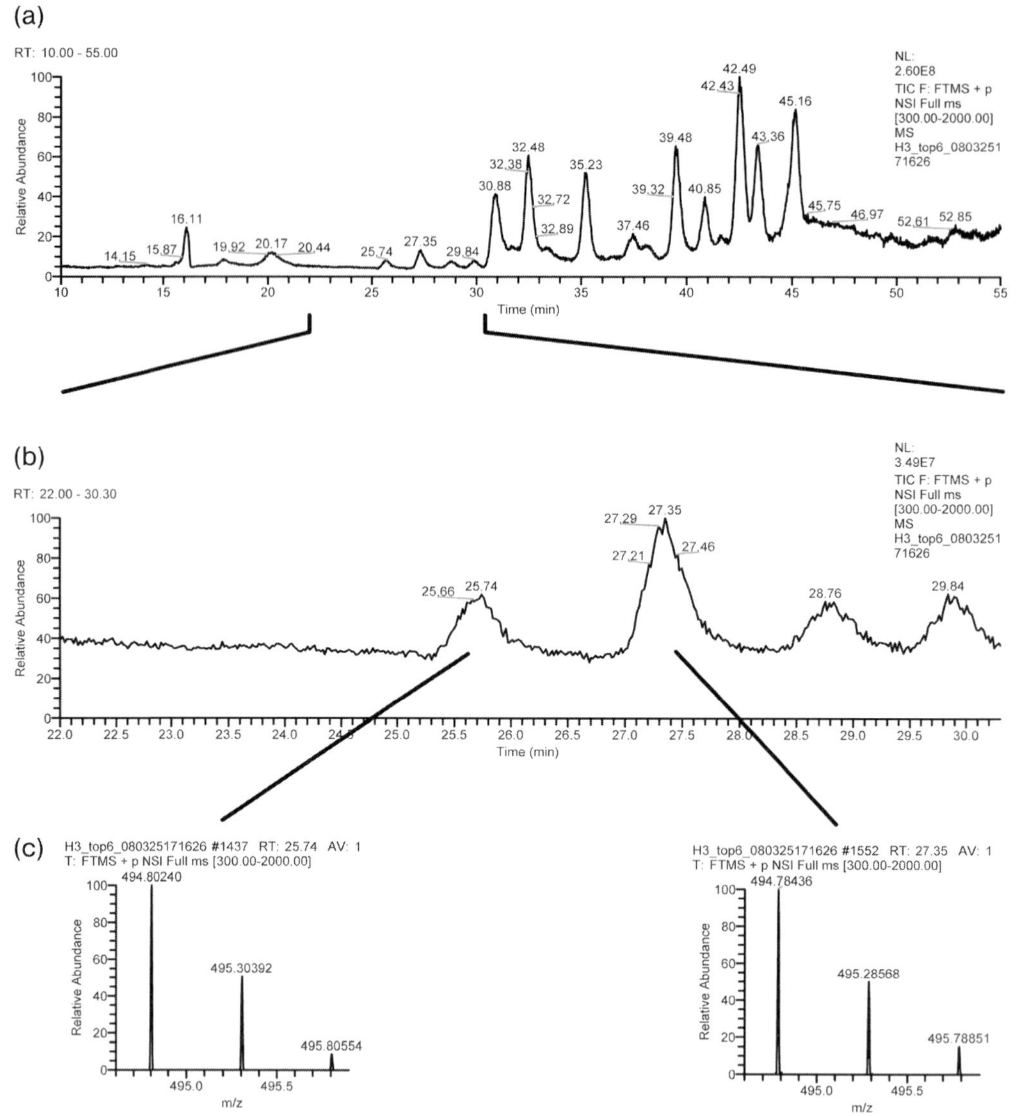

(d)

modification	expected *m/z*	found *m/z*	difference / ppm	retention time / min
trimethylation	494.8031	494.8024	-1.41	25.7
monoacetylation	494.7849	494.7846	-0.61	27.3

Figure 4.1 Separation of H3 9–17 trimethylated at K9 from H3 9–17 monoacetylated. Histone H3 isolated from *Drosophila melanogaster* was acylated with deuterated acetic anhydride and subsequently digested with trypsin. The resulting peptides were analyzed by LC-MS/MS employing LTQ-Orbitrap (Thermo Scientific) as detector. (a) Chromatogram of the analysis. The *y* axis

of using those enzymes is their low activity when used for "in gel" digestions, making a more laborious and less sensitive reversed phase HPLC purification of individual histones necessary [22, 26–28]. Another way to circumvent this problem that is used by many laboratories using mass spectrometry to analyze histones and histone modifications is the derivatization of lysines within the histone molecules using acid anhydrides [29–31]. This class of molecules reacts very efficiently with unmodified or monomethylated ε-amino groups of lysine residues, thereby preventing the tryptic cleavage C-terminal of the modified residue. As di- and trimethylation or acetylation of the lysine ε-amino group also prevent the trypsin cleavage, trypsin only cleaves the C-terminal of an arginine residue. The resulting peptides are much larger and can be analyzed by MALDI-TOF mass spectrometry more easily. Another advantage of this procedure is that the digestion with trypsin can be done in a gel slice from an SDS PAA gel, which allows a rapid, reliable and easy separation of the individual histone molecules. In addition to this effect the derivatization of lysine residues with isotopically labeled anhydrides can be used to quantitatively determine the acetylation status of a particular lysine.

However, especially when non-isotope-tagged molecules such as propionic anhydride are used, an additional complication has to be taken into account when analyzing the spectra. Propionylation of lysines leads to a mass shift of 56.0262, which is close to the addition of four methyl groups (56.0626). This is especially problematic if a peptide contains more than one lysine, such as the H3 peptides containing amino acids 9–17 or 27–40. An observed mass that corresponds to an unmodified peptide for example can also be explained by a peptide carrying one methyl group on one lysine and an acetyl group on the other. Therefore MS/MS experiments have to be performed in order to unambiguously assign a modification pattern to a particular peptide.

A related problem that is specific for the analysis of PTMs within histone molecules is the fact that several lysines within the histone tail (H3K9, H3K27) can carry either one, two or three methyl groups or one acetyl group. Whereas the mono- and dimethylated histones can be easily distinguished from an acetylated isoform, the mass shift generated by the addition of three methyl groups is very similar to that generated by an acetylation (42.0468 vs 42.0105) resulting in a mass difference of 0.036 Da or 36 ppm for a peptide with a $M_r = 1000$. This is particularly important as the two modifications have distinct biological outputs. Whereas H3K9me3 is a signal for gene repression and the silencing of a whole genomic locus, acetylation of the same residue indicates a transcriptionally active gene [12, 32]. Several ways have been used to distinguish between the two types of modifications using mass spectrometry.

represents the relative abundance of the total ion current for m/z values between 300 and 2000 for full MS spectra. (b) Zoom of the chromatogram displayed in (a). (c) Zooms of the full MS spectra acquired at 25.74 min (left) and 27.35 min (right). The observed masses indicate that at 25.74 min elutes the peptide 9–17 trimethylated at one lysine (K9 according to the MSMS spectra) whereas at 27.35 min elutes 9–17 with one natural acetyl group (K9/K14 according to the MSMS spectra). (d) The table summarizes what is shown in the other panels. The high resolution and accuracy of the spectrometer allows the distinction between acetylated peptides containing trimethylated lysine residues from those containing acetylated lysines.

One possibility is the recording of mass spectra with an accuracy of less than 5 ppm and a high resolution. This high mass accuracy can be achieved by using a high-resolution TOF mass analyzer in reflector mode and an internal calibration standard with a mass close to the one of interest [33]. However, with the development and increasing availability of high resolution FT mass spectrometer, a more elegant and direct way is frequently used to distinguish between the two modifications [26, 34]. A distinction between those two modifications can also be accomplished by studying the fragmentation behavior of the modified peptide in an MS/MS experiment. Very often the analysis of PTMs in histones makes use of the appearance of specific immonium ions that are generated after collision-induced decay of a modified molecule (precursor ion scan) or the loss of specific masses from a selected precursor ion after low-energy fragmentation (neutral loss). Both techniques have been applied to distinguish trimethylation from acetylation. In the case of a peptide carrying an acetylated lysine, high collision energy fragmentation leads to the formation of a specific ion with a m/z value of 126, which is not generated when the lysine is trimethylated [33]. In contrast, the fragmentation of a peptide where the same lysine is trimethylated results in a peptide characteristic of a neutral loss of 59 $[M + H-59]^+$, which can be explained by the loss of a trimethyl amine moiety ($N(CH_3)_3$). This loss is only observed in ions that carry the modified lysines and can therefore also be used to precisely map the modification in an MS/MS experiment. This is particularly useful when the two peptides analyzed have the same elemental composition and therefore the same monoisotopic mass, such as the H3 peptide 9–17 trimethylated at position 9 and acetylated at position 14 versus the peptide acetylated at position 9 and trimethylated at position 14 [33].

Finally, one of the biggest challenges in the analysis of protein molecules carrying complex modifications is the precise assignment of each modification within a single molecule. This interference between different modifications is of major biological interest as the modifications are often used to integrate various signals within a common pathway. However, when analyzing a mixture of molecules it is difficult to determine whether two modifications are located on the same molecule or exclude each other. A possible solution for this problem is the recent development of so-called "top down proteomics" that allows the sequence determination of intact proteins without prior proteolytic cleavage. As in the case for distinguishing methylated from acetylated lysines, the increased availability of high-resolution mass spectrometers permitted a rapid expansion of the methodological toolbox analyzing entire proteins. The high resolution of a Fourier transform mass spectrometer (FTMS) allows a reliable and precise assignment of multiply charged polypeptides and therefore greatly facilitates the interpretation of fragmentation spectra, which could otherwise not be deconvoluted using mass spectrometers with a lower resolution power. Fragmentation in a FTMS mass spectrometer is achieved by a process called electron capture dissection (ECD), in which multiply charged ions are trapped in a cyclotron and irradiated with a beam of low-energy electrons generated by an electron gun [35–37]. This fragmentation leads to an extensive cleavage of the N–C_α amine backbone bond resulting in a series of c and z ions (in contrast to the b/y fragmentation generated by CID) that can be used to deduce

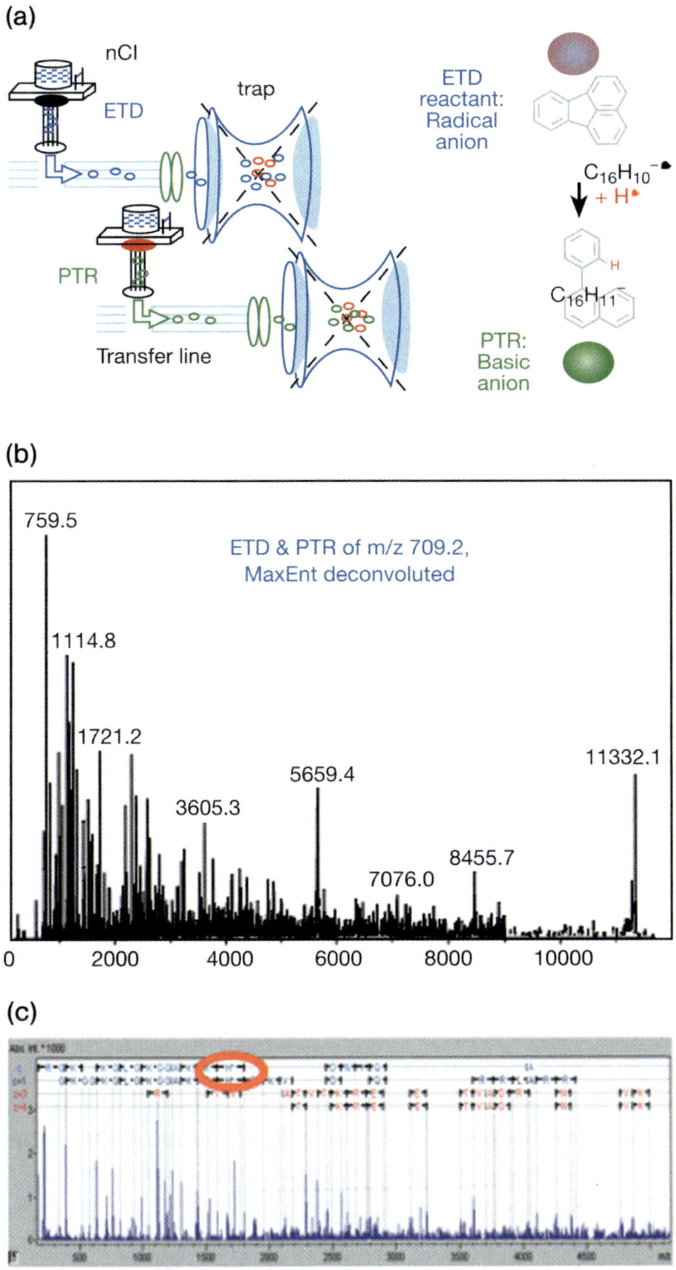

Figure 4.2 Top down mass spectrometry using ETD. (a) Setup of ETD and PTR in a 3D HCTultra ion trap (BDaltonics). ETD and PTR reactants are ionized in an additional nCI source and injected into the transfer line from the same reservoir. Switching nCI parameters decides whether the radical anion for ETD (fluoranthene) or its derivative, a basic anion, for PTR ($C_{16}H_{11}^{-}$) is extracted from the nCI source. (b) ETD/PTR-MS/MS spectrum of intact pH4 at 11 331 Da after MaxEnt deconvolution. Fragment ions all across the *m*/*z* range of 100–11 331 Da are visible. Since this is the deconvoluted result, noise is no longer visible. The sequence coverage is >80%. (c) Assignment of fragmentation peaks using Biotools reveals H18 as the most likely phosphorylation site in H4.

the primary sequence and the location of a specific PTM even within larger peptides such as the histones [38–40]. This then allows the analysis of complex modification patterns within the same molecule, thereby enabling the investigation of the interdependency of various modifications. In addition, due to the nature of fragmentation, ECD can also be used to detect the position of very labile modifications that are easily lost in other fragmentation methods [37].

An alternative method for top down sequencing that does not require expensive mass spectrometers was recently reported by Hunt and colleagues, also using histones as model proteins [41]. In their case complex fragmentation spectra are facilitated by collisions between radical anions and a protonated analyte. In this process, an electron is transferred to the positively charged ion. The radical anion then becomes a neutral aromatic hydrocarbon which is pumped away by the vacuum system, and the protonated peptide becomes a radical cation that then fragments at the amide backbone in a process analogous to that observed under electron capture conditions. This process results in the production of singly and doubly charged ion series that can be easily analyzed by low-resolution mass spectrometers such as an ion trap. This process has been termed electron transfer dissociation (ETD) coupled to a proton transfer reaction (PTR) and allows a top down proteomics approach without requiring expensive equipment (Figure 4.2a). ETD is especially well suited to study labile posttranslational modifications such as N-phosphorylation [42] as it keeps the labile bond intact while still giving rise to a fragmentation of the peptide backbone (Figure 4.2b, C).

The use of different approaches to study complex histone modification patterns ranging from the bottom up approach that allows a detailed and quantitative measurement of particular histone modifications to the top down methods that help the dissection of interdependencies between different modifications will greatly facilitate the analysis of complex modification patterns and provide a deeper insight into the biological role of these patterns.

Acknowledgements

We would like to thank Dr. XinLinZu and Dr. Arnd Ingendoh from Bruker Daltonics for providing the phosphorylated H4 and for performing the top down analysis using ETD/PTR. Work in A.I.'s laboratory is funded by the Deutsche Forschungsgemeinschaft (IM23/4-3). Parts of this chapter have been published in Ref. [43].

References

1 Walsh, C.T. (2005) *Posttranslational Modifications of Proteins*, Roberts & Company Publishers, p. 576.

2 Mann, M. and Jensen, O.N. (2003) Proteomic analysis of post-translational modifications. *Nature Biotechnology*, **21**, 255–261.

3 Wilkins, M.R., Gasteiger, E., Gooley, A.A., Herbert, B.R., Molloy, M.P., Binz, P.A., Ou, K., Sanchez, J.C., Bairoch, A.,

Williams, K.L. and Hochstrasser, D.F. (1999) High-throughput mass spectrometric discovery of protein post-translational modifications. *Journal of Molecular Biology*, **289**, 645–657.

4 Sickmann, A., Mreyen, M. and Meyer, H.E. (2003) Mass spectrometry – a key technology in proteome research. *Advances in Biochemical Engineering/Biotechnology*, **83**, 141–176.

5 Sickmann, A., Mreyen, M. and Meyer, H.E. (2002) Identification of modified proteins by mass spectrometry. *IUBMB Life*, **54**, 51–57.

6 Schlosser, A., Vanselow, J.T. and Kramer, A. (2005) Mapping of phosphorylation sites by a multi-protease approach with specific phosphopeptide enrichment and NanoLC-MS/MS analysis. *Analytical Chemistry*, **77**, 5243–5250.

7 Stensballe, A., Andersen, S. and Jensen, O.N. (2001) Characterization of phosphoproteins from electrophoretic gels by nanoscale Fe(III) affinity chromatography with off-line mass spectrometry analysis. *Proteomics*, **1**, 207–222.

8 Zhou, H., Watts, J.D. and Aebersold, R. (2001) A systematic approach to the analysis of protein phosphorylation. *Nature Biotechnology*, **19**, 375–378.

9 Posewitz, M.C. and Tempst, P. (1999) Immobilized gallium(III) affinity chromatography of phosphopeptides. *Analytical Chemistry*, **71**, 2883–2892.

10 Appella, E. and Anderson, C.W. (2000) Signaling to p53: breaking the posttranslational modification code. *Pathologie-Biologie*, **48**, 227–245.

11 Puri, P.L. and Sartorelli, V. (2000) Regulation of muscle regulatory factors by DNA-binding, interacting proteins, and post-transcriptional modifications. *Journal of Cellular Physiology*, **185**, 155–173.

12 Jenuwein, T. and Allis, C.D. (2001) Translating the histone code. *Science*, **293**, 1074–1080.

13 Wisniewski, J.R., Szewczuk, Z., Petry, I., Schwanbeck, R. and Renner, U. (1999) Constitutive phosphorylation of the acidic tails of the high mobility group 1 proteins by casein kinase II alters their conformation, stability, and DNA binding specificity. *The Journal of Biological Chemistry*, **274**, 20116–20122.

14 Moreno Diaz de la Espina, S., Alverca, E., Cuadrado, A. and Franca, S. (2005) Organization of the genome and gene expression in a nuclear environment lacking histones and nucleosomes: the amazing dinoflagellates. *European Journal of Cell Biology*, **84**, 137–149.

15 Wolffe, A.P. (1998) *Chromatin Structure and Function*, 3rd edn, Academic Press, San Diego, CA, p. 447.

16 Luger, K., Mader, A.W., Richmond, R.K., Sargent, D.F. and Richmond, T.J. (1997) Crystal structure of the nucleosome core particle at 2.8 A resolution. *Nature*, **389**, 251–260.

17 Ling, X., Harkness, T.A., Schultz, M.C., Fisher-Adams, G. and Grunstein, M. (1996) Yeast histone H3 and H4 amino termini are important for nucleosome assembly in vivo and in vitro: redundant and position-independent functions in assembly but not in gene regulation. *Genes and Development*, **10**, 686–699.

18 Urdinguio, R.G., Pino, I., Ropero, S., Fraga, M.F. and Esteller, M. (2007) Histone H3 and H4 modification profiles in a Rett syndrome mouse model. *Epigenetics*, **2**, 11–14.

19 Fraga, M.F., Ballestar, E., Villar-Garea, A., Boix-Chornet, M., Espada, J., Schotta, G., Bonaldi, T., Haydon, C., Ropero, S., Petrie, K., Iyer, N.G., Perez-Rosado, A., Calvo, E., Lopez, J.A., Cano, A., Calasanz, M.J., Colomer, D., Piris, M.A., Ahn, N., Imhof, A., Caldas, C., Jenuwein, T. and Esteller, M. (2005) Loss of acetylation at Lys16 and trimethylation at Lys20 of histone H4 is a common hallmark of human cancer. *Nature Genetics*, **37**, 391–400.

20 Lindner, H., Helliger, W. and Puschendorf, B. (1986) Histone separation by high-performance liquid chromatography on

C4 reverse-phase columns. *Analytical Biochemistry*, **158**, 424–430.

21 Aguilar, C., Hofte, A.J., Tjaden, U.R. and van der Greef, J. (2001) Analysis of histones by on-line capillary zone electrophoresis-electrospray ionisation mass spectrometry. *Journal of Chromatography. A*, **926**, 57–67.

22 Bonaldi, T., Imhof, A. and Regula, J.T. (2004) A combination of different mass spectroscopic techniques for the analysis of dynamic changes of histone modifications. *Proteomics*, **4**, 1382–1396.

23 Hake, S.B., Garcia, B.A., Duncan, E.M., Kauer, M., Dellaire, G., Shabanowitz, J., Bazett-Jones, D.P., Allis, C.D. and Hunt, D.F. (2006) Expression patterns and post-translational modifications associated with mammalian histone H3 variants. *The Journal of Biological Chemistry*, **281**, 559–568.

24 McKittrick, E., Gafken, P.R., Ahmad, K. and Henikoff, S. (2004) Histone H3.3 is enriched in covalent modifications associated with active chromatin. *Proceedings of the National Academy of Sciences of the United States of America*, **101**, 1525–1530.

25 Bonaldi, T., Regula, J.T. and Imhof, A. (2004) The use of mass spectrometry for the analysis of histone modifications. *Methods in Enzymology*, **377**, 111–130.

26 Freitas, M.A., Sklenar, A.R. and Parthun, M.R. (2004) Application of mass spectrometry to the identification and quantification of histone post-translational modifications. *Journal of Cellular Biochemistry*, **92**, 691–700.

27 Zhang, L., Freitas, M.A., Wickham, J., Parthun, M.R., Klisovic, M.I., Marcucci, G. and Byrd, J.C. (2004) Differential expression of histone post-translational modifications in acute myeloid and chronic lymphocytic leukemia determined by high-pressure liquid chromatography and mass spectrometry. *Journal of the American Society for Mass Spectrometry*, **15**, 77–86.

28 Zhang, K., Tang, H., Huang, L., Blankenship, J.W., Jones, P.R., Xiang, F., Yau, P.M. and Burlingame, A.L. (2002) Identification of acetylation and methylation sites of histone H3 from chicken erythrocytes by high-accuracy matrix-assisted laser desorption ionization-time-of-flight, matrix-assisted laser desorption ionization-postsource decay, and nanoelectrospray ionization tandem mass spectrometry. *Analytical Biochemistry*, **306**, 259–269.

29 Smith, C.M., Gafken, P.R., Zhang, Z., Gottschling, D.E., Smith, J.B. and Smith, D.L. (2003) Mass spectrometric quantification of acetylation at specific lysines within the amino-terminal tail of histone H4. *Analytical Biochemistry*, **316**, 23–33.

30 Taipale, M., Rea, S., Richter, K., Vilar, A., Lichter, P., Imhof, A. and Akhtar, A. (2005) hMOF histone acetyltransferase is required for histone H4 lysine 16 acetylation in mammalian cells. *Molecular and Cellular Biology*, **25**, 6798–6810.

31 Peters, A.H., Kubicek, S., Mechtler, K., O'Sullivan, R.J., Derijck, A.A., Perez-Burgos, L., Kohlmaier, A., Opravil, S., Tachibana, M., Shinkai, Y., Martens, J.H. and Jenuwein, T. (2003) Partitioning and plasticity of repressive histone methylation states in mammalian chromatin. *Molecular Cell*, **12**, 1577–1589.

32 Turner, B.M. (2002) Cellular memory and the histone code. *Cell*, **111**, 285–291.

33 Zhang, K., Yau, P.M., Chandrasekhar, B., New, R., Kondrat, R., Imai, B.S. and Bradbury, M.E. (2004) Differentiation between peptides containing acetylated or tri-methylated lysines by mass spectrometry: an application for determining lysine 9 acetylation and methylation of histone H3. *Proteomics*, **4**, 1–10.

34 Syka, J.E., Marto, J.A., Bai, D.L., Horning, S., Senko, M.W., Schwartz, J.C., Ueberheide, B., Garcia, B., Busby, S., Muratore, T., Shabanowitz, J. and Hunt, D.F. (2004) Novel linear quadrupole ion trap/FT mass spectrometer: performance

characterization and use in the comparative analysis of histone H3 post-translational modifications. *Journal of Proteome Research*, **3**, 621–626.

35 Ge, Y., Lawhorn, B.G., ElNaggar, M., Strauss, E., Park, J.H., Begley, T.P. and McLafferty, F.W. (2002) Top down characterization of larger proteins (45 kDa) by electron capture dissociation mass spectrometry. *Journal of the American Chemical Society*, **124**, 672–678.

36 McLafferty, F.W., Horn, D.M., Breuker, K., Ge, Y., Lewis, M.A., Cerda, B., Zubarev, R.A. and Carpenter, B.K. (2001) Electron capture dissociation of gaseous multiply charged ions by Fourier-transform ion cyclotron resonance. *Journal of the American Society for Mass Spectrometry*, **12**, 245–249.

37 Kelleher, N.L., Zubarev, R.A., Bush, K., Furie, B., Furie, B.C., McLafferty, F.W. and Walsh, C.T. (1999) Localization of labile posttranslational modifications by electron capture dissociation: the case of gamma-carboxyglutamic acid. *Analytical Chemistry*, **71**, 4250–4253.

38 Boyne, M.T. 2nd, Pesavento, J.J., Mizzen, C.A. and Kelleher, N.L. (2006) Precise characterization of human histones in the H2A gene family by top down mass spectrometry. *Journal of Proteome Research*, **5**, 248–253.

39 Siuti, N., Roth, M.J., Mizzen, C.A., Kelleher, N.L. and Pesavento, J.J. (2006) Gene-specific characterization of human histone H2B by electron capture dissociation. *Journal of Proteome Research*, **5**, 233–239.

40 Thomas, C.E., Kelleher, N.L. and Mizzen, C.A. (2006) Mass spectrometric characterization of human histone H3: a bird's eye view. *Journal of Proteome Research*, **5**, 240–247.

41 Coon, J.J., Ueberheide, B., Syka, J.E., Dryhurst, D.D., Ausio, J., Shabanowitz, J. and Hunt, D.F. (2005) Protein identification using sequential ion/ion reactions and tandem mass spectrometry. *Proceedings of the National Academy of Sciences of the United States of America*, **102**, 9463–9468.

42 Zu, X.L., Besant, P.G., Imhof, A. and Attwood, P.V. (2007) Mass spectrometric analysis of protein histidine phosphorylation. *Amino Acids*, **32**, 347–357.

43 Villar-Garea, A. and Imhof, A. (2006) The analysis of histone modifications. *Biochimica et Biophysica Acta*, **1764**, 1932–1939.

5
In Vitro Assays for Histone-Modifying Enzymes

Alexander-Thomas Hauser and Manfred Jung

5.1
Introduction

The major aim of medicinal chemistry is to provide small molecules that can be developed into new drugs. For the determination of potency and selectivity in both mono-target- and multi-target-based approaches, biochemical *in vitro* assays are very important, and mostly even indispensable tools. In this chapter, we want to review assay systems that are used to determine the activity of different histone-modifying enzymes. These assays can be used in high-throughput screening (HTS) for the identification of new lead structures as starting points for medicinal chemistry programs and the development of chemical tools. Such tools can help to elucidate the specific functions of epigenetic modifiers and the role of these in cellular processes. We focus in this chapter on the most important histone-modifying enzymes. We start with some general aspects on screening and assay setups commonly used for enzymes that carry out posttranslational modifications and then we present assays used for enzymes that affect reversible histone acetylation and methylation.

5.2
Screening Hierarchy

In any target-based drug discovery approach a whole set of assays is necessary for *in vitro* evaluation of potential drugs. Of course there is the need for an assay for the initial target in a cell-free system. Then cell- or (later) animal-based assays are used that: (i) may verify the inhibition of the target in a relevant range of concentration, (ii) link this target verification to a certain function and (iii) register the occurrence of a desired phenotype. Here, we limit the scope mostly to cell-free assay systems as cell-based assays are subject of other chapters in this book; but we point out applications of some of these assays in cellular systems. Generally, each type of assay may be used for the primary screening and several screening campaigns have led to inhibitors that target epigenetic modifiers by any one of these approaches.

Epigenetic Targets in Drug Discovery. Edited by Wolfgang Sippl and Manfred Jung

ISBN: 978-3-527-32355-5

While *in vitro* enzyme assays are probably the standard approach for the primary screen (for examples see Refs. [1–3]), other strategies have also been employed. Target verification for posttranslational modifications, like histone acetylation, is typically done by Western blots which suffer from low throughput. But ELISA-type variants that allow for a higher throughput can be performed [4–7]. As an example of functional assays, protein overexpression, for example p21 with histone deacetylase (HDAC) inhibitors [8], by Western blot or ELISA can either be measured or reporter gene assays [9–11] can be used. Finally, as phenotypic assays proliferation or differentiation can be applied in standard assays that also have led to the discovery of epigenetically active compounds [12, 13]. Each approach has its own advantages and disadvantages. No matter which assay was used for primary screening, eventually the other layers of testing have to follow before a new inhibitor may proceed to animal testing and finally clinical trials.

5.3
General Principles of Screening for Histone-Modifying Enzymes

As histone modifications are one example for posttranslational protein modifications, antibodies directed at these modifications may generally be used for the quantitation of the conversion by the enzyme. In these cases histones or peptides that derived from substrate sequences from histones or nonhistone proteins serve as substrates. The histone peptides might contain a tag (usually biotine) for immobilization or conjugation purposes. The antibody is usually detected with a secondary antibody against the F_C-part or protein A from *Staphylococcus aureus* that also binds the F_C-part [14]. The secondary antibody may be labeled with a fluorophor or for example lanthanides for final quantitation purposes. Generally one could avoid this procedure by labeling the primary antibody but this requires additional steps for each modification that is screened. With the secondary antibody strategy one such antibody can be applied in theory for all targets that eventually will be assayed. Antibody-based approaches are usually more specific if one detects the modification (i.e. acetylation or methylation of a certain amino acid) and not the unmodified form. For example, this may be used for both an acetyltransferase and a deacetylase. But only in the case of the acetyltransferase is the specific formation of the modification really measured. In the case of monitoring a deacetylase or demethylase with an antibody unspecific binding of the enzyme or other proteins during the course of the assay procedure may mask the modification and falsely mimic removal of the modification. It is very important to have robust inhibitors of the enzymes for control experiments as such masking effects are not affected by inhibitors as opposed to a decrease in the signal that is caused by the desired target.

Enzymes that cleave off modifications may be assayed by measuring the formation of either the protein or a protein-mimicking substrate or the small molecule product or byproducts (like acetate for histone deacetylases, or formaldehyde or hydrogen peroxide for histone demethylases). Transferases may generally be screened by measuring the conversion of the cosubstrate or quantitatin the formation of the metabolite of the cosubstrate (e.g. formation of CoA-SH from acetyl-CoA by acetyltransferases). Examples of these general procedures and additional screening assays are presented in the following sections in a target-based fashion (Table 5.1).

5.4
Histone Deacetylases

The equilibrium of reversible histone lysine acetylation is maintained by histone deacetylases (HDACs) on one hand and histone acetyltransferases on the other hand. Human histone deacetylases can be separated into four classes [15]. HDACs of class I, II and IV are zinc-dependent amidohydrolases, whereas class III HDACs, also referred to as sirtuins, have a mechanism that is dependent on NAD^+ [16]. As histone deacetylases have been widely studied, it is not surprising that there are also a large number of assays existing that have helped to characterize modulators of these enzymes and subsequently the enzymes themselves.

5.4.1
Radioactive Assays

Traditional radioactive HDAC assays are based on the measurement of released tritiated acetic acid from radiolabeled histones or oligopeptide substrates via extraction and scintillation counting. To determine enzyme activity, enzyme samples are mixed with pre-prepared acetate-labeled protein or oligopeptide. After incubation, extraction with ethyl acetate and centrifugation, an aliquot of the overlaying organic phase is added to a liquid scintillation cocktail and counted for radioactivity in a scintillation spectrophotometer [17]. The tritiated histones were originally gained by a complicated procedure, in which chicken were exposed to phenylhydrazine. The degree of acetylation of the radiolabeled core histones may differ from preparation to preparation, making it difficult to standardize the substrate properties. Therefore, efforts have been made to use chemically [^{3}H]acetylated oligopeptides with 8 [18] or 24 [19] amino acids derived from histone peptide sequences as HDAC substrates, which can be produced under defined standardized conditions. These radioactive assays have been widely used, but the requirement to separate the product from the substrate in the extraction step limits the assay throughput. A homogeneous version of the radioactive assay is the scintillation proximity assay (SPA) [20], where no extraction and separation are necessary. In the SPA, a [^{3}H]acetate radioactively labeled oligopeptide histone substrate is coupled via an N-terminal biotin group to streptavidine-coated SPA beads. The proximity of the radiolabel to the beads, which contain a scintillant, results in energy transfer and therefore emission of light. Incubation of the [^{3}H]acetylated substrate with histone deacetylases releases radioactively labeled acetate, leading to a decrease in light emission. This scintillation proximity assay is applicable for a number of target enzymes by altering the radiolabeled substrate and allows for a higher throughput, but like all other radioactive assay systems it leads to several problems, such as

Table 5.1 Overview over assays for histone modifying enzymes.

Target	Substrate	Detection	Principle	Remarks
HDACs (class I, II, IV)	Trifluoracetyl lysine derivative	NMR	Signal of released trifluoroacetate differs	Noninvasive cellular measurement, lower throughput
	Various acetylated substrates	Absorbance	Detection of acetate by a coupled enzymatic reaction	Absorbance not very sensitive and selective
	Thioacetylated oligopeptide	Absorbance	Detection of thioacetate by Ellman's reagent	Absorbance not very sensitive and selective
	[^{3}H]Acetate-labeled histones	Scintillation counting	Heterogeneous radioactive assay with an extraction step	Difficult standardization; "no batch-to-batch conformity"
	[^{3}H]Acetate-labeled oligopeptides	Scintillation counting	Heterogeneous radioactive assay with an extraction step	Substrate synthesis under standardized conditions
	[^{3}H]Acetate-labeled octapeptides	Scintillation counting	Scintillation proximity assay with beads or plates	Homogeneous radioactive assay
	MAL, also subtype selective variants	RP-HPLC, fluorescence detection	Heterogeneous assay with an extraction step	Not amenable for HTS due to the extraction step and the detection method
		Fluorescence intensity	Heterogeneous assay with an extraction step	Plate reader measurement
		Fluorescence intensity	Derivatization with NDA, quenching of metabolite	Homogeneous fluorescent assay
		Fluorescence intensity	Second incubation step with trypsin	Also with short oligopeptide substrates, homogeneous assay
	Not applicable	Fluorescence polarization	Competition assay with labeled inhibitor	Less sensitive towards compound fluorescence
	Not applicable	Quenching of FRET	FRET	Competition with fluorescent inhibitor

Sirtuins	ZMAL, labeled oligopeptides	Fluorescence intensity	Second incubation step with trypsin	ZMAL also for HDACs from various species (maize, human, mouse)
	Fluorescence labeled oligopeptide with quencher	FRET	Second incubation step with trypsin	Complicated substrate
	Biotinylated p53 peptide with fluorescence label	Fluorescence polarization	Incubation with streptavidine and trypsin cleavage	Complicated substrate, less interference with compound fluorescence
HATs	Radiolabeled acetyl CoA	Scintillation counting	Heterogeneous radioactive assay	Homogeneous version with FlashPlates available
	Histones or oligopeptides	Absorbance of NADH	Conversion of generated CoA-SH to succinyl-CoA/acetyl-CoA with α-KG- or pyruvate dehydrogenase	Interference with compound absorbance; coupled enzymatic assay
	Histones or oligopeptides	Fluorescence intensity	Chemical conversion of CoA-SH with CPM	Interference by other thiols (e.g. as enzyme buffer components)
	Biotinylated histone peptides	Chemoluminescence generated by thioxene	AlphaScreen, AlphaLisa	Homogeneous assay, commerically available components
PRMTs	Biotinylated oligopeptides	Time-resolved fluorescence	EuLISA; based on primary and Eu-labeled secondary antibody;	Heterogeneous assay, very low assay volume possible
	Biotinylated histone peptides	Absorbance	Based on primary and peroxidase-labeled secondary antibody	Heterogeneous assay
PKMTs	Biotinylated oligopeptides	Time-resolved fluorescence	EuLISA; based on primary and Eu-labeled secondary antibody;	Heterogeneous assay, very low assay volume possible
LSD1	Core histones or oligopeptides	Absorbance	Peroxidase-coupled assay	Coupled enzymatic assay
		Absorbance of NADH	Formaldehyde dehydrogenase-coupled assay	Coupled enzymatic assay
JmjC	Core histones	Absorbance of NADH	Formaldehyde dehydrogenase-coupled assay	Coupled enzymatic assay
	Core histones	Absorbance	Chemical formaldehyde detection	Sensitivity ?

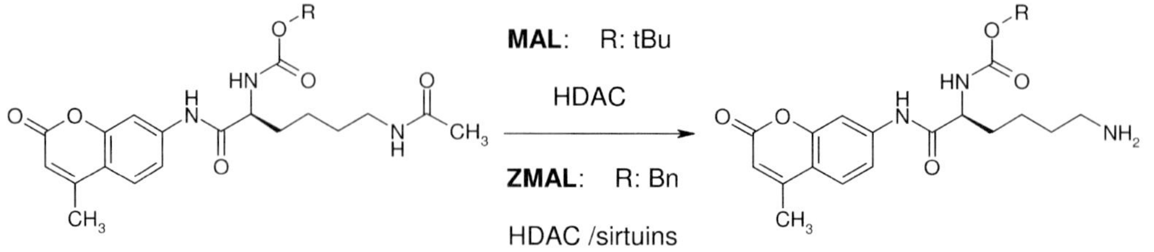

Figure 5.1 Structure of small molecule histone deacetylase substrates.

exposure of laboratory personnel to radioactivity, decontamination of screening equipment and disposal of radioactive waste. Therefore, attempts have been made to develop methods that use inexpensive substrates that are easy to obtain and allow nonradioactive *in vitro* determination of histone deacetylase activity.

5.4.2
Fluorescent Assays

In the search for nonisotopic HDAC substrates, different fluorescence-labeled substrates have been developed, allowing for a convenient nonradioactive assay. The first described fluorescence-based HDAC activity assay [21] uses the lysine-derived deacetylase substrate Boc(Ac)Lys-AMC, also called MAL (Figure 5.1). The incubation with a histone deacetylase preparation shows time-dependent conversion into its metabolite ML.

As this deacetylated metabolite shows the same fluorescence properties as the parent substrate, the conversion had to be monitored in the original assay by a protocol that includes an extraction step before using a reversed phase HPLC and fluorescence detection, which prohibited a high throughput. The precision of this method, concerning the extraction procedure, can be increased with the use of an internal standard [22], and a new protocol for the extraction procedure even allows for a plate reader measurement [23, 24]. The HPLC protocols may still be of value if selected highly fluorescent inhibitor candidates can be verified after initial plate reader screening with an independent method. Finally, a truly homogeneous assay version based on a derivatization reaction of MAL was realized [25]. In this so-called HDASH method, the fluorescence of the generated metabolite ML is quenched by the addition of the amine detection reagent naphthalene dicarboxaldehyde (NDA), whereas the amount of the remaining substrate MAL can be detected without any further separation steps (Figure 5.2).

Alternatively, MAL can also be determined using an assay procedure that makes use of a second incubation step with a detection reagent containing the endopeptidase trypsin [26]. This enzyme is able to recognize MAL as a substrate only if deacetylation by a deacetylase preparation has taken place. Upon cleavage by trypsin, the aminocoumarin is released and can be detected without extraction steps due to its fluorescent properties ($\lambda_{Ex} = 390$ nm, $\lambda_{Em} = 460$ nm) that differ from those of MAL. This homogenous assay protocol was originally used with tripeptide substrates that contained a C-terminal acetyl-lysine-coumarinylamide [27] and there also are

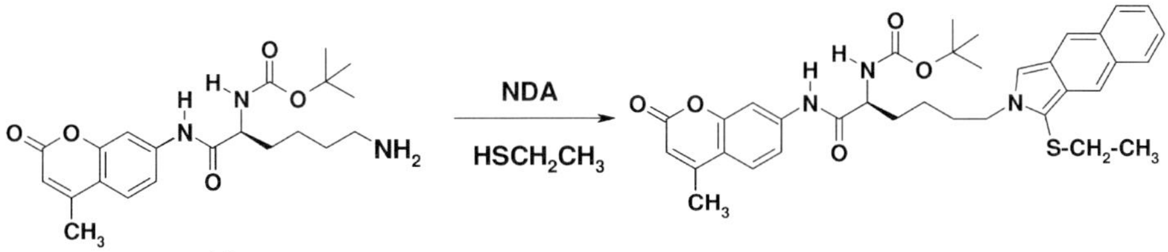

Figure 5.2 Quenching of HDAC metabolite ML by chemical derivatization.

commercial assay kits that work similarly and in part use larger peptide substrates. Z(Ac)Lys-AMC, also termed ZMAL (Figure 5.1) [28], is an optimized analog of MAL, whose conversion into its metabolite ZML by histone deacetylases takes place faster and to a greater extent. Fluorescence-labeled oligopeptides have also been used, for example in HPLC assays for HDACs [29] or in automated microfluidic assays for histone deacetylases and acetyltransferases [30].

Interestingly, ZMAL, in contrast to MAL, also is a good substrate for HDACs of class III (sirtuins). The NDA detection protocol does not work with sirtuins, but as ZML is a very good substrate for trypsin, a convenient homogenous sirtuin assay can be performed with the inexpensive ZMAL. While ZMAL is deacetylated equally well by HDAC1 as a histone deacetylase of class I and by HDAC6 as a class II deacetylase, MAL shows moderate subtype selectivity towards HDAC6. Similar substrates that show even greater selectivity towards certain subtypes of deacetylases (HDAC1, HDAC6, sirtuins) have also been described as helpful tools in order to elucidate the subtype selectivity of HDAC inhibitors [31]. For example it has been shown for HDAC8 that a trifluoroacetyl group instead of an acetyl moiety is important for good conversion [32]. A trifluoroacetyl lysine derivative without a fluorophore has been used for noninvasive HDAC activity detection in cells by ^{19}F nuclear magnetic resonance (NMR) [33]. As MAL is cell permeable it can be used to determine cellular HDAC activity not only from cell culture but also from patient material [34]. This can be used to monitor clinical studies with HDAC inhibitors.

There is also the possibility to detect the acetate released by HDACs during the deacetylase reaction [35, 36]. In this method, the acetate is converted to acetyl-CoA in the presence of acetyl-CoA synthetase, CoA and ATP. In a second step, this generated acetyl-CoA and oxaloacetate form citrate in a reaction catalyzed by citrate synthetase. The detection reaction in this assay is the generation of the required oxaloacetate from L-malate catalyzed by L-malate dehydrogenase, hereby reducing NAD^+ to $NADH^+$, whose absorption can be monitored at a wavelength of 340 nm. For HDAC8 a thioacetyl derivative is used that releases thioacetate which can be monitored by the thiol-sensitive Ellman's reagent and measurement of absorbance [37].

As the investigation of the interactions between HDAC inhibitors and the enzymes are an important issue, competition assay systems are helpful implements in facilitating the characterization of inhibitor binding. Such a competition binding assay that has been developed for histone deacetylases is based on fluorescence resonance energy transfer (FRET) between tryptophan residues of the histone deacetylase and a fluorescent HDAC inhibitor [38]. In competition with other

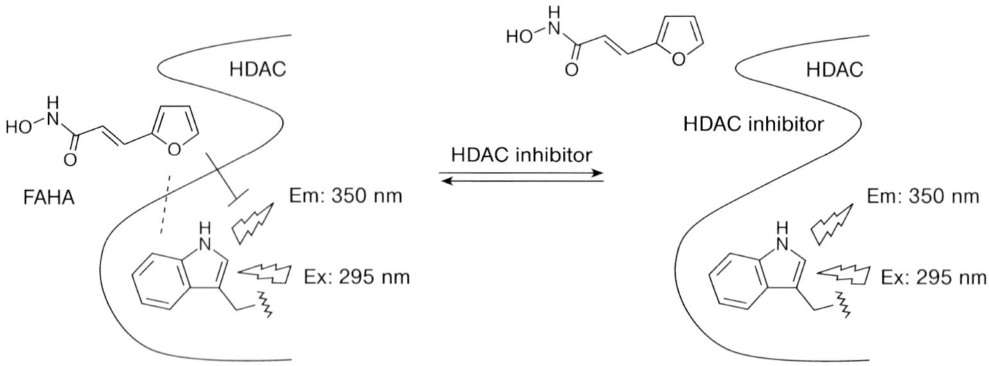

Figure 5.3 FRET competition assay for HDAC.

inhibitors, this fluorescent inhibitor FAHA (2-furylacryloylhydroxamate) is displaced, leading to a decrease in fluorescence resonance energy transfer (Figure 5.3). This decrease in FRET subsequently leads to a reduced quenching of fluorescence. This assay is applicable for screening with a high throughput, but is especially well suited for kinetic studies of inhibitor binding and displacement.

Another homogenous protocol that utilizes fluorescence resonance energy transfer [39] makes use of a peptide substrate based on p53, a known nonhistone substrate for sirtuins [40]. This peptide carries a single acetylated lysine residue, a fluorescent group near the C-terminal end and a nonfluorescent quenching group near the N-terminus. After deacetylation of the lysine residue by a preparation showing sirtuin activity, the peptide in a second step is cleaved by trypsin, resulting in a strongly increased fluorescence intensity of the fluorophor.

Intensity-based fluorescence assay systems are prone to false-negative or -positive results (depending on the assay design) by library components with intrinsic fluorescence or quenching properties. One way to avoid that is by the use of longer wavelength fluorophores, for example rhodamins in the case of sirtuins [41], instead of the coumarins that are used in most cases. Another approach to avoid these problems is an assay protocol that is based on fluorescence polarization (FP) [42]. FP makes use of linear polarized excitation light and measures the degree of polarization of the emitted light. The polarization increases with a decrease in molecular rotation, which correlates with the size of the fluorescent molecules [43]. So, FP assays are homogeneous systems which are less prone to quenching effects, which has made FP a widely applied technique. The assay protocol described to investigate sirtuin inhibition and activation [44] also utilizes a peptide substrate based on a segment of the sirtuin substrate p53. This peptide substrate is biotinylated on the N-terminal end and linked to a fluorescent tag on the C-terminal end. In this coupled enzyme assay, the first step is the deacetylation of the substrate and the second step is the cleavage by trypsin at the newly exposed lysine residue. Streptavidin is added in order to create a large difference in size between the uncleaved, still biotinylated and fluorescence-tagged substrate and the smaller cleavage product which still contains the fluorophore but not the biotin tag. Finally, fluorescence polarization is determined at 650 nm excitation wavelength and an emission wavelength of 680 nm. A high deacetylase turnover in this assay results in high polarization signals, because when the trypsin cleavage cannot take place, the whole streptavidin-bound fluorescent substrate is left, showing low molecular rotation. Another FP assay is based on the competition of inhibitors with a fluorescein-labeled derivative of the HDAC inhibitor suberoylanilide hydroxamic acid (SAHA, INN: Vorinostat) [45]

5.5 Histone Acetyltransferases

Histone acetyltransferases (HATs) catalyze the transfer of an acetyl moiety from acetyl-CoA to the ε-amino group of certain lysine residues within core histone proteins. This transferase reaction produces acetylated histones and the deacetylated cofactor CoA-SH. As HATs are important enzymes in the regulation of gene expression, there are also a number of assays available to detect acetyltransferases activity.

5.5.1 Radioactive Assays

Traditionally, HAT activity is measured with a discontinuous radioactive filter-binding assay, which uses $[^3H]$acetyl-*CoA* as a histone acetyltransferase substrate [46]. The transfer of $[^3H]$acetyl-groups to the histone substrate by histone acetyltransferases is detected by liquid scintillation counting of $[^3H]$acetylated histones, which are retained on a phosphocellulose disk. Due to its discontinuous character, this assay is technically problematic and not ideal for kinetic analysis. Hence, other assays that work with radiolabeled acetyl-CoA have been described that are suitable for a higher throughput. These work with streptavidin-covered beads [47] or a variant of the SPA with microtiter plates that contain a scintillant (FlashPlates) [48]. But as all these protocols are based on radioactively labeled substrates, they apparently show the same disadvantages that were described for the radioactive HDAC assay protocols. Therefore, nonradioactive assays have been developed to study histone acetyltransferase activity.

5.5.2 Assays Based on CoA-SH Detection

Several spectroscopic assays measure the amount of CoA-SH, which is generated by HATs during the acetyltransferase reaction [49, 50]. This determination of CoA-SH can be carried out by using a coupled enzyme system, utilizing the CoA-SH-dependent oxidation reaction of α-ketoglutarate dehydrogenase. This oxidation delivers succinyl-CoA, accompanied by the reduction of NAD^+ to NADH, which can be quantified photometrically at a wavelength of 340 nm (Figure 5.4).

Alternatively, pyruvate and pyruvate dehydrogenase can be used instead of α-ketoglutarate and its corresponding dehydrogenase. This oxidation reaction

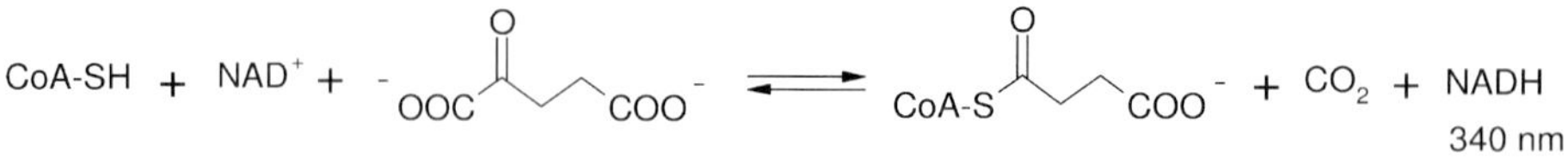

Figure 5.4 Oxidation reaction of α-ketoglutarate dehydrogenase.

provides acetyl-CoA, while NAD^+ still is reduced to NADH, which can be measured at 340 nm. As production of CoA-SH takes place at all histone acetyltransferase reactions, this methods are suitable for a wide variety of uses, independent of the nature of the substrate or the enzyme. But photometric determinations usually are not as sensitive as fluorescence-based assay systems and therefore larger amounts of substrate and enzyme are needed to perform the quantification.

Therefore, a way to determine the amounts of generated CoA-SH by fluorescence has been developed [50]. In this method the released CoA-SH is chemically transformed into a fluorescent product, as the maleinimide group of the coumarin-derived 7-diethylamino-3-(4′-maleimidylphenyl)-4-methylcoumarin (CPM) is able to react with the thiol group of CoA-SH in a Michael reaction (Figure 5.5). So the amount of transformed CPM can be determined as a function of generated CoA-SH ($\lambda_{Ex} = 390$ nm, $\lambda_{Em} = 469$ nm). This method is more sensitive than the photometric assays described above, but the very reactive maleinimide group of CPM can react with cysteine residues of other proteins and therefore causes high background emissions. Many proteins are stored in thiol-containing buffers, which makes the use of this method impossible. Another problem is that potential inhibitors of histone acetyltransferases that are able to react with thiol groups themselves, as shown for curcumin, cannot be tested in this kind of assay system.

5.5.3 Antibody-Based Assays

In order to avoid the described problems, antibody-based assays have been developed. As mentioned above, usually a primary antibody recognizes the modification, which in turn is then quantitated. One of these approaches is based on the technology of AlphaScreen (*A*mplified *L*uminescent *P*roximity *H*omogeneous *A*ssay) [51, 52], also known as *l*uminescent *o*xygen *c*hanneling *i*mmunoassay (LOCI) [53], a method that can be used to study protein–protein interactions in general. In this case the enzymatic transfer of acetyl groups to a histone peptide is determined.

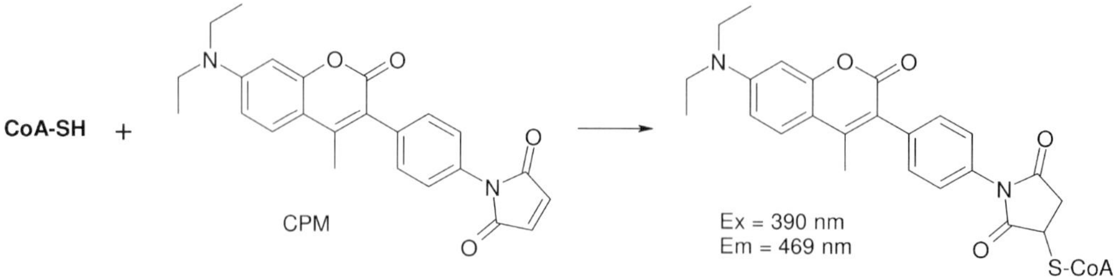

Figure 5.5 Detection of CoA-SH with CPM as fluorescent addition product.

The biotinylated histone peptide substrate is incubated with the HAT enzyme and acetyl-CoA. In a second vessel, the so-called donor beads and the acceptor beads are incubated together with an antibody that is directed against the acetylated histone lysine residue. The donor beads are streptavidin-coated and contain a photosensitizer, for example a phthalocyanine, that under certain conditions leads to the formation of singlet oxygen. The acceptor beads contain a thioxene derivative, which can react with singlet oxygen and the product spontaneously decays under chemoluminescence. These acceptor beads are coated additionally with protein A. As this protein is able to bind antibodies without affecting their binding capability, the antibody binds to the acceptor beads. After the two incubation batches are pooled, the biotinylated peptide substrate ligates to the donor beads because of their streptavidin coating and the antibodies that are linked to the acceptor beads are able to recognize the acetylated lysine residues. When exciting the preparation at 680 nm, singlet oxygen is generated. This singlet oxygen only has a limited lifetime of 4 μs which allow it to diffuse about 200 nm. Only when an acceptor bead is present within this distance does the thioxene react in a cycloaddition reaction with singlet oxygen and the resulting dioxetane decays under chemoluminescence, which can be monitored at a wavelength of 520–620 nm (Figure 5.6). This proximity is only possible when the antibody linked to the acceptor beads has recognized its substrate. We have set up such an assay for a homogeneous screening method for inhibitors of the histone acetyltransferase PCAF [54]. This assay is applicable to be used for other posttranslational modifications like histone lysine or arginine methylation simply by changing the antibody and possibly the histone peptide substrate.

Another antibody-based immunosorbent assay that can be used to determine HAT activity uses a secondary anti-IgG antibody, which is directed against the primary antibody and is labeled with the lanthanide Europium (Eu). After another washing step that removes all nonbound secondary antibody, one last incubation step is performed, which releases the lanthanide ion from the antibody, so that the final detection of time-resolved fluorescence (340/615 nm) caused by the released metal ion correlates with the acetylation level of the oligepeptide histone substrate, which is correlated with enzymatic activity. So far,

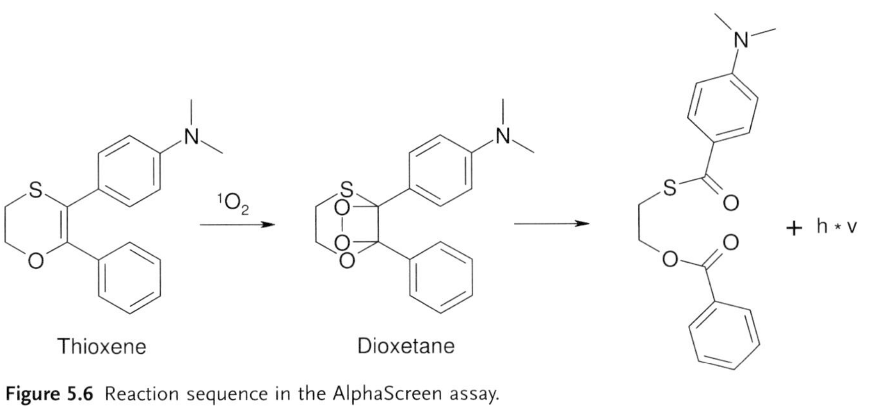

Figure 5.6 Reaction sequence in the AlphaScreen assay.

this assay has been used for the determination of cellular HAT activity [5] but it can also be used for *in vitro* assays.

5.6 Histone Methyltransferases

Histone methylation by methyltransferases is another widely described modification that also plays an important role in regulation of transcriptional activity. Methylation can occur either on arginine or on lysine residues in the N-termini of histones and therefore this group of enzymes can be separated into protein arginine methyltransferases (PRMTs) and lysine methyltransferases (KMTs).

5.6.1 Arginine Methyltransferases

Protein arginine methyltransferases (PRMTs) can be divided into two different groups. PRMTs of both groups are enzymes that catalyze the transfer of the methyl group from the cosubstrate S-adenosyl methionine (SAM) to the guanidine group of arginines in protein substrates [55]. Thus, monomethylated arginine residues and S-adenosyl homocysteine (SAH) are generated in all cases. The two groups of PRMTs, however, differ in the following reaction, which leads to dimethylated arginines. Type-I arginine methyltransferases catalyze the transfer of the second methyl group to the same nitrogen of the arginine guanidine, leading to an “asymmetric” dimethyl arginine, whereas the PRMTs of type II transfer the second methyl group to the other terminal nitrogen of the guanidine group forming a “symmetric” dimethylated arginine.

For methyltransferases mostly antibody-based assays have been used in order to determine the enzymatic activity. Again, the primary antibody is targeted towards the modification and serves as a starting point for the quantitation. One assay system uses a nonhistone protein substrate and a secondary antibody that is labeled with a peroxidase [56]. After all washing and incubation steps, a peroxidase substrate solution is added, in this case 2,2′-azino-bis(3-ethylbenzthiazoline-6-sulfonic acid) (ABTS). This compound is oxidized by the peroxidase to form stable radicals that can be detected photometrically at a wavelength of 415 nm. In a heterogeneous assay system again an Eu-labeled secondary antibody can be used both for *in vitro* assay and also for the detection of cellular hypomethylation [57]. As a homogeneous assay, the Alphascreen technology (see above) can be used for the arginine methyltransferase PRMT1 [54].

5.6.2 Lysine Methyltransferases

Lysine methyltransferases catalyze the transfer of methyl groups from the cosubstrate SAM to certain lysine residues in histone proteins. To characterize modulators of these transferases, the above-mentioned antibody-based assay protocols are also applicable.

Again, Eu-labeled secondary antibodies are used, for example in an *in vitro* assay for the PKMT G9a [58] or for cellular hypomethylation of the target of the lysine methyltransferase SET7/9 [59]. An alternative is a radioactive assay, in which the biotinylated synthetic peptide substrate is bound to the cavities of avidin-coated microplates. The methylation reaction is started by the addition of a methyltransferase preparation and the radioactively labeled cosubstrate S-adenosyl-[methyl-^{3}H] methionine ([^{3}H]AdoMet) [60]. During the methylation reaction, the radioactivity of the cosubstrate is transferred to the peptide substrate. After washing of the plates in order to remove the free [^{3}H]AdoMet, the bound radiolabeled peptide is released with the help of hydrochloric acid and finally radioactivity is quantified by scintillation counting. Although this protocol shows the disadvantage of using radioactivity, it is sensitive, inexpensive and allows for a high throughput and automation.

A coupled enyzmatic assay makes use of S-adenosylhomocysteine hydrolase (SAHH) which hydrolyzes the methyltransfer product SAH to homocysteine and adenosine. The homocysteine concentration can be determined by conjugation of its free sulfhydryl moiety to a thiol-sensitive fluorophore [61]. This could of course also be used for arginine methyltransferases.

5.7 Histone Demethylases

Until recently, histone methylation by methyltransferases had been thought to be an irreversible epigenetic modification, but now we know that histone demethylation takes place on both lysine and arginine residues, and therefore we can distinguish between histone lysine demethylases and histone arginine demethylases. Increasing efforts are pursued to further characterize both groups of enzymes and therefore *in vitro* assay systems play an important role in elucidating the specific functions of these chromatin-modifying enzymes in gene regulation.

5.7.1 Lysine Demethylases

In the case of lysine methylation, two different families of histone lysine demethylases with different mechanisms of action have been described. This has implication also for the assay design.

There are demethylases which act like amine oxidases that are dependent in their mechanism on their cosubstrate flavine adenine dinucleotide (FAD). So far, lysine-specific demethylase 1 (LSD1) is the only representative of this class [62]. LSD1, as an amine oxidase leads to oxidation of the methylated lysine residue, generating an imine intermediate, while the protein-bound cosubstrate FAD is reduced to $FADH_2$. In a second step, the imine intermediate is hydrolyzed to produce the demethylated histone lysine residue and formaldehyde. Importantly, the reduced cosubstrate is regenerated to its oxidized form by molecular oxygen, producing hydrogen peroxide (Figure 5.7) [62, 63].

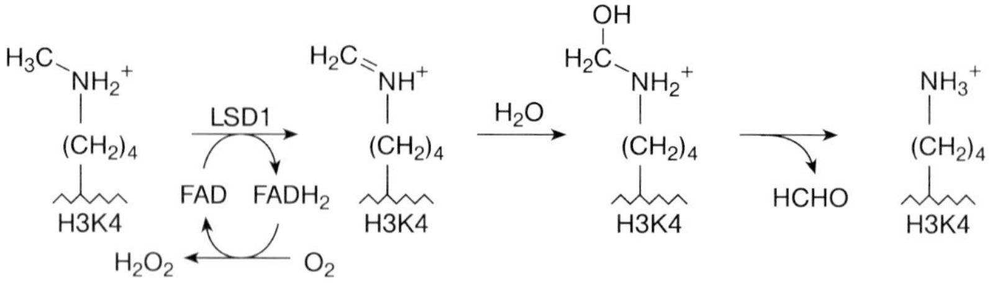

Figure 5.7 Lysine demethylation by the amino oxidase LSD1.

As equimolar amounts of formaldehyde and hydrogen peroxide are produced throughout the demethylase reaction, detection of these small molecules can be used to determine LSD1 activity. The amounts of released hydrogen peroxide can be detected in a peroxidase-coupled approach [64]. The detection makes use of the two substrates 4-aminoantipyrine and 3,5-dichloro-2-hydroxybenzenesulfonic acid. These substrates are oxidized in the presence of a peroxidase and hydrogen peroxide to generate a deeply red-colored product, whose production can be spectroscopically monitored at a wavelength of 515 nm. Alternatively, chemoluminescence generated by luminol and horseradish peroxidase in presence of hydrogen peroxide can be detected [65, 66]. In order to quantify the released formaldehyde, a formaldehyde dehydrogenase can be used. This dehydrogenase generates formic acid by oxidation of formaldehyde and thereby NAD^+ is reduced to NADH, whose absorbance can be measured at 340 nm [67].

The other class of histone lysine demethylases is a growing group of enzymes with a jumanjiC domain as catalytic core. These jumanjiC domain-containing (JmjC) enzymes are members of the cupin superfamily of α-ketoglutarate-dependent Fe(II) oxygenases. JmjC enzymes demethylate methylated lysines through hydroxylation of the methyl groups, forming an unstable hemi-aminal intermediate besides the α-ketoglutarate-derived products succinate and carbon dioxide. The hemi-aminal intermediate spontaneously decomposes to the demethylated lysine residue and formaldehyde (Figure 5.8) [68].

This release of formaldehyde can also be quantified by using formaldehyde dehydrogenase, as described above. An alternative way to determine demethylase activity by measuring the amounts of released formaldehyde is the use of the Nash reaction [68, 69]. This method is based on the formation of the colored 3,5-diacetyl-1,4-dihydropyridine by condensation of formaldehyde and acetylacetone in the

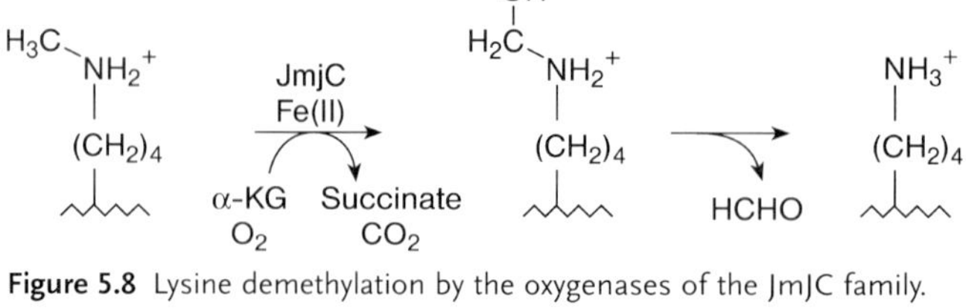

Figure 5.8 Lysine demethylation by the oxygenases of the JmjC family.

presence of ammonium. The generation of this heterocycle is monitored and quantified at a wavelength of 415 nm.

5.7.2 Arginine Demethylases

For a long time, removal of arginine methylation was thought to be possible only by arginine deimination. This means the conversion of arginine residues into citrulline residues [70]. But recently, a member of the above-mentioned jmjC oxygenases was shown to remove methyl groups from arginines, leaving unmethylated arginines [71]. There are no specific assay systems to identify modulators of histone arginine demethylases so far, but the mentioned antibody-based methods that are not specific for a certain target can of course also be used to determine arginine demethylase activity.

5.8 Conclusion

For the major epigenetic targets convenient homogeneous assays are now available. Whereas for acetylation and deacetylation simple procedures based on fluorescence are available for protein methylation, mostly antibody based assays are used. These assays are important tools in the characterization of new inhibitors that are interesting as tools for the investigation of cellular functions of epigenetic targets and also as potential drugs. Such assays also allow for the determination of enzymatic activity in immunoprecipitation experiments in order to study protein–protein interactions and are helpful in the characterization and purification of candidate proteins that are thought to be epigenetic modifiers. Thus, such *in vitro* assays will be important tools to further drive epigenetic research, especially in the field of drug discovery.

References

1. Wilson, K.J., Witter, D.J., Grimm, J.B., Siliphaivanh, P., Otte, K.M., Kral, A.M., Fleming, J.C., Harsch, A., Hamill, J.E., Cruz, J.C., Chenard, M., Szewczak, A.A., Middleton, R.E., Hughes, B.L., Dahlberg, W.K., Secrist, J.P. and Miller, T.A. (2008) Phenylglycine and phenylalanine derivatives as potent and selective HDAC1 inhibitors (SHI-1). *Bioorganic & Medicinal Chemistry Letters*, **18**, 1859–1863.
2. Cheng, D., Yadav, N., King, R.W., Swanson, M.S., Weinstein, E.J. and Bedford, M.T. (2004) Small molecule regulators of protein arginine methyltransferases. *The Journal of Biological Chemistry*, **279**, 23892–23899.
3. Stimson, L., Rowlands, M.G., Newbatt, Y.M., Smith, N.F., Raynaud, F.I., Rogers, P., Bavetsias, V., Gorsuch, S., Jarman, M., Bannister, A., Kouzarides, T., McDonald, E., Workman, P. and Aherne, G.W. (2005) Isothiazolones as inhibitors of PCAF and p300 histone acetyltransferase activity.

Molecular Cancer Therapeutics, **4**, 1521–1532.

4 Stockwell, B.R., Haggarty, S.J. and Schreiber, S.L. (1999) High-throughput screening of small molecules in miniaturized mammalian cell-based assays involving post-translational modifications. *Chemistry & Biology*, **6**, 71–83.

5 Wynne Aherne, G., Rowlands, M.G., Stimson, L. and Workman, P. (2002) Assays for the identification and evaluation of histone acetyltransferase inhibitors. *Methods (San Diego, Calif)*, **26**, 245–253.

6 Spannhoff, A., Heinke, R., Bauer, I., Trojer, P., Metzger, E., Gust, R., Schüle, R., Brosch, G., Sippl, W. and Jung, M. (2007) Target-based approach to inhibitors of histone arginine methyltransferases. *Journal of Medicinal Chemistry*, **50**, 2319–2325.

7 Haggarty, S.J., Koeller, K.M., Wong, J.C., Grozinger, C.M. and Schreiber, S.L. (2003) Domain-selective small-molecule inhibitor of histone deacetylase 6 (HDAC6)-mediated tubulin deacetylation. *Proceedings of the National Academy of Sciences of the United States of America*, **100**, 4389–4394.

8 Remiszewski, S.W. (2003) The discovery of NVP-LAQ824: from concept to clinic. *Current Medicinal Chemistry*, **10**, 2393–2402.

9 Su, G.H., Sohn, T.A., Ryu, B. and Kern, S.E. (2000) A novel histone deacetylase inhibitor identified by high-throughput transcriptional screening of a compound library. *Cancer Research*, **60**, 3137–3142.

10 Glaser, K.B., Li, J., Aakre, M.E., Morgan, D.W., Sheppard, G., Stewart, K.D., Pollock, J., Lee, P., O'Connor, C.Z., Anderson, S.N., Mussatto, D.J., Wegner, C.W. and Moses, H.L. (2002) Transforming growth factor beta mimetics: discovery of 7-[4-(4-cyanophenyl)phenoxy]-heptanohydroxamic acid, a biaryl hydroxamate inhibitor of histone deacetylase. *Molecular Cancer Therapeutics*, **1**, 759–768.

11 Lain, S., Hollick, J.J., Campbell, J., Staples, O.D., Higgins, M., Aoubala, M., McCarthy, A., Appleyard, V., Murray, K.E., Baker, L., Thompson, A., Mathers, J., Holland, S.J., Stark, M.J., Pass, G., Woods, J., Lane, D.P. and Westwood, N.J. (2008) Discovery, in vivo activity, and mechanism of action of a small-molecule p53 activator. *Cancer Cell*, **13**, 454–463.

12 Kim, Y.B., Lee, K.H., Sugita, K., Yoshida, M. and Horinouchi, S. (1999) Oxamflatin is a novel antitumor compound that inhibits mammalian histone deacetylase. *Oncogene*, **18**, 2461–2470.

13 Bedalov, A., Gatbonton, T., Irvine, W.P., Gottschling, D.E. and Simon, J.A. (2001) Identification of a small molecule inhibitor of Sir2p. *Proceedings of the National Academy of Sciences of the United States of America*, **98**, 15113–15118.

14 Forsgren, A. and Sjoquist, J. (1966) "Protein A" from S. aureus. I. Pseudo-immune reaction with human gamma-globulin. *Journal of Immunology (Baltimore, Md: 1950)*, **97**, 822–827.

15 Yang, X.J. and Seto, E. (2008) The Rpd3/Hda1 family of lysine deacetylases: from bacteria and yeast to mice and men. *Nature Reviews. Molecular Cell Biology*, **9**, 206–218.

16 Smith, J.S., Avalos, J., Celic, I., Muhammad, S., Wolberger, C. and Boeke, J.D. (2002) SIR2 family of NAD(+)-dependent protein deacetylases. *Methods in Enzymology*, **353**, 282–300.

17 Kolle, D., Brosch, G., Lechner, T., Lusser, A. and Loidl, P. (1998) Biochemical methods for analysis of histone deacetylases. *Methods (San Diego, Calif)*, **15**, 323–331.

18 Darkin-Rattray, S.J., Gurnett, A.M., Myers, R.W., Dulski, P.M., Crumley, T.M., Allocco, J.J., Cannova, C., Meinke, P.T., Colletti, S.L., Bednarek, M.A., Singh, S.B., Goetz, M.A., Dombrowski, A.W., Polishook, J.D. and Schmatz, D.M. (1996) Apicidin: a novel antiprotozoal agent that inhibits parasite histone deacetylase. *Proceedings of the National Academy of Sciences of the United States of America*, **93**, 13143–13147.

19 Taunton, J., Hassig, C.A. and Schreiber, S.L. (1996) A mammalian histone deacetylase related to the yeast transcriptional regulator Rpd3p. *Science*, **272**, 408–411.

20 Nare, B., Allocco, J.J., Kuningas, R., Galuska, S., Myers, R.W., Bednarek, M.A. and Schmatz, D.M. (1999) Development of a scintillation proximity assay for histone deacetylase using a biotinylated peptide derived from histone-H4. *Analytical Biochemistry*, **267**, 390–396.

21 Hoffmann, K., Brosch, G., Loidl, P. and Jung, M. (1999) A non-isotopic assay for histone deacetylase activity. *Nucleic Acids Research*, **27**, 2057–2058.

22 Hoffmann, K., Heltweg, B. and Jung, M. (2001) Improvement and validation of the fluorescence-based histone deacetylase assay using an internal standard. *Archiv der Pharmazie*, **334**, 248–252.

23 Heltweg, B. and Jung, M. (2002) A microplate reader-based nonisotopic histone deacetylase activity assay. *Analytical Biochemistry*, **302**, 175–183.

24 Heltweg, B. and Jung, M. (2002) Eosin Y as an internal standard for a plate reader based quantitation of a histone deacetylase substrate. *Archiv der Pharmazie and Pharmaceutical and Medicinal Chemistry*, **335**, 296–300.

25 Heltweg, B. and Jung, M. (2003) A homogeneous nonisotopic histone deacetylase activity assay. *Journal of Biomolecular Screening*, **8**, 89–95.

26 Heltweg, B., Trapp, J. and Jung, M. (2005) In vitro assays for the determination of histone deacetylase activity. *Methods (San Diego, Calif)*, **36**, 332–337.

27 Wegener, D., Wirsching, F., Riester, D. and Schwienhorst, A. (2003) A fluorogenic histone deacetylase assay well suited for high-throughput activity screening. *Chemistry & Biology*, **10**, 61–68.

28 Heltweg, B., Dequiedt, F., Verdin, E. and Jung, M. (2003) Nonisotopic substrate for assaying both human zinc and NAD+-dependent histone deacetylases. *Analytical Biochemistry*, **319**, 42–48.

29 Hoffmann, K., Söll, R.M., Beck-Sickinger, A.G. and Jung, M. (2001) Fluorescence-labeled octapeptides as substrates for histone deacetylase. *Bioconjugate Chemistry*, **12**, 51–55.

30 Blackwell, L., Norris, J., Suto, C.M. and Janzen, W.P. (2008) The use of diversity profiling to characterize chemical modulators of the histone deacetylases. *Life Sciences*, **82**, 1050–1058.

31 Heltweg, B., Dequiedt, F., Marshall, B.L., Brauch, C., Yoshida, M., Nishino, N., Verdin, E. and Jung, M. (2004) Subtype selective substrates for histone deacetylases. *Journal of Medicinal Chemistry*, **47**, 5235–5243.

32 Riester, D., Wegener, D., Hildmann, C. and Schwienhorst, A. (2004) Members of the histone deacetylase superfamily differ in substrate specificity towards small synthetic substrates. *Biochemical and Biophysical Research Communications*, **324**, 1116–1123.

33 Sankaranarayanapillai, M., Tong, W.P., Maxwell, D.S., Pal, A., Pang, J., Bornmann, W.G., Gelovani, J.G. and Ronen, S.M. (2006) Detection of histone deacetylase inhibition by noninvasive magnetic resonance spectroscopy. *Molecular Cancer Therapeutics*, **5**, 1325–1334.

34 Bonfils, C., Kalita, A., Dubay, M., Siu, L.L., Carducci, M.A., Reid, G., Martell, R.E., Besterman, J.M. and Li, Z. (2008) Evaluation of the pharmacodynamic effects of MGCD0103 from preclinical models to human using a novel HDAC enzyme assay. *Clinical Cancer Research*, **14**, 3441–3449.

35 Hildmann, C., Ninkovic, M., Dietrich, R., Wegener, D., Riester, D., Zimmermann, T., Birch, O.M., Bernegger, C., Loidl, P. and Schwienhorst, A. (2004) A new amidohydrolase from Bordetella or Alcaligenes strain FB188 with similarities to histone deacetylases. *Journal of Bacteriology*, **186**, 2328–2339.

36 Baumann, M., Sturmer, R. and Bornscheuer, U.T. (2001) A high-throughput-screening method for the identification of active and enantioselective hydrolases. *Angewandte Chemie-International Edition*, **40**, 4201–4204.

37 Fatkins, D.G. and Zheng, W. (2008) A spectrophotometric assay for histone deacetylase 8. *Analytical Biochemistry*, **372**, 82–88.

38 Riester, D., Hildmann, C., Schwienhorst, A. and Meyer-Almes, F.J. (2007) Histone deacetylase inhibitor assay based on fluorescence resonance energy transfer. *Analytical Biochemistry*, **362**, 136–141.

39 Marcotte, P.A., Richardson, P.L., Guo, J., Barrett, L.W., Xu, N., Gunasekera, A. and Glaser, K.B. (2004) Fluorescence assay of SIRT protein deacetylases using an acetylated peptide substrate and a secondary trypsin reaction. *Analytical Biochemistry*, **332**, 90–99.

40 Vaziri, H., Dessain, S.K., Ng Eaton, E., Imai, S.I., Frye, R.A., Pandita, T.K., Guarente, L. and Weinberg, R.A. (2001) hSIR2(SIRT1) functions as an NAD-dependent p53 deacetylase. *Cell*, **107**, 149–159.

41 Borra, M.T., Smith, B.C. and Denu, J.M. (2005) Mechanism of human SIRT1 activation by resveratrol. *The Journal of Biological Chemistry*, **280**, 17187–17195.

42 Burke, T.J., Loniello, K.R., Beebe, J.A. and Ervin, K.M. (2003) Development and application of fluorescence polarization assays in drug discovery. *Combinatorial Chemistry & High Throughput Screening*, **6**, 183–194.

43 Jameson, D.M. and Croney, J.C. (2003) Fluorescence polarization: past, present and future. *Combinatorial Chemistry & High Throughput Screening*, **6**, 167–173.

44 Milne, J.C., Lambert, P.D., Schenk, S., Carney, D.P., Smith, J.J., Gagne, D.J., Jin, L., Boss, O., Perni, R.B., Vu, C.B., Bemis, J.E., Xie, R., Disch, J.S., Ng, P.Y., Nunes, J.J., Lynch, A.V., Yang, H., Galonek, H., Israelian, K., Choy, W., Iffland, A., Lavu, S., Medvedik, O., Sinclair, D.A., Olefsky, J.M., Jirousek, M.R., Elliott, P.J. and Westphal, C.H. (2007) Small molecule activators of SIRT1 as therapeutics for the treatment of type 2 diabetes. *Nature*, **450**, 712–716.

45 Mazitschek, R., Patel, V., Wirth, D.F. and Clardy, J. (2008) Development of a fluorescence polarization based assay for histone deacetylase ligand discovery. *Bioorganic & Medicinal Chemistry Letters*, **18**, 2809–2812.

46 Tanner, K.G., Trievel, R.C., Kuo, M.H., Howard, R.M., Berger, S.L., Allis, C.D., Marmorstein, R. and Denu, J.M. (1999) Catalytic mechanism and function of invariant glutamic acid 173 from the histone acetyltransferase GCN5 transcriptional coactivator. *The Journal of Biological Chemistry*, **274**, 18157–18160.

47 Ait-Si-Ali, S., Ramirez, S., Robin, P., Trouche, D. and Harel Bellan, A. (1998) A rapid and sensitive assay for histone acetyl-transferase activity. *Nucleic Acids Research*, **26**, 3869–3870.

48 Turlais, F., Hardcastle, A., Rowlands, M., Newbatt, Y., Bannister, A., Kouzarides, T., Workman, P. and Aherne, G.W. (2001) High-throughput screening for identification of small molecule inhibitors of histone acetyltransferases using scintillating microplates (FlashPlate). *Analytical Biochemistry*, **298**, 62–68.

49 Kim, Y., Tanner, K.G. and Denu, J.M. (2000) A continuous, nonradioactive assay for histone acetyltransferases. *Analytical Biochemistry*, **280**, 308–314.

50 Trievel, R.C., Li, F.Y. and Marmorstein, R. (2000) Application of a fluorescent histone acetyltransferase assay to probe the substrate specificity of the human p300/CBP-associated factor. *Analytical Biochemistry*, **287**, 319–328.

51 Rouleau, N., Turcotte, S., Mondou, M.H., Roby, P. and Bosse, R. (2003) Development of a versatile platform for nuclear receptor screening using AlphaScreen. *Journal of Biomolecular Screening*, **8**, 191–197.

52 Warner, G., Illy, C., Pedro, L., Roby, P. and Bosse, R. (2004) AlphaScreen kinase HTS platforms. *Current Medicinal Chemistry*, **11**, 721–730.

53 Ullman, E.F., Kirakossian, H., Singh, S., Wu, Z.P., Irvin, B.R., Pease, J.S., Switchenko, A.C., Irvine, J.D., Dafforn, A., Skold, C.N. *et al.* (1994) Luminescent oxygen channeling immunoassay: measurement of particle binding kinetics by chemiluminescence. *Proceedings of the National Academy of Sciences of the United States of America*, **91**, 5426–5430.

54 Spannhoff, A., Valkov, V., Trojer, P., Bauer, I., Brosch, G. and Jung, M. (2009) In-vitro screening assays for histone acetyl- and methyltransferases using Alphascreen. (in preparation).

55 Gary, J.D. and Clarke, S. (1998) RNA and protein interactions modulated by protein arginine methylation. *Progress in Nucleic Acid Research and Molecular Biology*, **61**, 65–131.

56 Cheng, D., Yadav, N., King, R.W., Swanson, M.S., Weinstein, E.J. and Bedford, M.T. (2004) Small molecule regulators of protein arginine methyltransferases. *The Journal of Biological Chemistry*, **279**, 23892–23899.

57 Spannhoff, A., Heinke, R., Bauer, I., Trojer, P., Metzger, E., Gust, R., Schule, R., Brosch, G., Sippl, W. and Jung, M. (2007) Target-based approach to inhibitors of histone arginine methyltransferases. *Journal of Medicinal Chemistry*, **50**, 2319–2325.

58 Kubicek, S., O'Sullivan, R.J., August, E.M., Hickey, E.R., Zhang, Q., Teodoro, M.L., Rea, S., Mechtler, K., Kowalski, J.A., Homon, C.A., Kelly, T.A. and Jenuwein, T. (2007) Reversal of H3K9me2 by a small-molecule inhibitor for the G9a histone methyltransferase. *Molecular Cell*, **25**, 473–481.

59 Spannhoff, A., Machmur, R., Heinke, R., Trojer, P., Bauer, I., Brosch, G., Schule, R., Hanefeld, W., Sippl, W. and Jung, M. (2007) A novel arginine methyltransferase inhibitor with cellular activity. *Bioorganic & Medicinal Chemistry Letters*, **17**, 4150–4153.

60 Gowher, H., Zhang, X., Cheng, X. and Jeltsch, A. (2005) Avidin plate assay system for enzymatic characterization of a histone lysine methyltransferase. *Analytical Biochemistry*, **342**, 287–291.

61 Collazo, E., Couture, J.F., Bulfer, S. and Trievel, R.C. (2005) A coupled fluorescent assay for histone methyltransferases. *Analytical Biochemistry*, **342**, 86–92.

62 Shi, Y., Lan, F., Matson, C., Mulligan, P., Whetstine, J.R., Cole, P.A. and Casero, R.A. (2004) Histone demethylation mediated by the nuclear amine oxidase homolog LSD1. *Cell*, **119**, 941–953.

63 Shi, Y.J., Matson, C., Lan, F., Iwase, S., Baba, T. and Shi, Y. (2005) Regulation of LSD1 histone demethylase activity by its associated factors. *Molecular Cell*, **19**, 857–864.

64 Forneris, F., Binda, C., Vanoni, M.A., Mattevi, A. and Battaglioli, E. (2005) Histone demethylation catalysed by LSD1 is a flavin-dependent oxidative process. *FEBS Letters*, **579**, 2203–2207.

65 Wang, Y., Murray-Stewart, T., Devereux, W., Hacker, A., Frydman, B., Woster, P.M. and Casero, R.A. Jr. (2003) Properties of purified recombinant human polyamine oxidase, PAOh1/SMO. *Biochemical and Biophysical Research Communications*, **304**, 605–611.

66 Huang, Y., Greene, E., Stewart, T.M., Goodwin, A.C., Baylin, S.B., Woster, P.M. and Casero, R.A. Jr. (2007) Inhibition of lysine-specific demethylase 1 by polyamine analogues results in reexpression of aberrantly silenced genes. *Proceedings of the National Academy of Sciences of the United States of America*, **104**, 8023–8028.

67 Lizcano, J.M., Unzeta, M. and Tipton, K.F. (2000) A spectrophotometric method for determining the oxidative deamination of methylamine by the amine oxidases. *Analytical Biochemistry*, **286**, 75–79.

68 Tsukada, Y., Fang, J., Erdjument-Bromage, H., Warren, M.E., Borchers, C.H., Tempst, P. and Zhang, Y. (2006) Histone demethylation by a family of JmjC domain-containing proteins. *Nature*, **439**, 811–816.

69 Nash, T. (1953) The colorimetric estimation of formaldehyde by means of

the Hantzsch reaction. *The Biochemical Journal*, **55**, 416–421.

70 Cuthbert, G.L., Daujat, S., Snowden, A.W., Erdjument-Bromage, H., Hagiwara, T., Yamada, M., Schneider, R., Gregory, P.D., Tempst, P., Bannister, A.J. and Kouzarides, T. (2004) Histone deimination antagonizes arginine methylation. *Cell*, **118**, 545–553.

71 Chang, B., Chen, Y., Zhao, Y. and Bruick, R.K. (2007) JMJD6 is a histone arginine demethylase. *Science*, **318**, 444–447.

6
Epigenetic Targets in Drug Discovery: Cell-Based Assays for HDAC Inhibitor Hit Validation

Mira Jung, Kwon-Jeong Yong, Alfredo Velena, and Sung Lee

6.1
Introduction

Inhibitors of histone deacetylases (HDACs) are emerging as novel potential therapeutic agents for patients with cancers and/or neurological diseases. A number of HDAC inhibitors (HDACIs) have already entered clinical trials; and recently the hydroxamic acid derivative Vorinostat, suberoylanilide hydroxamic acid (SAHA), received FDA approval for the treatment of patients with cutaneous T-cell lymphoma. Furthermore, improved understanding of the roles of various HDAC isoforms in cell processes and in diseases contribute to the strategies for developing second generation inhibitors offering enhanced target specificity and improved toxicity profiles. Reports presenting new classes of HDAC inhibitors with isoform specificity have been developed utilizing *in vitro* enzymatic screening assays. However, *in vitro* enzyme activities have limitations and full assessment of isoform specificities of HDACIs requires the application of assays based on functions of multiprotein complexes that may include HDACs and/or other cofactors. In this setting, cell-based assays are needed to permit selective profiling and screening of HDACIs for relative HDAC isoform inhibitory activities for rational drug discovery. The approaches that have been used to assess molecular and biological actions of HDACIs in cells and tissues are reviewed in this chapter.

Histone deacetylases are metalloenzymes that catalyze the deacetylation of the ε-lysine of acetylated substrates, including histones and nonhistone proteins. Eighteen human HDACs have been identified to date and these are divided into four classes, based on structure, sequence homology, and domain organization. Class I consists of HDACs 1, 2, 3 and 8. These HDACs are homologous to yeast RPD3 [1, 2]. Class I HDACs are expressed primarily in the nucleus and play a role in cell proliferation [3, 4]. Class II HDACs include isoforms 4, 5, 6, 7, 9 and 10 and are further subdivided into IIa (HDACs 4, 5, 7, 9) and IIb (HDACs 6, 10) [5]. These enzymes are characterized by a large NH_2-terminal domain or a second catalytic site and play roles in cellular differentiation and development [6]. Class III HDACs were originally

Epigenetic Targets in Drug Discovery. Edited by Wolfgang Sippl and Manfred Jung

ISBN: 978-3-527-32355-5

found in yeast, include the SIRTs (sirtuins) or Sir2-related proteins and are NAD-dependent [3, 7]. Class III HDACs are not affected by TSA or by other hydroxamate inhibitors. Class IV comprises of HDAC 11, based on a phylogenetic analysis and is the least characterized to date [8].

Inhibitors of HDACs have been discovered and developed as promising anticancer drugs based on their actions in cell growth arrest, anti-angiogenesis, apoptosis and cellular differentiation [3, 9]. Various approaches have been used for screening candidate ligands, including *in vitro* enzyme assays and cell-based assays. However, accumulated recent reports reveal large variations in data obtained using different assays relying on various preparations of HDAC proteins and artificial substrates which do not reflect the cellular situation. Such variations make data interpretation difficult, underscoring the need for suitable assay systems that permit the identification of promising drug candidates with specificity and clinical relevance.

6.2 *In Vitro* Assays for HDAC Inhibitors

Primary screenings of candidate HDACIs are generally performed using *in vitro* assays consisting of sources of HDACs (i.e. cell extracts or rat liver) and substrates (i.e. radiolabeled acetylated histones or synthetic peptides with a fluorophor). Isoform selective studies are performed using purified recombinant, immunoprecipitated proteins using antibodies against selected HDACs and computer-based virtual prediction assays.

6.2.1 *In Vitro* Enzymatic Assay and Substrate Specificity

Commonly, *in vitro* determination of HDAC activity is a manual assay utilizing a coupled two-step process, including enzymatic deacetylation of a substrate followed by reaction termination and readout [10]. Assays utilize nuclear extracts and substrates containing labeled (radioactive or fluorescent) acetylated histones. For the isotope-based assays, the enzymes are incubated with acetate-radiolabled histones prepared from chicken reticulocytes or chemically [^{3}H]acetylated peptide substrates, and the enzymatic activity is determined by liquid scintillation counting [11]. Alternatively, histones may be obtained from cells following treatment with [^{3}H]acetyl-CoA [12]. The caveats of these approaches include the variability of prelabeled acetylated core histones within preparations, potential high costs, their labor-intensive nature and the presence of radioactive waste.

Non-isotopic assays have been developed using synthetic acetylated forms of fluorescein-labeled substrates. A number of artificial substrates containing acetylated lysines based on some proteins, such as histones, p53 and p300/CBP, are available for HDAC enzyme activities [11–14]. These include the generic peptides (Fluor-de-Lys), Ac-GA-(NH-Ac-K)-amino-4-methylcoumarin (AMC), Boc-K(Ac)-7-AMC, Ac-NH-GGK(Ac)-AMC [12] and Ac-NH-RHK(Ac)K(Ac)-AMC [14]. The generic peptide

(Fluor-de-Lys) trade marked by BioMol is used for pan-HDACs, while Ac-GA-(NH-Ac-K)-AMC, Ac-NH-GGK(Ac)-AMC and Ac-NH-RHK(Ac)K(Ac)-AMC have been advanced for HDAC1, 3, 6 and 8 specificity [13, 14]. Limitations of this approach include detection of fluorescence, less favorable substrates due to steric hindrance caused by the bulky fluorescein group, low solubility and low reactivity.

6.2.2 *In Vitro* High-Throughput Assays

The recent development of automation and high-throughput methods for measuring enzyme activities has been implemented to overcome the limitations of manual assays for drug screening. Hassig *et al.* [15] reported the use of a miniaturized high-throughput robot (i.e. the proprietary Kalypsys uHTS screening robot) for screening a 600 000 small molecule compound library using HeLa nuclear extract with a fluorescent acetyl-lysine substrate (BioMol). Another approach incorporates robotic screening that measures target inhibition in a cellular context for compound profiling as proposed by Ciossek *et al.* using the substrate Boc-K(Ac)-7-AMC, a cell-permeable HDAC substrate [16]. However, optimization of the assay for suitable HDAC substrates, kinetics of substrate cleavage in specific cells and reaction conditions appear to be under development.

6.2.3 *In Vitro* Isoform-Specificity Assays

With the commercial availability of purified recombinant HDAC proteins, the number of reports claiming development of isoform-specific HDACIs has increased. FK228, a natural product HDACI in clinical trials, shows strong inhibitory activities toward HDACs 1 and 2 and weak activities toward HDACs 4 and 6 [17]. The hydroxamate, Tubacin, was identified through the screening of a rationally designed chemical library, and was found to be relatively selective for the inhibition of tubulin deacetylase (TDAC) HDAC6, based on the high concentrations required to induce histone acetylation [18]. The recently identified inhibitor, SB-379 278-A, shows selectivity for HDAC8 and also fails to affect cellular histone acetylation [17]. MS275 belongs to the benzamide class of drugs and is reported to inhibit HDAC1 ($IC_{50} = 300$ nM) as compared to HDAC3 (8 μM) and does not inhibit HDAC8 (IC50 > 100 μM). A novel series of (aryloxopropenyl)pyrrolyl hydroxamates have been described as HDAC inhibitors and some of these have been found to select for maize HD1-A, a mammalian Class II (IIa) HDAC homolog.

However, various assays utilizing nonstandardized sources of HDAC protein preparations and substrates appear to generate large variations in the resulting data. As an example, Table 6.1 summarizes the observed variations in the recently reported *in vitro* data for the effects of SAHA on individual HDAC isoforms [14, 19–23]. HDAC isoforms used for *in vitro* screening assays have been expressed in *Escherichia coli* (HDAC1, 3), *Picchia*, SF9 insect cells (HDAC1–11) or mammalian cells (recombinant HDAC1, 3); these sources may lead to differential enzyme activities.

Table 6.1 Summary of the observed variations in the *in vitro* data for the effects of SAHA on individual HDAC isoforms.

Isoforms	IC$_{50}$ inhibition activity (nM)						
	BPS	Andrianov [19]	Balasubramanian [20]	Beckers [14]	Kozikowski [21]	Li [22]	Richon [23]
HDAC1	40.6	68.1	28	21	68	148	10
HDAC2	134	163.6	60		164		
HDAC3	46.5	67.1	44	37	48	119	20
HDAC4	>30 000	100.9					
HDAC5	~15 000	107.3					
HDAC6	17.7	110.6	22	25	90		
HDAC7	21 000	102.4					
HDAC8	76.9	1374.7	410	1200	1524		
HDAC9	>30 000	107.2					
HDAC10	57.5		40				
HDAC11	133						

Bioscience (BPS) used recombinant HDACs prepared in baculovirus systems; Andrianov *et al.* used batch-mode capture for recombinant HDAC preparations; Balasubramanian *et al.* performed continuous protease-coupled enzyme assays for recombinant HDAC activity; Kozikowski *et al.* used a microfluid method for activities; Li *et al.* and Richon *et al.* used immunoprecipitated HDAC proteins for reactions.

These differences may reflect difficulties in obtaining equivalent enzymatic activities of recombinant HDAC isoforms.

Another factor affecting the action of drugs is related to the substrate specificity of individual HDACs and possible cofactors, which may stabilize the protein or direct the enzyme to its biological targets [12, 24]. For example, purified recombinant HDAC6 has been shown to be extremely active by itself, while HDAC3 exhibits poor enzymatic activity unless it is prepared in the presence of SMART/N-CoR, which serves to stabilize the protein [24]. Furthermore, the kinetic variables (K_m, K_i) of these purified enzymes need to be considered for a baseline of enzyme activity prior to use in isoform-specific inhibition assays. Some reported studies have used semi-purified epitope-tagged proteins and immunoprecipitated proteins for measuring *in vitro* inhibition activity [22, 23]. However, the endogenous biologically active multiprotein complex may also confer less potency than a recombinant protein. Therefore, claims of isoform specificity based on *in vitro* assays should be interpreted with caution.

6.3
Cell-Based Assays

Histone deacetylases mediate the extent of acetylation of nuclear and cytoplasmic proteins, leading to regulation of key cellular processes, including cell growth, differentiation and death. Understanding the biological mechanisms of HDACs within the context of the cell provides a rational basis for selectivity profiles. Although histone deacetylases are known to be associated with transcriptional repression, accumulated studies have revealed a broad range of HDAC functions (reviewed in Ref. [25]). Class I HDACs are mainly in the nucleus of most cell types and contributes to cancer cell proliferation and apoptosis [26]. However, a recent report has demonstrated that HDAC8 is a prominently cytosolic marker of smooth muscle differentiation, associates with cytoskeletal proteins and plays a role in smooth muscle contractility [27]. HDAC8 also associates with the inv(16) fusion protein, a frequent chromosomal translocations found in acute myeloid leukemia (AML) [28]. Class II HDACs are characterized by subcellular localization, their expression is more restricted and they play important roles in cellular differentiation and development. These HDACs are not directly involved in processes that control proliferation and apoptosis in tumor cells. Class IIa enzymatic activity is not intrinsic, but is derived from its association with HDAC3 [24]. Recent studies have shown that the Class IIb HDAC6 is a deacetylase of tubulin and Hsp90 and its inhibition decreases cell motility, but does not affect cell cycle progression [29, 30].

6.3.1 HDAC Activity Assays in Cultured Cells

To determine isoform selectivity of HDAC inhibitors, epitope-tagged HDAC cDNAs are expressed in cells, and pull-downs using antibodies to epitope-tags are affinity purified and used for assays. However, the pull-down products often contain protein complexes with multiple HDACs and/or other cofactors, presenting an obstacle to HDACI selectivity assays. Investigations of nuclear preparations by anion exchange chromatography revealed complexes that contained predominantly HDAC1 and 2, but not HDAC3 [31]. Furthermore, purification of Class II HDACs has also been difficult for similar reasons. HDACs 4, 5 and 7 have been shown to be enzymatically active in the presence of HDAC3 [32]. Taking such caveats into consideration, inhibitor potency and selectivity against different recombinant forms of HDACs need to be optimized within the context of these complex form preparations. Identifying the distinct role of protein cofactors in the biological activity of deacetylases should provide the strategies for potential clinical applicability with selectivity profile.

6.3.2 Detection of Acetylated Histones and Nonhistone Proteins

The first functional cell-based assay for the determination of pan-histone deacetylase activity was achieved by detecting hyperacetylated histones by Western blotting. The histone acetylation level in cells offers a measure of candidate HDACI activity and has been linked to antiproliferative and cytotoxic effects. Beckers *et al.* used a cellular histone hyperacetylation assay for quantification of the cellular efficacy of HDACIs using the Cellomics Array Scan II platform in 96 wells [14]. The program identifies cells by nuclear staining with Hoe33342 and by nuclear fluorescence of Alexa Fluor 488, which quantifies nuclear histone acetylation levels with the mitotic index normalized with nuclear fluorescence intensity. However, recent studies demonstrated that the chelating moieties of HDAC inhibitors are major determinants of tubulin deacetylase activity (the TDAC site is one of two catalytic sites on HDAC6) that is observed in cellular systems as accumulation of acetylated α-tubulin [33]. SAHA and TSA cause accumulation of acetylated tubulin, but other HDACIs (e.g. trapoxin B, sodium butyrate, FK-228) do not, suggesting the selectivity at the cellular level with these HDACIs.

The accumulation of acetylated histone and acetylated tubulin are also used as surrogate measures for inhibition of tumor cell growth and induction of apoptosis. Pharmacokinetics and pharmacodynamics of HDACIs have been determined by evaluating expression levels and kinetics of acetylation of histones or nonhistone target proteins, including α-tubulin, Hsp90, p53 and p21. Hyperacetylations of α-tubulin and Hsp90 have also been tightly linked to HDAC6 inhibition. The data shown in Figure 6.1 demonstrate kinetics of acetylating histone H4 and α-tubulin in response to some HDACIs [34, 35]. Other approaches have been developed in cell-based high-throughput assay formats to monitor competitive binding of HDAC inhibitors to cellular HDACs. One approach is by staining cells with an HDACI-derived fluorophor (K-trap-coumarin dye) to visualize nuclei by fluorescence microscopy [36]. Using a genetic-like approach, a miniaturized "cytoblot" assay, has also been developed to understand cellular pathways in mammalian systems

Structure	IC50 [nM]						Cpd
	pan	HD1	HD2	HD6	HD8	HD10	
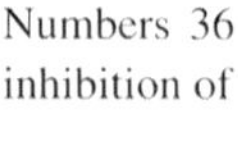	80	52	193	16	2660	70	7c[36]
	44	3220	7380	95.3	6120	10700	10b[37]
	4	4	27	3	1950	4	17b[36]

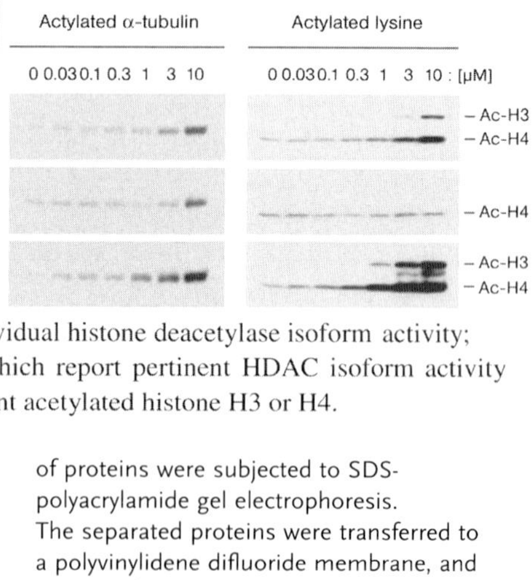

Pan = Total histone deacetylase activities; HD(#) = Individual histone deacetylase isoform activity; Numbers 36 and 37 correspond to citation references which report pertinent HDAC isoform activity inhibition of compounds (Cpd); ac-H3 and Ac-H4 represent acetylated histone H3 or H4.

Figure 6.1 Effects of various concentrations of HDAC inhibitors on acetylation of α-tubulin and histone in MCF7 human breast carcinoma cells. MCF7 cells were incubated for 5 h with various HDAC inhibitors at the indicated concentrations. The total cell extracts were isolated by scraping cells into SDS-lysis buffer. Protein concentrations were determined by performing Bradford assay using bovine serum albumin as a standard. Equal amounts of proteins were subjected to SDS-polyacrylamide gel electrophoresis. The separated proteins were transferred to a polyvinylidene difluoride membrane, and nonspecific IgG binding sites were blocked by incubation with 5% nonfat dry milk for 1 h at room temperature. The membranes were then incubated overnight at 4 °C with primary antibodies. Immune complexes were detected by enhanced chemiluminescence (Amersham Biosciences).

using small molecules [37]. Another approach utilizes an ELISA type methodology after fixation and permeabilization, which is suitable for screening libraries of compounds for inhibitors of acetylase or deacetylase activity [38]. It is anticipated that further identification of nonhistone proteins as individual HDAC isoform substrates may advance the capacity for selectivity profiling of candidate isoform-specific HDACIs.

6.4 Biological Function-Based Assays

6.4.1 Cell Proliferation Assays

HDAC Inhibitors promote cell growth arrest, differentiation and cell death. Particularly, HDACIs induce growth arrest in proliferating cancer cells and normal cells are considerably more resistant to these inhibitors than are malignant cells [3]. Inhibition of cell proliferation can be assessed by determining the IC_{50} concentrations of HDAC inhibitors, for example using the CellTiter 96 AQueous one solution cell proliferation assay kit (Promega), which is a colorimetric method for determining the number of viable cells in proliferation or cytotoxicity assays. Various numbers of cells are added to the wells of a 96-well plate and allowed to equilibrate with 20 μl/well of CellTiter 96 AQueous one solution reagent. After incubation for 1 h at 37 °C, the absorbance at 490 nm is recorded using an ELISA plate reader. The antiproliferative effects of HDACIs on a panel of cancer cell lines complement the *in vivo* enzyme inhibition assays.

6.4.2 Reporter Systems

HDAC family members play as important regulators of gene transcription that control biological processes. As such, *in vitro* and *in vivo* reporter systems have been developed to characterize HDACIs targeting specific signaling pathways by using a target promoter linked to a reporter gene (i.e. luciferase or GFP), known as reverse chemical genetics [31]. This approach utilizes cell lines with reporter constructs for a given signaling pathway, which provides information on changes in cellular phenotype [39]. For example, the promoter of cyclin-dependent kinase inhibitor p21 contains six SP1 binding sites, some of which are directly associated with HDAC-mediated gene activation [40]. A number of sequence-specific DNA-binding proteins (e.g. NCoR, SMART, MEF, MeCP2, sin3A) utilize HDACs to repress transcription and block tumor suppressor gene functions, resulting in antiproliferative effects *in vitro* and *in vivo* [41, 42]. The functional importance of recruiting HDACs for B-lymphocyte maturation protein (Blimp-1)-dependent repression of c-myc transcription has been demonstrated by using Gal4-fusion protein assays [43]. Tumor necrosis factor (TNF)-induced NFκB-dependent gene expression, such as interleukin-8 gene, has been shown to be regulated by HDAC1 and HDAC2 by which TSA treatment results in an increase in both basal and TNF-induced expression of the NFκB-regulated IL-8 gene [44].

Stable integrated reporter constructs targeting signaling pathways, including TGFβ tumor-suppressor- or NFκB-mediated, have been used for high-throughput assays [45]. The reporter construct was engineered to contain repeats of factor-binding elements linked to a minimal SV40 or CMV promoter and the reporter gene. A genetically integrated cell model system with ErbB2 promoter-reporter has also been used for a breast cancer-specific cell screen [46]. Therefore, the reporter assay system is useful to study unknown molecular basis for antitumor selectivity of candidate HDACIs. Furthermore, considering the finding that Class II HDACs regulate transcription by bridging the enzymatically active SMART/N-CoR-HDAC3 complex [24], intrinsic HDAC activity via the transcriptional coprepressor may be deciphered by this approach.

Another approach involves the use of a phenotypic selection-based yeast model [47]. This model utilizes genetic modification by silencing ura3 inserted into the telomere region of yeast chromosomal DNA where yeast cells can grow in the presence of thymidine analog 5-fluoroorotic acid (5-FOA). In the presence of inhibitors, however, cells die because of the desilencing of ura3 and the subsequent conversion of 5-FOA to toxic fluorouracil by URA3. This assay has been successfully used to identify Sir2 inhibitors in high-throughout screening [47].

6.4.3 High-Throughput Gene Expression Analysis

Growing evidence support the premise that there are fundamental epigenetic differences between normal and tumor cells that alter transcriptional responses following exposure to HDAC inhibitors. Transcriptional responses may be cell type-specific, or HDACI-specific. HDACs utilize histone and nonhistone proteins as substrates, including key modulators of oncogenesis (e.g. p53, Hsp90, STAT, Bax, NFκB) [9]. Acetylation of these molecules by HDAC inhibition results in the modulation of signaling cascades and cellular processes. However, little is known of the cellular and molecular factors that determine sensitivity or resistance to HDACIs. Therefore, high-throughput gene expression analysis generates a global view of gene regulation in response to stimuli. Advanced bioinformatics programs allow extraction of vital information from vast amounts of microarray data.

Expression profiling studies have shown that HDACi treatment of cells alters the expression of 2–10% of cellular genes [48]. Upregulated genes include tumor suppressors (i.e. p21, p16, gelsolin, TBP2, etc.) and downregulated genes include those coding for invasion and angiogenesis (i.e. Her2/Neu, VEGF, cyclin proteins). Microarray technology has been applied to characterize structurally different HDACIs using clustering algorithms. Recent studies have demonstrated HDAC inhibitor-specific profiles in response to structurally different compounds (SAHA, TSA, MS-275) in T24 bladder and MDA breast carcinoma cells and revealed the core regulated genes predominantly involved in cell cycle/apoptosis and DNA synthesis [49]. MS-275 produces a gene expression pattern significantly different from the hydroxamate HDAC inhibitors, SAHA and TSA, probably due to its subtype profile.

HDACs appear to function in concert with multiprotein complexes that are recruited to specific regions in the genome that generate the unique spectrums of expressed and silenced genes [50]. HDACIs are able to depress gene expression, resulting in antiproliferative effects *in vitro* and antitumor effects *in vivo*. Which HDAC(s) are involved, resulting in antiproliferative and antitumoral phenotypes can be addressed. There is compelling data on potential species-specific and tissue-specific roles of HDACIs. Gene expression profiling of HDACIs may be used to identify acetylation patterns of HDAC substrates and for optimal selectivity patterns of candidate HDACIs (e.g. α-tubulin or p53) in selective assays. Identifying biomarkers and/or substrates specific for HDAC isoforms should advance development of selective HDACIs.

6.4.4
Flow Cytometry Analysis

The action of HDACIs attributes to cell growth arrest and apoptosis. HDACIs have shown to disrupt cell cycle progression, arresting cells mainly in G1 phase. In parallel, quantification of acetylated lysines of histones and G1 checkpoint proteins, such as p53 and p21, has been used to determine the effect of HDACIs on cell cycle progression. Cell cycle arrest following HDACI treatment correlates with the induction of p21 expression in a p53-independent manner. As shown in Figure 6.2,

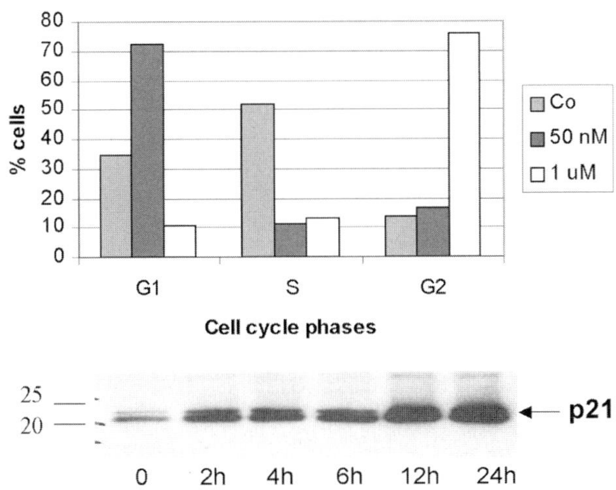

Figure 6.2 Cell cycle distributions of MCF-7 cells after treatment with TSA for 24 hours were determined by performing flow cytometric analysis. Following treatment of cells with 50 nM and 1 μM of TSA, the samples were analyzed on a Becton-Dickinson FACStar^{plus} instrument and the percentage of nuclei with G_1, S, and G_2/M DNA content was determined. p21 protein was also correspondingly increased at various intervals.

MCF-7 cells exposed to 50 nM TSA were in G1 phase (>70%). However, cells treated with 1 μM TSA arrested cells predominantly in G2/M phase, suggesting a dose-dependent fashion. With either dose, cells accumulated least in the S phase. In addition to accumulation of hyperacetylated nucleosome core histones, TSA enhanced p21 expression. Therefore, flow cytometry (FACS) offers an efficient tool for analyzing the action of HDACIs in cell proliferation. This method is particularly useful for application to clinical samples, where cell numbers may be small. The effects of HDACIs on the cell cycle are dose-dependent.

Furthermore, since the cell growth arrest is often linked to cell death, The annexin V staining positive cell or the amount of DNA fragmentation assessed by TUNEL and FACS analysis has been interpreted as indicative of apoptosis. The HDACI-induced apoptosis can also be determined by Western blotting of target proteins, detection of mitochondrial membrane potentials, activation of caspases and their substrate cleavages in a dose- and time-dependent manner.

6.5 HDAC Isoform Functional Assays

Inhibition of HDACs has become an interesting approach for anticancer therapy. Therefore, two approaches, gene knockdown in cells and knockout in animals, have been developed and widely used for functional studies of specific HDAC isoforms.

6.5.1 Depletion of Target Genes in Cells

Gene knockdown approaches using small interfering double-stranded RNA (siRNA) targeting specific molecules has provided insights into HDAC containing protein complexes. Reduction of Class I HDAC levels resulted in a phenotype similar to that observed following exposure of cells to small molecule HDAC inhibitors. The knockdowns of Class I HDACs (HDAC1, HDAC3) exhibit significant morphological phenotype similar to that observed with HDACI (SAHA) treatment of cells, whereas knockdowns of Class II HDACs (HDAC4. HDAC7) in HeLa cells show no changes in cell morphology and proliferation [39]. HDAC7 has a specific role in the clonal expansion of T cells by suppressing Nur77-dependent apoptosis [36] and in vascular integrity through suppression of MMP10 [51]. HDAC6 is a deacetylase known to act on tubulin, which promotes independent cell movement as occurs in metastasis [52, 53]. Tubulin deacetylation is also required for disposal of misfolded proteins in aggresomes [54]. HDAC6 also deacetylates heat shock protein 90. Disruption of its chaperon function is crucial to cancer cell stress response [55–57]. Therefore, the gene knockdown approach supports the development of selective inhibitors designed against the Class I HDACs for the treatment of cancers, perhaps reducing potential dose-limiting toxicities.

6.5.2 Knockout Animal Models

Recent studies using genetically manipulated animal models offer physiological roles of HDAC isoforms. HDAC1 knockout mice die during embryonic development [58], implicating its involvement in development and cell proliferation. HDAC4 knockout mice have a pronounced chondrocyte hypertrophy and die of aberrant ossification [59]. HDAC9 knockout mice show cardiac hypertrophy [60] that is further exacerbated in HDAC9 and HDAC5 double-knockout animals [61]. Recently, Olsen *et al.* reported that global deletion of HDAC2 results in peri-natal lethality in mice due to severe cardiac defects [62]. HDAC1 and HDAC2 are functionally redundant in cardiac growth and development and maintain cardiomyocyte identity and function, at least in part, through repression of genes encoding skeletal muscle specific myofibrillar proteins and calcium channels. Mice lacking HDAC7 die during embryogenesis from abnormalities in endothelial cell development [63]. As such, Class II HDACs are associated with pathological cardiac growth and maintenance of normal cardiac size and function, suggesting that strategies for normalizing gene expression in the failing heart (by regulating HDAC phosphorylation and function) represent potentially powerful therapeutic approaches [52]. Taken together, these knockout models provide physiological functions for HDACs *in vivo*.

6.6 Anticancer Activity

Consistent with early clinical findings in trials using HDACIs in patients to demonstrate that HDACI treatment leads to tumor regression and symptomatic improvement in a broad spectrum of human malignancies, histone deacetylation affects the expression of numerous genes implicated in oncogenesis, including angiogenesis, cellular differentiation, migration, invasion and adhesion. Cell-based assays have demonstrated that the action of HDACIs inhibiting angiogenesis is a mechanism underlying *in vivo* antitumor activity in xenograft models [64].

6.6.1 Antiangiogenic Assays

Multiple HDAC inhibitors have been shown to prevent new vessel formation in other models of angiogenesis [65–67]. Approaches include a molecular link between angiogenic factors (i.e. transcriptional activity, acetylation, polyubiquitination, degradation) and HDACIs, determining capillary tube-like structures and migration. In the presence of high concentrations of VEGF, endothelial cells form tube and capillary-like structures on the surface of basement membrane matrices. The zangiogenesis inhibitory activity of HDACIs has been measured using *in vitro* assays with endothelial cells (HUVECs) or rat aortic ring, freshly isolated from Sprague–Dawley rats and embedded in fibrin gel clots in six-well plates [64, 67].

Recent studies have demonstrated that overexpression of HDAC1 represses the tumor suppressors, p53 and von Hippel–Lindau (VHL), but induces the hypoxia-responsive genes, hypoxia inducible factor alpha (HIF-1α) and vascular endothelial growth factor (VEGF) and increases angiogenesis. Conversely, HDAC inhibitors derepress the tumor suppressors, p53 and VHL, and repress HIF-1α and VEGF [68, 69].

Class II HDAC4 and HDAC6 have also been shown to be associated with HIF-1α protein. Silencing these HDACs reduced HIF-1α protein expression and transcriptional activity [70]. Class II HDAC7 knockdown in endothelial cells altered cell morphology, migration and capacity to form capillary tube-like structures *in vitro* but did not affect cell adhesion, proliferation or apoptosis [71]. Alteration of angiogenesis factors, including platelet-derived growth factor B and its receptor (PDGFR-β) were unregulated following HDAC7 silencing, suggesting that HDAC7 may be a rational therapeutic target for cancer treatment.

6.6.2
Invasion Assay

HDACIs exhibit anti-invasion activities [70]. LBH589 attenuates VEGF-induced signaling in endothelial cells and reduces endothelial cell chemotaxis and invasion. Class I HDACs have been shown to directly regulate the expression of E-cadherin, a gene important for cell–cell adhesion, by which loss of E-cadherin expression causes epithelial invasion and the repressor Snail recruits HDAC1 and HDAC2 and the co-repressor mSin3A to the E-cadherin promoter. Others have shown that combined treatment of prostate cancer cells with a peroxisome proliferator-activated receptor-γ (PPARγ) agonist and the HDAC inhibitor VPA reduces the invasiveness of these cells while increasing expression of E-cadherin mRNA and protein [72]. Since E-cadherin expression often is lost in prostate cancer, combination therapy may reduce the metastatic potential of prostate cancer. HDAC1 has also been shown to repress cystatin, a peptidase inhibitor that suppresses tumor invasion [70]. Knockdown of HDAC1 or overexpression of cystatin reduces cellular invasion [73].

6.6.3
Tumor Xenograft Models

The finding that inhibitors of HDACs preferentially kill transformed cells at doses that confer little effect on normal cell growth has been a largely attractive rationale for developing HDACI inhibitors as anticancer agents. Some of HDACIs are currently in phase I and II clinical trials. Whether the selectivity profile of HDACI inhibitors has a major consequence on their clinical activity remains unknown. Accumulated studies have shown antitumor activities of HDACIs against solid (e.g. breast, colon, lung, prostate, ovarian, lung) and hematological (e.g., acute lymphoblastic leukemia, acute myeloid leukemia, chronic lymphoblastic leukemia, chronic myeloid leukemia, lymphoma, myeloma) malignancies by using cultured cancer cells and tumor xenograft animal models. A range of HDACIs has been administered via oral, intraperineal, intravenous and subcutaneous routes [14, 64]. The pharmacological doses are HDACI-dependent, ranging within micrograms to milligrams per kilogram of body weight per day for 5–28 days. Duration of treatment varies based on the administration routes. The compound can be administrated once daily intravenously for five consecutive days, while oral and i.p. administration can be delivered daily over 30 days without obvious toxicity. The maximum tolerated dose (MTD) is defined as the maximum dose that results in no death when the compound is administered with doses from 10 mg/kg to 200 mg/kg depending on HDACIs to animals once daily for compound-based scheduled days. MTD is often evaluated by measuring body weight loss or death following treatment. The levels of acetylated histones or nonhistone proteins (e.g. α-tubulin, p21, p53) have also been assessed as surrogates for efficacy of HDACIs in target tissues.

6.7 Perspective

The actions of HDAC inhibitors on cell cycle, apoptosis, angiogenesis, cellular differentiation and cellular transformation suggest the potential for their use in treating various tumor types, by affecting different mechanisms. Understanding which HDAC isoforms are most important for tissue type-specific cancer biology may lead to predictive markers and insights into clinical applications. As such, drug discovery efforts for HDAC inhibitors with isoform specificity should offer the potential for tissue type-specific cancer therapy and an improved therapeutic window by modulating a small set of disease-focused genes.

Findings that not all HDACIs can function as chemosensitizing agents suggest that HDACIs may target specific HDAC isoforms, or more likely, nonhistone proteins to varying degrees, the end result being changed chemosensitivity. Recent reports have shown that a number of HDAC isoforms are associated with breast cancer carcinoma. Significantly, strikingly different amounts of some HDAC isoforms were observed in different stages of breast cancer carcinoma. HDAC1, 3 and 5 were abundant in ductal and invasive lobular carcinoma whereas detectable levels were not observed in metastatic carcinoma. Therefore, it is of particular interest that there are cell line-dependent differences in the chemosensitizing effectiveness of the tested compounds, suggesting potential cancer-specific effects. These differences may support the potential for identifying HDAC-specific inhibitors for use alone or in combinations with hormonal therapy to achieve tumor-specific sensitivity.

Although HDACIs have generated significant interest as anticancer agents due to their ability to cause growth arrest, terminal differentiation and/or apoptosis in carcinoma cells, identification of the compound as an inhibitor of selected HDACs is still a major challenge. It has become evident that HDACs are present as multiprotein complexes and, in some cases, multiHDAC-containing complexes in their active forms. This suggests that any selectivity determinations would have to be considered in the context of these complexes. Although rapid progress has been made toward understanding the functions of individual HDACs, a remaining question is how the activities of these enzymes actually coordinate in the cell. Therefore, increased understanding of how HDACIs work will continue to aid our ability to establish new paradigms for rational drug design with broad clinical implications-continually improving the design of drugs for targeted human cancer therapies.

Without understanding biological functions, it is difficult to assess the relative contribution of individual or classes of HDACs to the therapeutic benefit of HDAC inhibition. Assessing HDACI selectivity *in vitro* must be approached with caution since active enzymes consist of a multiprotein complex containing other HDACs and cofactors. Endogenous biologically active multiprotein complexes confer less potency than a recombinant protein. Furthermore, lack of selectivity observation by HDACIs may be due to the use of a generic HDAC substrate, "Fluor-de-Lys." Thus, isoform specific substrates need to be developed. Another caveat is pertinent to physicochemistry of the selected compounds. Although containing potent enzymatic and cellular activity, the pharmacoproperties of compounds, such as a half-life *in vivo*, pharmacokinetics/dynamics and antitumor effects with toxicity, are critical parameters to be considered for the selection of lead compounds. As such, pharmacodynamic response and its relationship to pharmacokinetics will guide optimal dose selection and regimen in human use.

Acknowledgments

We thank Dr. Anatoly Dritschilo for scientific discussion and J. Tuturea for technical assistance. This work was supported by grant P02 CA74175 (to A.D. and M.J.) from the National Cancer Institute.

References

1 Rundlett, S.E., Carmen, A.A., Kobayashi, R., Bavykin, S., Turner, B.M. and Grunstein, M. (1996) HDA1 and RPD3 are members of distinct yeast histone deacetylase complexes that regulate silencing and transcription. *Proceedings of the National Academy of Sciences of the United States of America*, **93**, 14503–14508.

2 Yang, X.J. and Seto, E. (2008) The Rpd3/Hda1 family of lysine deacetylases: from bacteria and yeast to mice and men. *Nature Reviews. Molecular Cell Biology*, **9**, 206–218.

3 Marks, P., Rifkind, R.A., Richon, V.M., Breslow, R., Miller, T. and Kelly, W.K. (2001) Histone deacetylases and cancer: causes and therapies. *Nature Reviews. Cancer*, **1**, 194–202.

4 Bolden, J.E., Peart, M.J. and Johnstone, R.W. (2006) Anticancer activities of histone deacetylase inhibitors. *Nature Reviews. Drug Discovery*, **5**, 769–784.

5 Verdin, E., Dequiedt, F. and Kasler, H.G. (2003) Class II histone deacetylases: versatile regulators. *Trends in Genetics*, **19**, 286–293.

6 Kouzarides, T. (1999) Histone acetylases and deacetylases in cell proliferation. *Current Opinion in Genetics & Development*, **9**, 40–48.

7 Luo, J., Nikolaev, A.Y., Imai, S., Chen, D., Su, F., Shiloh, A., Guarente, L. and Gu, W. (2001) Negative control of p53 by Sir2alpha promotes cell survival under stress. *Cell*, **107**, 137–148.

8 Gregoretti, I.V., Lee, Y.M. and Goodson, H.V. (2004) Molecular evolution of the histone deacetylase family: functional implications of phylogenetic analysis. *Journal of Molecular Biology*, **338**, 17–31.

9 Marks, P.A. (2007) Discovery and development of SAHA as an anticancer agent. *Oncogene*, **26**, 1351–1356.

10 Wegener, D., Hildmann, C. and Schwienhorst, A. (2003) Recent progress in the development of assays suited for histone deacetylase inhibitor screening. *Molecular Genetics and Metabolism*, **80**, 138–147.

11 Kolle, D., Brosch, G., Lechner, T., Lusser, A. and Loidl, P. (1998) Biochemical methods for analysis of histone deacetylases. *Methods (San Diego, Calif)*, **15**, 323–331.

12 Ito, K., Barnes, P.J. and Adcock, I.M. (2000) Glucocorticoid receptor recruitment of histone deacetylase 2 inhibits interleukin-1beta-induced histone H4 acetylation on lysines 8 and 12. *Molecular and Cellular Biology*, **20**, 6891–6903.

13 Schultz, B.E., Misialek, S., Wu, J., Tang, J., Conn, M.T., Tahilramani, R. and Wong, L. (2004) Kinetics and comparative reactivity of human class I and class IIb histone deacetylases. *Biochemistry*, **43**, 11083–11091.

14 Beckers, T., Burkhardt, C., Wieland, H., Gimmnich, P., Ciossek, T., Maier, T. and Sanders, K. (2007) Distinct pharmacological properties of second generation HDAC inhibitors with the benzamide or hydroxamate head group. *International Journal of Cancer*, **121**, 1138–1148.

15 Hassig, C.A., Symons, K.T., Guo, X., Nguyen, P.M., Annable, T., Wash, P.L., Payne, J.E., Jenkins, D.A., Bonnefous, C., Trotter, C., Wang, Y., Anzola, J.V., Milkova, E.L., Hoffman, T.Z., Dozier, S.J., Wiley, B.M., Saven, A., Malecha, J.W., Davis, R.L., Muhammad, J., Shiau, A.K., Noble, S.A., Rao, T.S., Smith, N.D. and Hager, J.H. (2008) KD5170, a novel mercaptoketone-based histone deacetylase inhibitor that exhibits broad spectrum antitumor activity in vitro and in vivo. *Molecular Cancer Therapeutics*, **7**, 1054–1065.

16 Ciossek, T., Julius, H., Wieland, H., Maier, T. and Beckers, T. (2008) A homogeneous cellular histone deacetylase assay suitable for compound profiling and robotic screening. *Analytical Biochemistry*, **372**, 72–81.

17 Hu, E., Dul, E., Sung, C.M., Chen, Z., Kirkpatrick, R., Zhang, G.F., Johanson, K., Liu, R., Lago, A., Hofmann, G., Macarron, R., de los Frailes, M., Perez, P., Krawiec, J., Winkler, J. and Jaye, M. (2003) Identification of novel isoform-selective inhibitors within class I histone deacetylases. *The Journal of Pharmacology and Experimental Therapeutics*, **307**, 720–728.

18 Catley, L., Weisberg, E., Kiziltepe, T., Tai, Y.T., Hideshima, T., Neri, P., Tassone, P., Atadja, P., Chauhan, D., Munshi, N.C. and Anderson, K.C. (2006) Aggresome induction by proteasome inhibitor bortezomib and alpha-tubulin hyperacetylation by tubulin deacetylase (TDAC) inhibitor LBH589 are synergistic in myeloma cells. *Blood*, **108**, 3441–3449.

19 Andrianov, V., Gailite, V., Lola, D., Loza, E., Semenikhina, V., Kalvinsh, I., Finn, P., Petersen, K.D., Ritchie, J.W., Khan, N., Tumber, A., Collins, L.S., Vadlamudi, S.M., Bjorkling, F. and Sehested, M. (2008) Novel amide derivatives as inhibitors of histone deacetylase: Design, synthesis and SAR. *European Journal of Medicinal Chemistry*. .

20 Balasubramanian, S., Ramos, J., Luo, W., Sirisawad, M., Verner, E. and Buggy, J.J. (2008) A novel histone deacetylase 8 (HDAC8)-specific inhibitor PCI-34051 induces apoptosis in T-cell lymphomas. *Leukemia*, **22**, 1026–1034.

21 Kozikowski, A.P., Tapadar, S., Luchini, D.N., Kim, K.H. and Billadeau, D.D. (2008) Use of the nitrile oxide cycloaddition (NOC) reaction for molecular probe generation: a new class of enzyme selective histone deacetylase inhibitors (HDACIs) showing picomolar activity at HDAC6. *Journal of Medicinal Chemistry*, **51**, 4370–4373.

22 Li, J., Staver, M.J., Curtin, M.L., Holms, J.H., Frey, R.R., Edalji, R., Smith, R., Michaelides, M.R., Davidsen, S.K. and Glaser, K.B. (2004) Expression and functional characterization of recombinant human HDAC1 and HDAC3. *Life Sciences*, **74**, 2693–2705.

23 Richon, V.M., Emiliani, S., Verdin, E., Webb, Y., Breslow, R., Rifkind, R.A. and Marks, P.A. (1998) A class of hybrid polar inducers of transformed cell differentiation inhibits histone deacetylases. *Proceedings of the National Academy of Sciences of the United States of America*, **95**, 3003–3007.

24 Fischle, W., Dequiedt, F., Hendzel, M.J., Guenther, M.G., Lazar, M.A., Voelter, W. and Verdin, E. (2002) Enzymatic activity associated with class II HDACs is dependent on a multiprotein complex containing HDAC3 and SMRT/N-CoR. *Molecular Cell*, **9**, 45–57.

25 Wolffe, A.P. and Guschin, D. (2000) Review: chromatin structural features and targets that regulate transcription. *Journal of Structural Biology*, **129**, 102–122.

26 Xu, W.S., Parmigiani, R.B. and Marks, P.A. (2007) Histone deacetylase inhibitors: molecular mechanisms of action. *Oncogene*, **26**, 5541–5552.

27 Waltregny, D., De Leval, L., Glenisson, W., Ly Tran, S., North, B.J., Bellahcene, A., Weidle, U., Verdin, E. and Castronovo, V. (2004) Expression of histone deacetylase 8, a class I histone deacetylase, is restricted to cells showing smooth muscle differentiation in normal human tissues. *The American Journal of Pathology*, **165**, 553–564.

28 Durst, K.L., Lutterbach, B., Kummalue, T., Friedman, A.D. and Hiebert, S.W. (2003) The inv(16) fusion protein associates with corepressors via a smooth muscle myosin heavy-chain domain. *Molecular and Cellular Biology*, **23**, 607–619.

29 Martin, M., Kettmann, R. and Dequiedt, F. (2007) Class IIa histone deacetylases: regulating the regulators. *Oncogene*, **26**, 5450–5467.

30 Zhang, Y., Li, N., Caron, C., Matthias, G., Hess, D., Khochbin, S. and Matthias, P. (2003) HDAC-6 interacts with and deacetylates tubulin and microtubules in vivo. *The EMBO Journal*, **22**, 1168–1179.

31 Curtin, M. and Glaser, K. (2003) Histone deacetylase inhibitors: the Abbott experience. *Current Medicinal Chemistry*, **10**, 2373–2392.

32 de Ruijter, A.J., van Gennip, A.H., Caron, H.N., Kemp, S. and van Kuilenburg, A.B. (2003) Histone deacetylases (HDACs): characterization of the classical HDAC family. *The Biochemical Journal*, **370**, 737–749.

33 Glaser, K.B., Li, J., Pease, L.J., Staver, M.J., Marcotte, P.A., Guo, J., Frey, R.R., Garland, R.B., Heyman, H.R., Wada, C.K., Vasudevan, A., Michaelides, M.R., Davidsen, S.K. and Curtin, M.L. (2004) Differential protein acetylation induced by novel histone deacetylase inhibitors. *Biochemical and Biophysical Research Communications*, **325**, 683–690.

34 Kozikowski, A.P., Chen, Y., Gaysin, A.M., Savoy, D.N., Billadeau, D.D. and Kim, K.H. (2008) Chemistry, biology, and QSAR studies of substituted biaryl hydroxamates and mercaptoacetamides as HDAC inhibitors-nanomolar-potency inhibitors of pancreatic cancer cell growth. *ChemMedChem*, **3**, 487–501.

35 Kozikowski, A.P., Chen, Y., Gaysin, A., Chen, B., D'Annibale, M.A., Suto, C.M. and Langley, B.C. (2007) Functional differences in epigenetic modulators-superiority of mercaptoacetamide-based histone deacetylase inhibitors relative to hydroxamates in cortical neuron neuroprotection studies. *Journal of Medicinal Chemistry*, **50**, 3054–3061.

36 Kwon, H.J., Owa, T., Hassig, C.A., Shimada, J. and Schreiber, S.L. (1998) Depudecin induces morphological reversion of transformed fibroblasts via the inhibition of histone deacetylase. *Proceedings of the National Academy of Sciences of the United States of America*, **95**, 3356–3361.

37 Stockwell, B.R., Haggarty, S.J. and Schreiber, S.L. (1999) High-throughput screening of small molecules in miniaturized mammalian cell-based assays involving post-translational modifications. *Chemistry & Biology*, **6**, 71–83.

38 Wynne Aherne, G., Rowlands, M.G., Stimson, L. and Workman, P. (2002) Assays for the identification and evaluation of histone acetyltransferase inhibitors. *Methods (San Diego, Calif)*, **26**, 245–253.

39 Glaser, K.B., Li, J., Staver, M.J., Wei, R.Q., Albert, D.H. and Davidsen, S.K. (2003) Role of class I and class II histone deacetylases in carcinoma cells using siRNA. *Biochemical and Biophysical Research Communications*, **310**, 529–536.

40 Lin, Y.C., Lin, J.H., Chou, C.W., Chang, Y.F., Yeh, S.H. and Chen, C.C. (2008) Statins increase p21 through inhibition of histone deacetylase activity and release of promoter-associated HDAC1/2. *Cancer Research*, **68**, 2375–2383.

41 Johnstone, R.W. (2002) Histone-deacetylase inhibitors: novel drugs for the treatment of cancer. *Nature Reviews. Drug Discovery*, **1**, 287–299.

42 Ng, H.H. and Bird, A. (2000) Histone deacetylases: silencers for hire. *Trends in Biochemical Sciences*, **25**, 121–126.

43 Yu, J., Angelin-Duclos, C., Greenwood, J., Liao, J. and Calame, K. (2000) Transcriptional repression by blimp-1 (PRDI-BF1) involves recruitment of histone deacetylase. *Molecular and Cellular Biology*, **20**, 2592–2603.

44 Ashburner, B.P., Westerheide, S.D. and Baldwin, A.S. Jr. (2001) The p65 (RelA) subunit of NF-kappaB interacts with the histone deacetylase (HDAC) corepressors HDAC1 and HDAC2 to negatively regulate gene expression. *Molecular and Cellular Biology*, **21**, 7065–7077.

45 Wegener, D., Wirsching, F., Riester, D. and Schwienhorst, A. (2003) A fluorogenic histone deacetylase assay well suited for high-throughput activity screening. *Chemistry & Biology*, **10**, 61–68.

46 Scott, G.K., Marden, C., Xu, F., Kirk, L. and Benz, C.C. (2002) Transcriptional repression of ErbB2 by histone deacetylase inhibitors detected by a genomically integrated ErbB2 promoter-reporting cell screen. *Molecular Cancer Therapeutics*, **1**, 385–392.

47 Grozinger, C.M. and Schreiber, S.L. (2002) Deacetylase enzymes: biological functions and the use of small-molecule inhibitors. *Chemistry & Biology*, **9**, 3–16.

48 Cao, Z.A., Bass, K.E., Balasubramanian, S., Liu, L., Schultz, B., Verner, E., Dai, Y., Molina, R.A., Davis, J.R., Misialek, S., Sendzik, M., Orr, C.J., Leung, L., Callan, O., Young, P., Dalrymple, S.A. and Buggy, J.J. (2006) CRA-026440: a potent, broad-spectrum, hydroxamic histone deacetylase inhibitor with antiproliferative and antiangiogenic activity in vitro and in vivo. *Molecular Cancer Therapeutics*, **5**, 1693–1701.

49 Glaser, K.B., Staver, M.J., Waring, J.F., Stender, J., Ulrich, R.G. and Davidsen, S.K. (2003) Gene expression profiling of multiple histone deacetylase (HDAC) inhibitors: defining a common gene set produced by HDAC inhibition in T24 and MDA carcinoma cell lines. *Molecular Cancer Therapeutics*, **2**, 151–163.

50 Glaser, K.B. (2007) HDAC inhibitors: clinical update and mechanism-based potential. *Biochemical Pharmacology*, **74**, 659–671.

51 Dequiedt, F., Kasler, H., Fischle, W., Kiermer, V., Weinstein, M., Herndier, B.G. and Verdin, E. (2003) HDAC7, a thymus-specific class II histone deacetylase, regulates Nur77 transcription and TCR-mediated apoptosis. *Immunity*, **18**, 687–698.

52 Chang, S., Young, B.D., Li, S., Qi, X., Richardson, J.A. and Olson, E.N. (2006) Histone deacetylase 7 maintains vascular integrity by repressing matrix metalloproteinase 10. *Cell*, **126**, 321–334.

53 Hubbert, C., Guardiola, A., Shao, R., Kawaguchi, Y., Ito, A., Nixon, A., Yoshida, M., Wang, X.F. and Yao, T.P. (2002) HDAC6 is a microtubule-associated deacetylase. *Nature*, **417**, 455–458.

54 Matsuyama, A., Shimazu, T., Sumida, Y., Saito, A., Yoshimatsu, Y., Seigneurin-Berny, D., Osada, H., Komatsu, Y., Nishino, N., Khochbin, S., Horinouchi, S. and Yoshida, M. (2002) In vivo destabilization of dynamic microtubules by HDAC6-mediated deacetylation. *The EMBO Journal*, **21**, 6820–6831.

55 Kawaguchi, Y., Kovacs, J.J., McLaurin, A., Vance, J.M., Ito, A. and Yao, T.P. (2003) The deacetylase HDAC6 regulates aggresome formation and cell viability in response to misfolded protein stress. *Cell*, **115**, 727–738.

56 Yu, X., Guo, Z.S., Marcu, M.G., Neckers, L., Nguyen, D.M., Chen, G.A. and Schrump, D.S. (2002) Modulation of p53, ErbB1, ErbB2, and Raf-1 expression in lung cancer cells by depsipeptide FR901228. *Journal of the National Cancer Institute*, **94**, 504–513.

57 Kovacs, J.J., Murphy, P.J., Gaillard, S., Zhao, X., Wu, J.T., Nicchitta, C.V., Yoshida, M., Toft, D.O., Pratt, W.B. and Yao, T.P. (2005) HDAC6 regulates Hsp90 acetylation and chaperone-dependent activation of glucocorticoid receptor. *Molecular Cell*, **18**, 601–607.

58 Bali, P., Pranpat, M., Bradner, J., Balasis, M., Fiskus, W., Guo, F., Rocha, K., Kumaraswamy, S., Boyapalle, S., Atadja, P., Seto, E. and Bhalla, K. (2005) Inhibition of histone deacetylase 6 acetylates and disrupts the chaperone function of heat shock protein 90: a novel basis for antileukemia activity of histone deacetylase inhibitors. *The Journal of Biological Chemistry*, **280**, 26729–26734.

59 Lagger, G., O'Carroll, D., Rembold, M., Khier, H., Tischler, J., Weitzer, G., Schuettengruber, B., Hauser, C., Brunmeir, R., Jenuwein, T. and Seiser, C. (2002) Essential function of histone deacetylase 1 in proliferation control and CDK inhibitor repression. *The EMBO Journal*, **21**, 2672–2681.

60 Zhang, C.L., McKinsey, T.A., Chang, S., Antos, C.L., Hill, J.A. and Olson, E.N. (2002) Class II histone deacetylases act as signal-responsive repressors of cardiac hypertrophy. *Cell*, **110**, 479–488.

61 Vega, R.B., Matsuda, K., Oh, J., Barbosa, A.C., Yang, X., Meadows, E., McAnally, J., Pomajzl, C., Shelton, J.M., Richardson, J.A., Karsenty, G. and Olson, E.N. (2004) Histone deacetylase 4 controls chondrocyte hypertrophy during skeletogenesis. *Cell*, **119**, 555–566.

62 Chang, S., McKinsey, T.A., Zhang, C.L., Richardson, J.A., Hill, J.A. and Olson, E.N. (2004) Histone deacetylases 5 and 9 govern responsiveness of the heart to a subset of stress signals and play redundant roles in heart development. *Molecular and Cellular Biology*, **24**, 8467–8476.

63 Montgomery, R.L., Davis, C.A., Potthoff, M.J., Haberland, M., Fielitz, J., Qi, X., Hill, J.A., Richardson, J.A. and Olson, E.N. (2007) Histone deacetylases 1 and 2 redundantly regulate cardiac morphogenesis, growth, and contractility. *Genes and Development*, **21**, 1790–1802.

64 Chang, S., Bezprozvannaya, S., Li, S. and Olson, E.N. (2005) An expression screen reveals modulators of class II histone deacetylase phosphorylation. *Proceedings of the National Academy of Sciences of the United States of America*, **102**, 8120–8125.

65 Arts, J., Angibaud, P., Marien, A., Floren, W., Janssens, B., King, P., van Dun, J., Janssen, L., Geerts, T., Tuman, R.W., Johnson, D.L., Andries, L., Jung, M., Janicot, M. and van Emelen, K. (2007) R306465 is a novel potent inhibitor of class I histone deacetylases with broad-spectrum antitumoral activity against solid and haematological malignancies. *British Journal of Cancer*, **97**, 1344–1353.

66 Michaelis, M., Michaelis, U.R., Fleming, I., Suhan, T., Cinatl, J., Blaheta, R.A., Hoffmann, K.,

Kotchetkov, R., Busse, R., Nau, H. and Cinatl, J. Jr. (2004) Valproic acid inhibits angiogenesis in vitro and in vivo. *Molecular Pharmacology*, **65**, 520–527.

67 Kwon, H.J., Kim, M.S., Kim, M.J., Nakajima, H. and Kim, K.W. (2002) Histone deacetylase inhibitor FK228 inhibits tumor angiogenesis. *International Journal of Cancer*, **97**, 290–296.

68 Qian, D.Z., Wang, X., Kachhap, S.K., Kato, Y., Wei, Y., Zhang, L., Atadja, P. and Pili, R. (2004) The histone deacetylase inhibitor NVP-LAQ824 inhibits angiogenesis and has a greater antitumor effect in combination with the vascular endothelial growth factor receptor tyrosine kinase inhibitor PTK787/ ZK222584. *Cancer Research*, **64**, 6626–6634.

69 Kim, M.S., Kwon, H.J., Lee, Y.M., Baek, J.H., Jang, J.E., Lee, S.W., Moon, E.J., Kim, H.S., Lee, S.K., Chung, H.Y., Kim, C.W. and Kim, K.W. (2001) Histone deacetylases induce angiogenesis by negative regulation of tumor suppressor genes. *Nature Medicine*, **7**, 437–443.

70 Deroanne, C.F., Bonjean, K., Servotte, S., Devy, L., Colige, A., Clausse, N., Blacher, S., Verdin, E., Foidart, J.M., Nusgens, B.V. and Castronovo, V. (2002) Histone deacetylases inhibitors as anti-angiogenic agents altering vascular endothelial growth factor signaling. *Oncogene*, **21**, 427–436.

71 Qian, D.Z., Kachhap, S.K., Collis, S.J., Verheul, H.M., Carducci, M.A., Atadja, P. and Pili, R. (2006) Class II histone deacetylases are associated with VHL-independent regulation of hypoxia-inducible factor 1 alpha. *Cancer Research*, **66**, 8814–8821.

72 Mottet, D., Bellahcene, A., Pirotte, S., Waltregny, D., Deroanne, C., Lamour, V., Lidereau, R. and Castronovo, V. (2007) Histone deacetylase 7 silencing alters endothelial cell migration, a key step in angiogenesis. *Circulation Research*, **101**, 1237–1246.

73 Annicotte, J.S., Iankova, I., Miard, S., Fritz, V., Sarruf, D., Abella, A., Berthe, M.L., Noel, D., Pillon, A., Iborra, F., Dubus, P., Maudelonde, T., Culine, S. and Fajas, L. (2006) Peroxisome proliferator-activated receptor gamma regulates E-cadherin expression and inhibits growth and invasion of prostate cancer. *Molecular and Cellular Biology*, **26**, 7561–7574.

7
Chromatin Immunoprecipitation ChIP: Wet Lab Meets *In Silico*

Martin Seifert and Robert Schneider

7.1
Background and Overview

7.1.1
Chromatin and DNA Organization

All eukaryotes face the same challenge: they have to fit approximately 2 m of DNA within their nucleus. This has two implications: (i) a high compaction of the DNA is required and (ii) the DNA has to be accessible for processes like transcription, DNA repair and replication. Eukaryotic cells solve these issues by organizing DNA into chromatin. The basic elements of chromatin are the nucleosomes. A nucleosomal core particle consists of a histone octamer (two of each of the histones H3, H4, H2A, H2B) around which 1.75 turns of DNA are wrapped. With the help of the linker histone H1 and additional chromatin-associated proteins, higher-order chromatin structures are formed. The histone proteins are highly covalently modified (such as lysine acetylation, serine and threonine phosphorylation, arginine and lysine methylation; for a recent review see Ref. [1]). These posttranscriptional modifications can directly alter chromatin structure for example, by neutralizing the positive charge of histones. In addition, the huge combinatorial potential of these modifications can be read out – according to the so-called histone "code" hypothesis – by proteins that bind to specific modifications (or combinations of modifications) [2, 3]. Although it is still under discussion whether these modifications form a true "code", it is now well established that they are fundamental for the regulation of gene expression [4].

Inactive and active chromatin domains can be defined at the molecular level by the presence (or absence) of specific histone modifications (or combinations of modifications), by the degree of chromatin compaction and the presence of chromatin associated proteins. Several earlier studies focusing on specific genes or loci showed that active chromatin is generally more accessible and enriched in acetylated forms of histones H3, H4, H2A [5] and histone H3 methylated at lysine 4 (H3/K4) [6]. H3/K4 di- and tri-methylation and H3 acetylation correlate globally with open chromatin [7].

Epigenetic Targets in Drug Discovery. Edited by Wolfgang Sippl and Manfred Jung

ISBN: 978-3-527-32355-5

In contrast to this, inactive chromatin is characterized by histone hypoacetylation and the enrichment of histone H3 lysine 9 (H3/K9) methylation [6].

More recent genome-wide mapping studies of histone modifications allowed high-resolution and mapping of many histone marks [8, 9] These new studies showed that actively transcribed regions are preferentially enriched in H3/K4 mono-, di- or tri-methylation, H3/K36 tri-methylation and mono-methylation of H3/K9, H3/K27 and H4/K20. Interestingly, the distribution of these marks over genes is not equal; for example tri-methylation of H3/K4 is commonly enriched at the 5′ end of transcribed regions and can serve as an indicator for transcription start sites, whereas the H3/K36 methylation mark tends to be enriched at the 3′ end. In contrast tri-methylation of H3/K9 and H3/K27 is linked with transcriptional repression [8]. Active promoters and enhancers are found to be associated with H3/K4 methylation and H3/K9 mono-methylation. These criteria, therefore, can be used to identify and define genomic elements.

However, this quite simple "black and white" picture of active and repressive marks turns out to be an oversimplification. Some activating marks are not only found on genes that are transcribed, but also on genes that are poised for transcription [10]. Additionally, some modifications that were initially considered to be repressing, such as H3/K9 di-methylation, can be found in the body of certain active genes. Furthermore, in so-called "bivalent chromatin domains" repressive marks (H3/K27 tri-methylation) and activating marks (H3/K4 tri-methylation) can co-exist [8, 11–13]. These finding suggests that the histone "code" is likely more complex than it was initially thought and that not individual modifications but rather the combination of modifications is the real indicator for the transcriptional state.

General or specific transcription factors can activate or repress transcription – at least partially – by altering the chromatin structure. Many transcription factors have been shown to recruit specific chromatin-modifying enzymes. Recent studies allowing the genome-wide mapping of transcription factors have resulted in the identification of new target genes [14].

7.1.2
Chromatin Immunoprecipitation as a Powerful Method to Study Chromatin

The fascinating results described above were all obtained using the chromatin immunoprecipitation method (ChIP). ChIP is a very powerful and widely applied technique that has many variations on a common theme. All these variations have in common the fact that they can be used to analyze not only the dynamics of modifications of histones but also the spatial and temporal association of specific proteins (transcription factors, receptors, etc.) with DNA. The ChIP technique enables the precise mapping of temporal changes at specific promoters, genes or other genomic regions of interest at a unique resolution of up to the single nucleosome level (approx. 170 base pairs). Additionally, using ChIP it is possible to follow their distribution, for example transcription factors or histone modifications over entire genomes (see below). Importantly, the application of the ChIP technique allows one to gain unique insight into how genes are regulated in their native context.

The basic principle behind the ChIP method is relatively simple: It is based on the selective enrichment of a chromatin fraction containing a specific antigen (e.g. transcription factors, DNA binding proteins, modified histones, etc.) by an immunoprecipitation step. Specific (important, see below!) antibodies that recognize a protein of interest or the modified form of a protein can be used to determine the relative abundance of it within DNA regions.

Here we provide insight into the ChIP technique, the most important steps and some trouble-shooting guidelines. We describe the variations of ChIP and recent new developments, especially for genome-wide studies. We also focus on the data analysis, since in silico data analysis becomes more and more central for successful ChIP experiments. In the last section we discuss two examples for data analysis based on recent publications. For detailed ChIP protocols we refer the reader to the excellent protocols database freely available at: http://www.epigenome-noe.net/researchtools/protocols.php.

7.2 The Basic Principle of ChIP

Nowadays ChIP is a standard technique to determine whether a protein of interest (or a modification of the protein) is present at a specific DNA sequence *in vivo*. Figure 7.1 shows the basic steps of the "standard" ChIP protocol. It consists of

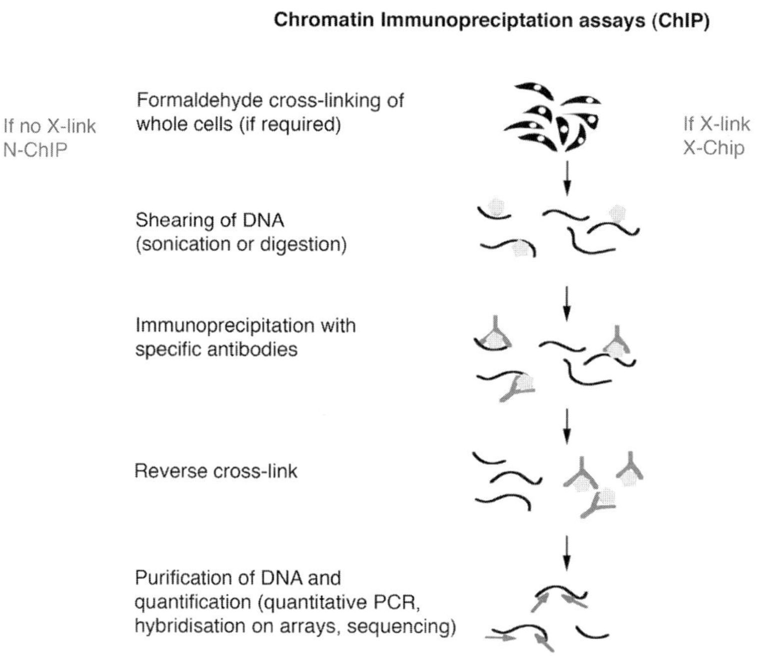

Figure 7.1 The basic steps of ChIP. For details see text.

an initial immunoprecipitation step (for the antigen and the bound chromatin), followed by analysis of the DNA which is attached to the immunoprecipitated proteins. The analyses of the DNA varies depending upon which questions are to be addressed, such as Southern blot, PCR, quantitative real-time PCR, hybridization on microarrays, or deep sequencing (see below for details). Subsequent to the wet-lab steps, enriched DNA regions can be mined by bioinformatics methods.

Often a cross-linking step is applied to stabilize the interactions between proteins and DNA. Thus, ChIP can be divided into: (i) native ChIP ("N-ChIP") without cross-linking and (ii) "X-ChIP" with cross-linking. Here we discuss briefly these two ways of performing ChIP.

7.2.1
N-ChIP

The N-ChIP method was initially described by Gilmour and colleagues. They showed a preferential association of RNA polymerase II and topoisomerase I with active genes in *Drosophila* [15, 16]. In 1988 the Crane–Robinson laboratory at Portsmouth University published the first account of an antibody against a histone modification applied in ChIPs [17]. They applied an acetyl lysine-specific antibody to immunoprecipitate and to enrich chicken nucleosomes containing acetylated histones. In their study, they demonstrated a positive *in vivo* correlation between histone hyperacetylation and an active transcriptional state of the analyzed genes. The advantage of the N-ChIP method is that potential antigens cannot be obscured (e.g. by irreversibly cross-linking a binding protein onto it, or by fixing it in an inaccessible position) by cross-linking. However, a tight association with chromatin is essential and therefore N-ChIP is usually limited to the analysis of histone, histone modifications, or strongly chromatin-associated proteins (such as MeCP2 or HP1; for a review see Ref. [18]).

7.2.2
X-ChIP

The aim of the cross-linking step in ChIP protocols is to fix the proteins of interest stably to their chromatin binding sites. Proteins with lower affinity to DNA or proteins with high mobility (such as most transcription factors) require cross-linking for stabilization. Therefore, X-ChIPs (compared to N-ChIP) allows the analysis of a significantly broader range of chromatin-associated factors. In 1993, Orlando and Paro established a ChIP protocol using formaldehyde as a cross-linking agent [19]. Formaldehyde (together with UV treatment) is still the most common cross-linker for ChIPs (at the concentrations used it efficiently cross-links proteins to DNA). The choice of the proper cross-linker and/or cross-linking conditions (e.g. time, concentration) is crucial for the success of the ChIP. However, changes in the epitope or epitope occlusion may occur due to the cross-linking process and, according to our experience, often higher relative enrichments may be obtained with N-ChIP.

7.2.3 Choice of DNA Fragmentation Method

Before the immunopreciptation step the chromatin has to be fragmented in order to make interactions accessible and to increase the resolution of the ChIP. Two different methods are commonly used: fragmentation via sonication of the chromatin, or an enzymatic digestion with micrococcal nuclease.

Enzymatic digestion is preferentially used in combination with N-ChIP protocols, since cross-linking can affect the accessibility for micrococcal nuclease and the resulting digestion of cross-linked chromatin can be relatively inefficient. The advantage is that enzymatic digestion is possible up to mono-nucleosomes (approx. 170 base pairs) and these mono-nucleosomes can be further purified using a sucrose gradient. These pure mono-nucleosomes allow very high resolution and can be stored at $-80\,^{\circ}C$ for years. However, enzymatic digestion is not completely random as it favors certain sequences and is not digesting the entire genome equally. Thus, some genomic loci may be over- or under-represented. In contrast to this, sonication is thought to generate randomly sized DNA fragments, with no particular sequences being preferentially fragmented. Typically the fragments obtained by sonication are longer (2–3 nucleosomes), decreasing the resolution of the ChIP.

7.2.4 Choice of Antibodies

Polyclonal (or more and more monoclonal) antibodies are used to immunoprecipitate proteins together with the interacting DNA. The most crucial step for a successful ChIP experiment is the choice of the right antibody. The antibody should be fully characterized to avoid the risk of chipping artefacts. But what does it mean to be "fully characterized?" Usually, the antibodies should be purified using affinity chromotography and be tested for their ability to immunoprecipitate the epitope they are raised against under the immunoprecipitation conditions to be used in the subsequent experiment (e.g. Western blot or mass spectrometry). Especially for antibodies against modifications, it is of central importance to check the specificity of the antibodies thoroughly. Many of the antibodies raised against modified histones cross-react upon further testing with other epitopes. Our standard antibody testing procedure involves screening the antibodies in ELISA, dot blots and Western blot (using the specific and unspecific antigens as competitor) to demonstrate specific epitope recognition. Immunofluorescence, combined with antigen competition, can be used to verify that antigen recognition also occurs under more native conditions. The best test is to perform parallel ChIP experiments in wild-type cells and a cell line mutant for the target antigen, or alternatively lacking the enzyme that adds the modification, in order to show that the observed enrichment is indeed only due to the expected target antigen. This technique, however, is often not possible for histone modifications. Frequently, polyclonal antibodies immunoprecipitate better than monoclonal ones, (although several companies now offer good rabbit monoclonal antibodies) since polyclonal antibodies usually contain several populations of antibodies that recognize different epitopes (e.g. in the case that some epitopes are masked due to cross-linking). In our experience many commercially available antibodies are not thoroughly tested, and significant batch to batch variation can occur (in particular if the antibody is raised in different animals), necessitating additional batch to batch quality control.

Unfortunately, the conditions for the immunoprecipitations (especially the stringency of the binding and wash buffers) have to be determined experimentally for each antibody. These stringent conditions, on the one hand, can help to reduce the background, but on the other hand, can result in a loss of signal.

7.3
Different Variations of ChIP

Different variations of ChIP experiments are now rapidly evolving. This is mainly due to the rapid progress in the field of microarrays and next-generation sequencing that can be used for the analysis of the immunopreciptated DNA. We discuss here the most important variations of the standard ChIP protocol with a focus on ChIP-on-chip and ChIP-sequencing technologies.

7.3.1
ChIP-On-Chip

The combination of chromatin immunoprecipitation with DNA microarrays allows the genome-wide analysis of the distribution of an antigen. The immunoprecipitated DNA is quantitatively amplified, labeled and used to probe DNA microarrays. In principle ChIP-on-chip methods can be divided into two basic groups, depending on the content of the microarrays which are used: (i) microarrays/promoter tiling arrays and (ii) genome tiling arrays.

In microarrays the probes are designed with a focus on specific genomic elements such as promoters. These promoter tiling arrays have the advantage that costs are reduced, but they are biased since array design relies on known annotation. Thus, relevant regions may not be covered [20].

Genome tiling arrays have a probe content covering entire genomes. These arrays allow a global genome-wide analysis. However, experimental costs can be high as the entire genomic content has to be distributed on several arrays. In addition, from a cost perspective, one has to consider that a statistically sound basis is only achieved if experiments are done in replicates.

7.3.2
ChIPDSL

Based on ChIP-on-chip, ChIP DSL (DNA selection and ligation) is aimed at the improvement of specificity and sensitivity. It was first published by Kwon *et al.* [21]. Its advantages are the avoidance of repetitive sequences and a significantly improved sensitivity due to PCR amplification of ligated oligonucleotides in an unbiased manner, as all amplicons contain the same pair of primers. The clear disadvantage of this technology is that only predefined sequences can be measured.

7.3.3
ChIP-Sequencing

ChIP-sequencing, also known as ChIP-Seq, is the next generation of technology for chromatin research. Rather than individual DNAs, millions of DNA molecules are sequenced in parallel with next-generation sequencing methods. ChIP-Seq combines chromatin immunoprecipitation (ChIP) with deep sequencing methods provided by 454, Illumina or ABI. With these next-generation sequencing technologies (NGS), the production of several million sequence reads during each run becomes feasible. ChIP-Seq can be used to precisely and cost-effectively map global chromatin positions.

ChIP-Seq has distinct advantages over ChIP-on-chip. Compared to whole genome tiling approaches, the advantages are lower costs, minimal hands-on processing, a requirement for fewer replicate experiments and a requirement for less input material [22]. In addition ChIP-Seq offers the first real opportunity to work in a totally unbiased way, as no predefined content (as is necessary for the design of probes) is applied. This allows the discovery of unexpected genomic elements (e.g. from integrated viral genomes) and provides the ability to perform analysis in organisms where little or no genomic sequence information is available. Additional advantages are increased sensitivity and scalability of sensitivity: Increasing the number of sequencing runs performed improves the signal to noise ratio, until saturation is reached. In addition, as each DNA is sequenced without hybridization, there are no issues with cross-hybridization.

As the data obtained are sequence reads, ChIP-seq offers a rapid analysis pipeline (as long as a high-quality genome sequence is available for read mapping), as well as the potential to detect mutations in binding-site sequences which may directly support any observed changes in protein binding and gene regulation. However, the huge amount of data produced with each sequencing run (in the terabyte range) requires sophisticated methods for data handling and analysis (see Section 7.5).

7.3.4
Re-ChIP

For re-ChIP (or double ChIP), two sequential rounds of immunoprecipitations are performed using two different antibodies. Re-ChIP allows one to determine whether two antigens occur together on the same chromatin fragment or on different fragments and can be used to assemble proteins in complexes [23].

7.3.5
ChIP-Chop

ChIP-chop allows one to determine if the DNA that is associated with an antigen of interest is highly CpG-methylated. The *Escherichia coli* enzyme McrBC is used to hydrolyze ("chop") the DNA that is methylated specifically at purine/cytosine sites. Hydrolysis within the target DNA sequence prevents detection of the DNA by PCR [24].

7.3.6
Methyl-DNA Immunoprecipitation (MeDIP)

Methyl-DNA immunoprecipitation (MeDip) can be used to identify methylated CpG islands in the genome. MeDip utilizes either antibodies against methylated CpG or the MBD (CpG methylation binding) proteins for immunoprecipitation of methylated DNA. Analysis of the DNA by tiling arrays or sequencing makes DNA methylation mapping across the genome possible [25].

7.4
Analysis of ChIP Data

The generation of massive amounts of raw data by the methods described above requires advanced bioinformatic and biostatistic tools for a successful analysis. The ChIP data analysis (regardless of the wet lab method used) is comprised of three generic steps:

1. Detection and definition of enriched regions;
2. Annotation of enriched regions;
3. Analysis of enriched regions.

Currently, for many laboratories, data analysis is the limiting step. Therefore we discuss here the basic principles of ChIP data analysis (see also Figure 7.2).

7.4.1
Detection and Definition of Enriched Regions in ChIP-on-Chip Experiments

The first step in defining enriched regions in ChIP-on-chip is a statistical analysis, the aim of which is to identify probes and clusters of probes which are significantly changed compared to background. This can be done by statistical testing algorithms like T-tests, ANOVA, SAM [26], or by model-based algorithms like MAT [27]. The common data sets used for comparison are replicated probes with specific enrichment that are compared to replicates of input DNA (or unspecific enrichment) controls. Regions are then defined by a sliding window or peak-finding algorithms. The output of this analytical step is the identification of chromosomal positions with a start and end position (so called BED file format), plus a measure for significance and ratio.

7.4.2
Detection and Definition of Enriched Regions in ChIP-Seq Experiments

ChIP-Seq analysis starts with the mapping of raw read sequences to a reference genome. Mapping reads from a next-generation sequencing platform present an obvious challenge: several millions of reads have to be mapped to large (mammalian) genomes within a reasonable amount of time. Short-read mapping algorithms are

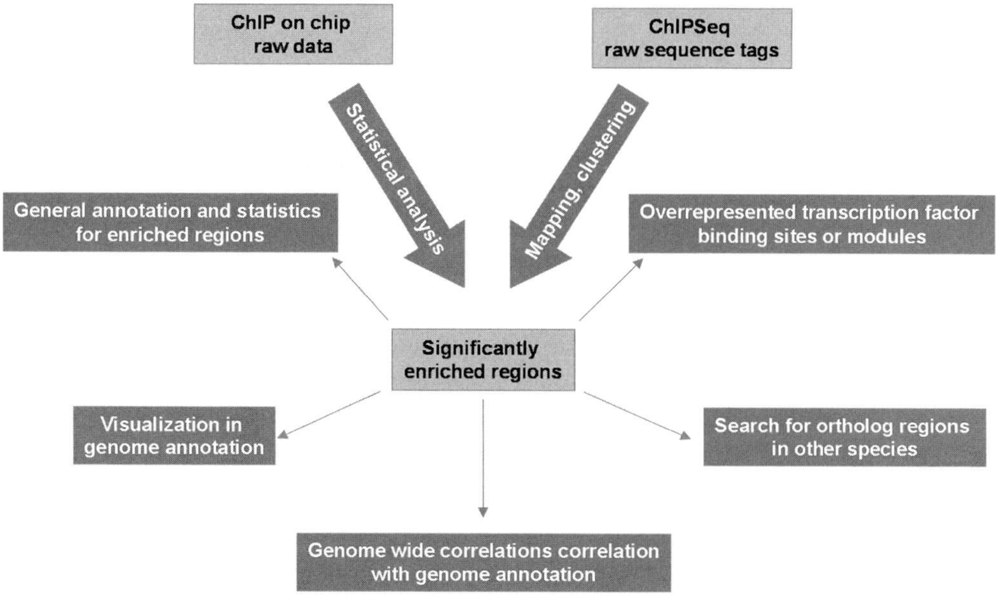

Figure 7.2 Data analysis strategies for ChIP data.

available that are effective in particular contexts. Here we describe some of the most commonly used mapping algorithms:

1. The efficient large-scale alignment of nucleotide databases (ELAND) algorithm is part of the Illumina sequencing analysis pipeline. ELAND is optimized to map very short reads, with the longest read possible being 32 bp in length, and ignores the additional bases when the sequenced reads are longer. ELAND allows maximally two mismatches between the read and the genomic background sequence, which may not be sufficient for longer reads. However, ELAND is very useful for many mapping tasks because it is extremely efficient.

2. The SXOligoSearch algorithm (by Synamatix) can quickly map reads of varying length, using different criteria, with performance varying depending on both the read length and the mapping criteria. SXOligoSearch depends on the use of the proprietary SynaBASE data structure. This data structure is a heavily compressed and annotated index for the reference genome that retains all nonredundant information. The gains in mapping speed by using such a data structure come at a cost in terms of the memory required for the SynaBASE data structure (www.synamatix.com). The extreme memory requirements of the data structure make SXOligoSearch unsuitable for use on the hardware that is available in most laboratories.

3. Recently, the RMAP algorithm was published by Smith *et al.* [28]. It efficiently uses two different mapping criteria, both based on approximate matching of the read and the reference genome.
4. The Genomatix Mining Station contains a mapping algorithm based on the Genomatix Genome Thesaurus, a library of shortest unique sub-words in the

genome. The Genome Thesaurus allows to find anchors very fast, subsequently alignments of the reads are carried out. In the mapping process, also information about SNPs can be obtained.

After the mapping to a reference genome, a clustering step is performed to define regions with a higher read density. The simplest way is to apply a sliding window. Recently, more sophisticated model-based algorithms for clustering have became available (http://www.liulab.dfci.harvard.edu/MACS/). The output of ChIP-Seq is also chromosomal position, for example in a BED file format that can be directly compared to ChIP-on-chip data.

Finally, if no reference genome is available, one can try to assemble the raw read sequences to regions of enrichment. A combination of Sanger sequencing and next-generation sequencing may be helpful here.

7.4.3
Annotation of Enriched Regions

The first step towards a biological interpretation of data is the data visualization. For this purpose raw reads, as well as the output files with the chromosomal positions of the enriched clusters (BED files) can be uploaded into current genome annotations. Public domain genome annotations like the genome browsers of UCSC (http:www.genome.ucsc.edu/) and Ensembl (http://www.ensembl.org/index.html), as well as commercial solutions like ElDorado (http://www.genomatix.de/products/ElDorado/) can be used for data upload. For regions which are not directly overlapping with annotated genomic regions, the next upstream and downstream elements can be searched and a distance can be assigned on the plus and minus strand. Additional information that can be obtained includes looking for phylogenetic conservation of regions of interest. To annotate the regions, public domain as well as commercial software packages are available. The Cis regulatory annotation system (CEAS) package is available at http://www.ceas.cbi.pku.edu.cn/. RegionMiner can be obtained at http://www.genomatix.de/regionminer. The correlation with available annotation allows a general annotation plus basic statistics (for the localization) of the enriched regions. In addition, the knowledge of overlapping or closest annotation (loci) opens new possibilities for subsequent pathway mining.

7.4.4
Analysis of Enriched Regions

The logical next step following the annotation of the enriched regions is to look deeper into the regions from a sequence perspective. Several options are possible depending on the type of ChIP. If the immunoprecipitation was performed against a certain transcription factor (TF), the enriched sequence can be scanned for the sequence binding motif of this TF. A calculation determining if the specific transcription factor binding site (TFBS) is overrepresented in the enriched region compared to the entire genomic background or a specific genomic element (e.g. promoters) is possible. Additionally, co-occurring binding motifs which are found in close proximity to the motif of interest can be identified and their degree of representation can be evaluated.

If the immunoprecipitation was performed against a chromatin binding factor with an as yet unknown binding motif, enriched sequences can be used to retrieve the binding motif. In the same way, previously known binding motifs can be modified.

7.5 Data Analysis Examples

Currently, many different possibilities for data analysis are available. Common data analysis strategies are illustrated by two examples, one based on ChIP-on–chip and the other on ChIP-Seq; and we discuss them here in more detail. Both datasets are publicly available:

1. ChIP-on-chip data analysis based on estrogen receptor and RNAPolII enrichments in MCF7 cells [20].
2. ChIP-Seq of histone modifications correlated with DNAse Seq of open chromatin in CD4 cells [8, 29].

Example 1: Transcription Factor Specific ChIP

The data for this example was derived from the supplementary material of the estrogen receptor (ER) ChIP-on-chip publication of Carroll *et al.* [20]. The dataset consists of three replicates of specific enrichments for the estrogen receptor alpha and RNA Polymerase II versus input controls. All three replicates were performed on the Affymetrix human tiling 1.0 microarrays (14-chip set).

- *Task:* Statistical analysis for regions significantly enriched in estrogen receptor binding.
- *Method:* As the first step in the data analysis strategy, a statistical analysis is performed. This can be done with different programs (e.g. MAT or ChipInspector [30]).
- *Result:* If the analysis is performed with ChipInspector with a false discovery rate (FDR) of 1% and a sliding window of 3 probes and a window of 300 bp, 4708 enriched regions are obtained. MAT, after BLAT analysis (to eliminate redundant sequences), identifies a final set of 3665 unique estrogen receptor binding sites and 3629 unique RNA Pol II binding sites using a threshold FDR of 1%. Figure 7.3 shows the correlation between the two methods. Over 70% of regions are overlapping. The significant regions are provided in a BED file format.
- *Task:* General annotation of significantly enriched regions.
- *Method:* For this task the enriched regions are mapped onto the genome under study and correlated with the available genome annotation using the program RegionMiner With this method, it is possible to determine if enriched regions

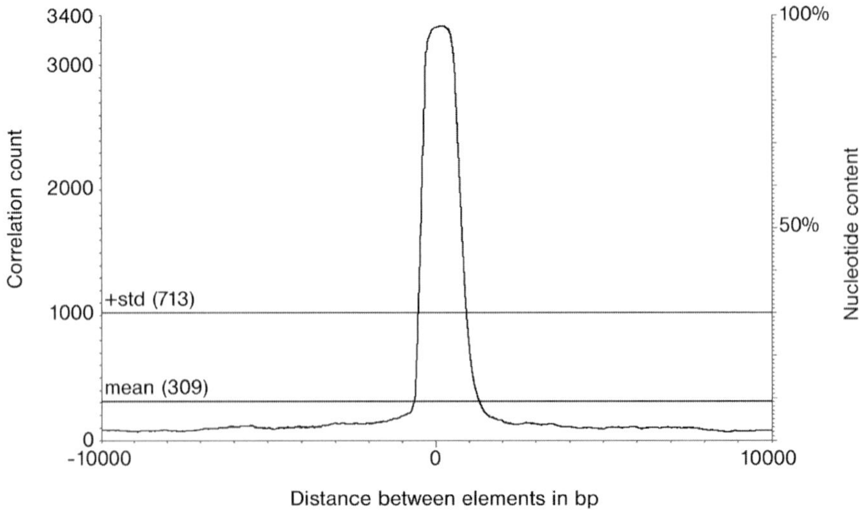

Figure 7.3 Correlation between MAT and ChipInsector results. All enriched regions identified by MAT are aligned at the zero position and correlated by all enriched regions identified by ChipInspector within a window of −10 000 to +10 000 bp. The curve shows the correlation histogram. The two lines give the mean count (309) and the standard deviation of counts (713) in the entire window.

overlap with annotated regions or, if not, what is the next upstream and downsteam annotation on the plus and minus strand of the genome.

- *Results:* Table 7.1 shows the general statistic of the annotation for the enriched regions. It is obvious that only a small percentage of the ER binding occurs within known promoter regions.
- *Task:* Visualization in the genome annotation.
- *Method:* BED files can be uploaded into current genome browsers such as the UCSC (http://www.genome.ucsc.edu/), Ensembl (www.ensembl.org), or ElDorado (http://www.genomatix.de/ElDorado) genome browsers.
- *Result:* Figure 7.4 shows region 582 (as an example) and the flanking genomic regions in ElDorado.
- *Task:* Identification of overrepresented transcription factor binding sites (TFBS and modules of TFBS on sequence level).
- *Method:* To evaluate if certain TFBS are overrepresented compared with the entire genomic background, or compared to promoter sequence background. It is necessary to have a library of binding site descriptions (e.g. TRANSFAC (http://www.biobase-international.com/pages/index.php?id=transfacdatabases) or MatBase (http://www.genomatix.de/matbase) and to be able to count the number of binding sites in the enriched regions and the entire genome. It is

Table 7.1 Annotation and general statistics of enriched regions.

Statistics of Regions

4708 regions given in input

Number of input regions	Percentage input regions	Description
2622	55.69%	regions overlap with at least one locus
2086	44.31%	regions overlap with intergenic regions
296	6.29%	regions overlap with at least one promoter
428	9.09%	regions overlap with at least one transcriptional start region (TSR)
36	0.76%	regions overlap with at least one repeat
286	6.07%	regions overlap with exon 1
135	2.87%	regions overlap with exon 2
85	1.81%	regions overlap with exon 3
78	1.66%	regions overlap with exon 4
63	1.34%	regions overlap with exon 5
52	1.10%	regions overlap with exon 6
60	1.27%	regions overlap with exon 7
1110	23.58%	regions overlap with intron 1
703	14.93%	regions overlap with intron 2
473	10.05%	regions overlap with intron 3
352	7.48%	regions overlap with intron 4
250	5.31%	regions overlap with intron 5
216	4.59%	regions overlap with intron 6
211	4.48%	regions overlap with intron 7

then possible to calculate a random expectation value which gives the probability for a binding site per basepair. This allows one to calculate not only the degree of representation of a TFBS in an enriched sequence, but also a p-value or z-score. These calculations can be done with CEAS or RegionMiner.

- *Result:* Transcription factor binding sites for the ER-enriched regions (calculated with RegionMiner and CEAS; Tables 7.2 and 7.3).

From the RegionMiner analysis it is clear that estrogen receptor elements (EREs) are strongly overrepresented in enriched regions. ER is found at 2116 sequences. The random expectation would be only 825 matches. This results in

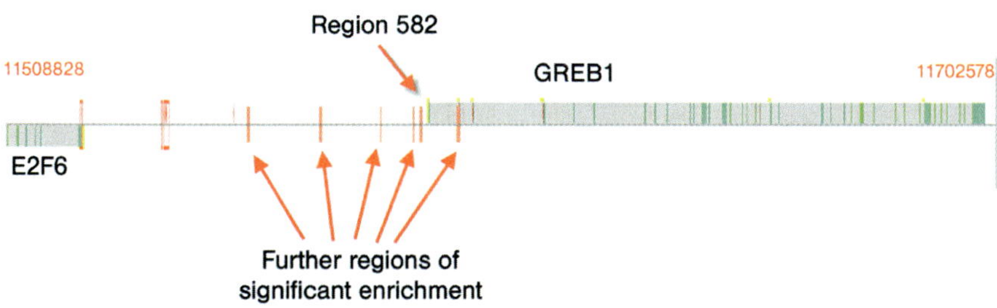

Figure 7.4 Visualization of enrichment. Color code: yellow = promoter; green = exon; gray = primary transcript; orange = enriched region; red = TSS; red box = promoter prediction.

Table 7.2 Overrepresentation of TFBS motifs from RegionMiner ranked by genome wide z-scores.

Listing of all TF Matrices

TF Matrices	#Sequences	#Matches	Expected (genome) ± Std.dev.	Overrepresentation (genome)	Z-Score (genome)	Expected (promoters) ± Std.dev.	Overrepresentation (promoters)	Z-Score (promoters)	Promoter association
V$ER.02	2116	3202	825.29±28.73	3.88	82.72	879.26±29.65	3.64	78.32	no
V$ER.01	2351	3392	1118.35±33.44	3.03	67.98	1040.18±32.25	3.26	72.91	no
V$AP2.02	1847	2925	1130.29±33.62	2.59	53.37	2984.75±54.62	0.98	-1.10	yes
V$AP2.01	1687	2348	979.56±31.30	2.40	43.71	3083.38±55.52	0.76	-13.26	yes
V$CTCF.01	1308	2285	1059.62±32.55	2.16	37.63	9635.67±98.09	0.24	-74.94	yes
V$ZNF76_143.01	1924	2862	1375.82±37.09	2.08	40.06	4260.13±65.25	0.67	-21.44	yes
V$HIC1.01	1479	2013	971.05±31.16	2.07	33.42	3121.73±55.86	0.64	-19.86	yes
V$SP1.01	2029	3950	1928.35±43.91	2.05	46.03	12875.87±113.36	0.31	-78.74	yes
V$HEN1.02	1051	1856	908.23±30.13	2.04	31.43	2205.93±46.96	0.84	-7.46	yes
V$SP1.02	1344	2190	1082.48±32.90	2.02	33.65	10568.77±102.72	0.21	-81.57	yes
V$NRSE.01	1056	1385	685.43±26.18	2.02	26.70	4011.72±63.32	0.35	-41.49	yes
V$ZF9.01	1753	3006	1547.99±39.34	1.94	37.05	10700.99±103.36	0.28	-74.45	yes
V$GC.01	2218	4324	2241.80±47.34	1.93	43.97	12002.91±109.46	0.36	-70.16	yes
V$HEN1.01	1062	1868	970.98±31.16	1.92	28.77	2071.03±45.50	0.90	-4.47	yes
V$AP1.03	2004	4305	2252.33±47.45	1.91	43.25	2100.60±45.83	2.05	48.09	no
V$OLF1.02	2374	3793	1996.07±44.67	1.90	40.21	4513.10±67.16	0.84	-10.73	yes
V$EGR1.02	1243	1941	1019.19±31.92	1.90	28.86	10402.09±101.91	0.19	-83.03	yes
V$PAX5.01	2150	3156	1700.73±41.23	1.86	35.28	4040.95±63.55	0.78	-13.93	yes
V$SP2.01	1948	2883	1565.63±39.56	1.84	33.29	6476.66±80.44	0.45	-44.68	yes
V$MAZR.01	2086	4105	2235.97±47.28	1.84	39.52	9876.37±99.31	0.42	-58.12	yes
V$MYOGENIN.02	1625	2279	1252.05±35.38	1.82	29.01	2215.92±47.07	1.03	1.33	no

Table 7.3 Overrepresentation of TFBS motifs from CEAS ranked by p-value.

Motif Enrichment Analysis

Motif	Hits	Fold Change	pValue	Sequence	Logo
M00959.ER	2317	2.4474	3.867398E-309	download	download
M00191.ER	1095	3.8689086	1.229611E-294	download	download
AP2alpha	4132	1.7973605	2.268544E-259	download	download
M00986.Churchill	6035	1.582923	9.400205E-242	download	download
M00470.AP-2gamma	2599	1.9283794	5.448819E-201	download	download
M00428.E2F-1	4909	1.5819421	1.238175E-196	download	download
M00174.AP-1	4406	1.5053428	3.394483E-143	download	download
M00716.ZF5	3744	1.5235138	1.066206E-128	download	download
M00517.AP-1	2434	1.6804174	1.617692E-123	download	download
M00111.CF1	1828	1.7906728	7.792856E-115	download	download
M00803.E2F	2376	1.6426023	3.070259E-111	download	download
M00199.AP-1	1833	1.728383	6.426613E-103	download	download
M00172.AP-1	2739	1.5369053	2.043652E-98	download	download
M00008.Sp1	2001	1.6608882	7.099554E-98	download	download
M00431.E2F-1	1892	1.6366961	6.648989E-88	download	download
M01034.Ebox	2218	1.517586	6.553403E-76	download	download
M00193.NF-1	1716	1.5707296	2.441923E-68	download	download
M00188.AP-1	1884	1.505885	1.152274E-62	download	download
SP1	1458	1.5960401	3.683946E-62	download	download
M00490.Bach2	590	2.0965207	2.469983E-58	download	download
M00511.ERR	1001	1.736152	4.292337E-58	download	download
RORalfa-1	768	1.8536465	7.6337E-55	download	download
Ahr-ARNT	1216	1.5944847	5.055873E-52	download	download
M00187.USF	1281	1.5729676	7.073158E-52	download	download
M00796.USF	1070	1.6266023	1.385096E-49	download	download

an over-representation of 3.88 with a z-score of 82.72. CEAS results can be seen in Table 7.3.

Additionally, we can now address the question as to which other factors are co-occurring with the most overrepresented ER-binding motif (ERE family). This can be done by setting the ERE family as a mandatory factor. RegionMiner then searches for which TFBSs occur in proximity to the EREs and whether the motif of two TFBS (ERE + X) is also overrepresented. (Table 7.4) The module representation analysis show on the first three positions the co-occurrence of AP1, RXR and FKHD (forkhead domain) factors. The co-localization of ERE and FKHD is experimentally verified [31].

Example 2: Data Analysis for Epigenetic Modifications Based on ChIP-Seq

The data for this example is derived from the publication of Barski *et al.* [8]: "*High-resolution profiling of histone methylations in the human genome*" [8] and Boyle *et al.* [29]: "*High-resolution mapping and characterization of open chromatin across the genome*" [29]. Both datasets were done on CD4 cells. The raw sequence reads were mapped and clustered according to a proprietary Genomatix NGS protocol. 36 sequence tags in a 100 bp window were used as the significance threshold for the clustering of the mapped reads.

Table 7.4 Overrepresentation of TFBS family modules. ERE is set as mandatory factor.

Listing of all Modules with V$EREF

Modules with V$EREF	#Sequences	#Matches	Expected (genome) ± Std.dev.	Overrepresentation (genome)	Z-Score (genome)	Expected (promoters) ± Std.dev.	Overrepresentation (promoters)	Z-Score (promoters)	Promoter association
V$AP1R-V$EREF	543	1071	158.76±12.60	6.75	72.36	155.56±12.47	6.88	73.36	no
V$EREF-V$RXRF	888	1765	375.85±19.38	4.70	71.64	390.42±19.76	4.52	69.55	no
V$EREF-V$FKHD	664	1229	360.75±18.99	3.41	45.69	222.01±14.90	5.54	67.55	no
V$EREF-V$NR2F	728	1333	261.27±16.16	5.10	66.28	264.87±16.27	5.03	65.61	no
V$EREF-V$HOXF	753	1519	581.61±24.11	2.61	38.85	371.81±19.28	4.09	59.47	no
V$EREF-V$GATA	516	888	261.60±16.17	3.39	38.70	179.42±13.39	4.95	52.86	no
V$EREF-V$NKXH	573	1193	399.04±19.97	2.99	39.73	291.17±17.06	4.10	52.83	no
V$EREF-V$PERO	405	662	109.14±10.45	6.07	52.87	112.86±10.62	5.87	51.65	no
V$EREF-V$PARF	437	863	280.19±16.74	3.08	34.79	180.80±13.45	4.77	50.70	no
V$AP1F-V$EREF	224	485	87.75±9.37	5.53	42.35	68.55±8.28	7.07	50.24	no
V$EREF-V$SORY	539	928	308.44±17.56	3.01	35.25	207.45±14.40	4.47	50.00	no
V$EREF-V$RORA	437	714	165.79±12.88	4.31	42.54	135.04±11.62	5.29	49.78	no
V$EREF-V$OCT1	516	882	313.64±17.71	2.81	32.07	196.12±14.00	4.50	48.94	no

- *Task:* Global correlation of histone modification with genomic elements, for example, the correlation of H3K4me3 histone methylation with transcription start regions (TSR).
- *Method:* Use RegionMiner to compare the annotated TSR with the modifications in a window of −10 000 to +10 000 bp around the enriched regions (Figure 7.5).
- *Result:* There are two distinct peaks of tri methyl H3K4 enrichments around the TSR (which are aligned at the zero position) with a most frequent distance of 176 bp, indicating that H3K4tri-methylation occurs at a preferred distance to the TSR.
- *Task:* Correlation between several datasets.
- *Method:* Instead of comparing one ChIP dataset with pre-existing annotation, two or more ChIP datasets can be compared using RegionMiner. In this case we show

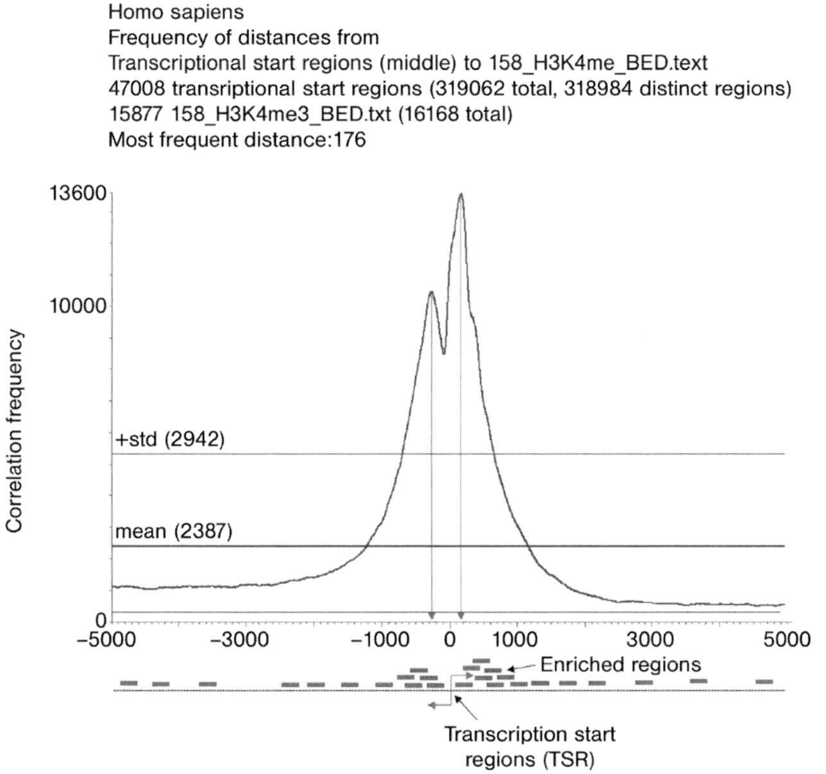

Figure 7.5 Correlation of the H3K4me3 enriched regions with TSR. All transcription start regions are aligned at the zero position and correlated with the regions enriched in H3K4me3. The two lines give the mean count (2387) and the standard deviation of counts (2942) in the entire window. The gray bars symbolize the enriched regions relative to the TSR.

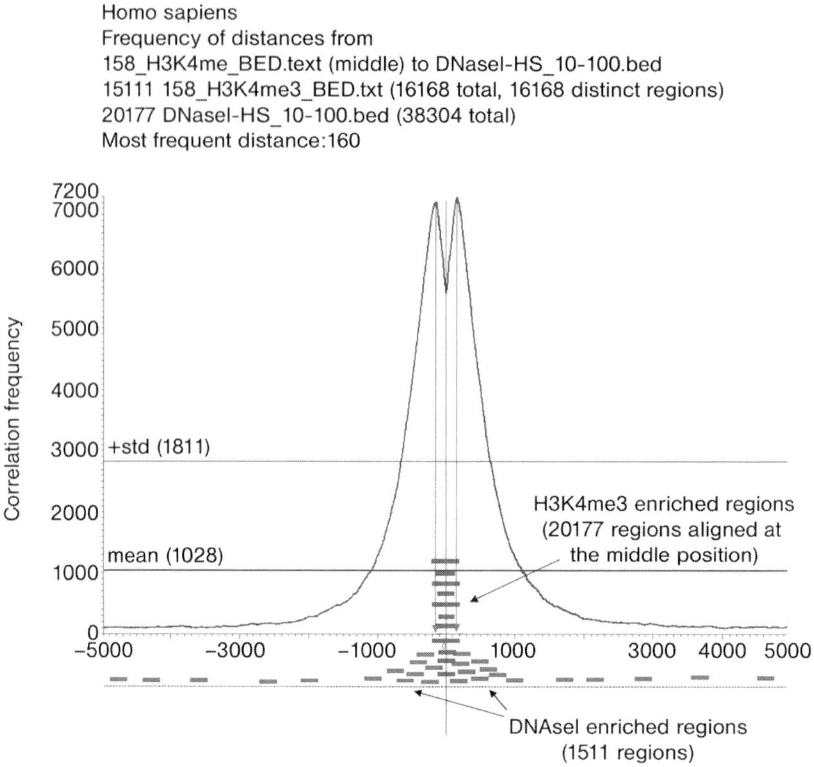

Figure 7.6 Correlation of open chromatin IP (DNaseI hypersensitivity data) with H3K4me3 enrichment. All H3K4me3 enriched regions (symbolized as gray bars) are aligned at the zero position and correlated with the open chromatin regions from the DNaseI hypersensitivity screen (symbolized as dark-gray bars). The two lines give the mean count (1028) and the standard deviation of counts (1811) in the entire window.

the comparison of the H3K4me3 enrichments with the open chromatin data (DNAse Seq) from Boyle *et al.* [29] (Figure 7.6).

- *Results:* Two distinct peaks for the correlation of H3K4me3 enrichment and DNAse accessibility are obtained with a most frequent distance of 160 bp, indicating that open chromatin occurs with a specific distance of approximately 160 bp to regions with H3K4me3 methylation. Two peaks are obtained because the measurement procedure of the open chromatin data and the histone modifications are not strand-specific.

7.6 The Future of ChIP

Currently the number of ChIP grade antibodies available is rapidly increasing, allowing the analysis of more and more new antigens. The use of alternative, more specific and faster cross-linking reagents, along with the automation of the ChIP protocol will enable us to improve the temporal resolution in response to specific signals. At the moment, array-based profiling approaches are getting more and more substituted by next-generation sequencing approaches. Recent and future advances in direct sequencing of immunoprecipitated DNA will significantly increase the resolution of genome-wide analyses and will make this method widely accessible. In the next few years, comprehensive reference maps will be available that will help to interpret and integrate the obtained results. The immense amount of data generated by deep sequencing will require new bioinformatics and, increasingly, biostatistic tools. One current shortfall is the fact that repeated genomic regions cannot be analyzed by ChIP sequencing, or by ChIP-on-chip. To solve this issue, further improvements in the ChIP protocols and the data analysis will be necessary. For the future, a combination of ChIP and mass spectrometry analysis will enable not only the analysis of single antigens, but also the identification of protein complexes bound to specific DNA sequences. One might speculate that at some point new, innovative, non-invasive imaging technologies might replace ChIP, but until then, ChIP will remain the most powerful technique available for the study of protein interactions with DNA.

References

1 Kouzarides, T. (2007) Chromatin modifications and their function. *Cell*, **128** (4), 693–705.

2 Turner, B.M. (1993) Decoding the nucleosome. *Cell*, **75** (1), 5–8.

3 Strahl, B.D. and Allis, C.D. (2000) The language of covalent histone modifications. *Nature*, **403** (6765), 41–45.

4 Turner, B.M. (2007) Defining an epigenetic code. *Nature Cell Biology*, **9** (1), 2–6.

5 Davie, J.R. and Candido, E.P. (1978) Acetylated histone H4 is preferentially associated with template-active chromatin. *Proceedings of the National Academy of Sciences of the United States of America*, **75** (8), 3574–3577.

6 Litt, M.D., Simpson, M., Gaszner, M., Allis, C.D. and Felsenfeld, G. (2001) Correlation between histone lysine methylation and developmental changes at the chicken beta-globin locus. *Science*, **293** (5539), 2453–2455.

7 The Encode Project Consortium (2007) Identification and analysis of functional elements in 1% of the human genome by the ENCODE pilot project. *Nature*, **447**, 799–816.

8 Barski, A., Cuddapah, S., Cui, K., Roh, T.Y., Schones, D.E., Wang, Z., Wei, G., Chepelev, I. and Zhao, K. (2007) High-resolution profiling of histone methylations in the human genome. *Cell*, **129** (4), 823–837.

9 Bernstein, B.E., Meissner, A. and Lander, E.S. (2007) The mammalian epigenome. *Cell*, **128** (4), 669–681.

10 Foster, S.L., Hargreaves, D.C. and Medzhitov, R. (2007) Gene-specific control of inflammation by TLR-induced chromatin modifications. *Nature*, **447**, 972–978.

11 Azuara, V., Perry, P., Sauer, S., Spivakov, M., Jorgensen, H.F., John, R.M., Gouti, M., Casanova, M., Warnes, G., Merkenschlager, M. and Fisher, A.G. (2006) Chromatin signatures of pluripotent cell lines. *Nature Cell Biology*, **8** (5), 532–538.

12 Bernstein, B.E., Mikkelsen, T.S., Xie, X., Kamal, M., Huebert, D.J., Cuff, J., Fry, B.,

Meissner, A., Wernig, M., Plath, K., Jaenisch, R., Wagschal, A., Feil, R., Schreiber, S.L. and Lander, E.S. (2006) A bivalent chromatin structure marks key developmental genes in embryonic stem cells. *Cell*, **125** (2), 315–326.

13 Lee, T.I., Jenner, R.G., Boyer, L.A., Guenther, M.G., Levine, S.S., Kumar, R.M., Chevalier, B., Johnstone, S.E., Cole, M.F., Isono, K., Koseki, H., Fuchikami, T., Abe, K., Murray, H.L., Zucker, J.P., Yuan, B., Bell, G.W., Herbolsheimer, E., Hannett, N.M., Sun, K., Odom, D.T., Otte, A.P., Volkert, T.L., Bartel, D.P., Melton, D.A., Gifford, D.K., Jaenisch, R. and Young, R.A. (2006) Control of developmental regulators by Polycomb in human embryonic stem cells. *Cell*, **125** (2), 301–313.

14 Dietz, S.C. and Carroll, J.S. (2008) Interrogating the genome to understand oestrogen-receptor-mediated transcription. *Expert Rev Mol Med*, 10.1017/S1462399408000653.

15 Gilmour, D.S. and Lis, J.T. (1985) In vivo interactions of RNA polymerase II with genes of Drosophila melanogaster. *Molecular and Cellular Biology*, **5**, 2009–2018.

16 Gilmour, D.S., Pflugfelder, G., Wang, J.C. and Lis, J.T. (1986) Topoisomerase I interacts with transcribed regions in Drosophila cells. *Cell*, **44**, 401–407.

17 Hebbes, T.R., Thorne, A.W. and Crane-Robinson, C. (1988) A direct link between core histone acetylation and transcriptionally active chromatin. *The EMBO Journal*, **7**, 1395–1402.

18 O'Neill, L.P. and Turner, B.M. (2003) Immunoprecipitation of native chromatin: NChIP. *Methods (San Diego, Calif)*, **31**, 76–82.

19 Orlando, V. and Paro, R. (1993) Mapping Polycomb-repressed domains in the bithorax complex using in vivo formaldehyde cross-linked chromatin. *Cell*, **75**, 1187–1198.

20 Carroll, J.S., Meyer, C.A., Song, J., Li, W., Geistlinger, T.R., Eeckhoute, J., Brodsky, A.S., Krasnickas Keeton, E., Fertuck, K.C., Hall, G.F., Wang, Q., Bekiranov, W., Sementchenko, V., Fox, E.A., Silver, P.A., Gingeras, T.R., Liu, X.S. and Brown, M. (2006) Genome.wide analysis of estrogen receptor binding sites. *Nature Genetics*, **38**, 1289–1297.

21 Kwon, Y.S., Garcia-Bassets, I., Hutt, K.R., Cheng, C.S., Jin, M., Liu, D., Benner, C., Wang, D., Ye, Z., Bibikova, M., Fan, J.B., Duan, L., Glass, C.K., Rosenfeld, M.G. and Fu, X.D. (2007) Sensitive ChIP-DSL technology reveals an extensive estrogen receptor alpha-binding program on human gene promoters. *Proceedings of the National Academy of Sciences*, **104**, 4852–4857.

22 Mardis, E.R. (2007) ChIP-seq: welcome to the new frontier. *Nature Methods*, **4**, 613–614.

23 Metivier, R., Penot, G., Hubner, M.R., Reid, G., Brand, H., Kos, M. and Gannon, F. (2003) Estrogen receptor-alpha directs ordered, cyclical, and combinatorial recruitment of cofactors on a natural target promoter. *Cell*, **115**, 751–763.

24 Lawrence, R.J., Earley, K., Pontes, O., Silva, M., Chen, Z.J., Neves, N., Viegas, W. and Pikaard, C.S. (2004) A concerted DNA methylation/histone methylation switch regulates rRNA gene dosage control and nucleolar dominance. *Molecular Cell*, **13**, 599–609.

25 Fraga, M.F., Ballestar, E., Montoya, G., Taysavang, P., Wade, P.A. and Esteller, M. (2003) The affinity of different MBD proteins for a specific methylated locus depends on their intrinsic binding properties. *Nucleic Acids Research*, **31**, 1765–1774.

26 Cui, X. and Churchill, G.A. (2003) Statistical tests for differential expression in cDNA microarray experiments. *Genome Biology*, **4**, 210.

27 Johnson, W.E., Li, W., Meyer, C.A., Gottardo, R., Carroll, J.S., Brown, M. and Liu, X.S. (2006) Model-based analysis of tiling-arrays for ChIP-chip. *PNAS*, **103**, 12457–12462.

28 Smith, A.D., Xuan, Z. and Zhang, M.Q. (2008) Using quality scores and longer reads improves accuracy of Solexa read mapping. *BMC Bioinformatics*, **9**.

29 Boyle, A.P., Davis, S., Shulha, H.P., Meltzer, P., Margulies, E.H., Weng, Z., Furey, T.S. and Crawford, G.E. (2008) High-resolution mapping and characterization of open chromatin across the genome. *Cell*, **132**, 311–322.

30 Gehrig, A., Langmann, T., Horling, F., Janssen, A., Bonin, M., Walter, M., Poths, S. and Weber, B.H. (2007) Genome-wide expression profiling of the retinoschisin-deficient retina in early postnatal mouse development. *Ophthalmology and Vision Science*, **42**, 891–900.

31 Lupien, M., Eeckhoute, J., Meyer, C.A., Wang, Q., Zhang, Y., Li, W., Carroll, J.S., Liu, X.S. and Brown, M. (2008) FoxA1 translates epigenetic signatures into enhancer driven lineage-specific transcription. *Cell*, **132** (6), 958–970.

Part Two
Epigenetic Target Classes and Inhibitor Development

Epigenetic Targets in Drug Discovery. Edited by Wolfgang Sippl and Manfred Jung

ISBN: 978-3-527-32355-5

8
DNA Methyltransferase Inhibitors

Wolfgang Sippl and Manfred Jung

8.1
Introduction

The major two biochemical pathways of epigenetic regulation of transcription are DNA methylation and posttranslational modifications of amino acid side-chains in histones. The latter actually comprise a whole set of different biochemical modifications, such as reversible acetylation of lysines, methylation of arginines and lysines, phosphorylation, but also large molecule modifications such as sumoylation or ubiquitinylation. Those histone modifications interact with each other and constitute a pattern of alterations in the chromatin structure, the so-called histone code. Multiple enzymes are involved and the same modification on different amino acids in the histone proteins may lead to opposing effects of transcription [1]. The various modifications on histones and their biological consequences are outlined in other chapters in this book. DNA methylation refers to the enzymatic addition of a methyl group to nucleotide bases. There are three known types of base methylation: (i) adenine can be modified at the N-6 position (in bacteria, also in most eukaryotes) and cytosine can be modified (ii) at the N-4 position (mostly thermophilic bacteria) and (iii) at the C-5 position. The latter modification is the most common form of DNA alteration among all organisms [2]. Cytosine is methylated by DNA nucleotide methyltransferases (DNMTs) to 5-methylcytosine. The differences in biological significance of various patterns of methylation result from the stretch of DNA where the methylation takes place. Usually methylation of the promoter regions of genes results in repression of transcription. For DNMTs the first inhibitors are already approved for clinical use but there is much less work published that deals with novel inhibitors or structure–activity relationships [3], as compared to other epigenetic modulators, for example histone deacetylases.

8.2
DNA Methylation

DNMTs catalyze the methylation of cytosines located 5′ to a guanosine as part of a CpG dinucleotide (CpG) in DNA to 5-methylcytosines using S-adenosyl methionine

Epigenetic Targets in Drug Discovery. Edited by Wolfgang Sippl and Manfred Jung

ISBN: 978-3-527-32355-5

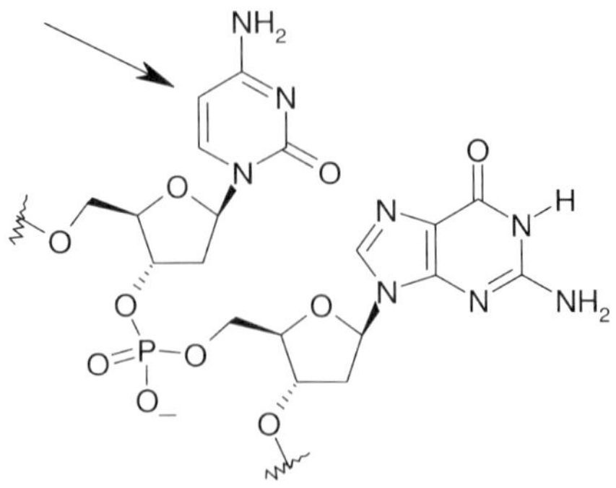

Figure 8.1 CpG dinucleotide as part of the DNA. The arrow indicates the methylation site.

(SAM) as the methyl donor (Figure 8.1) [2, 4]. Therefore, DNA actually contains five and not only four different bases (i.e. adenine, thymine, guanine, cytosine, 5-methylcytosine). At first this seems to be a contradiction to the conserved genetic code and the definition of epigenetics. In a narrower sense, epigenetics is regarded as "somatically inherited changes in gene expression that occur without a change in the genetic code" [5]. In the case of DNA methylation, the biochemical modification occurs directly on the DNA but the base pairing of cytosine to the guanine on the complementary DNA strand is not altered upon methylation (Figure 8.2) and thus the genetic code is preserved. Frequently, longer hypermethylated stretches of CpG sequences are observed which are recognized by proteins with methyl-CpG-binding domain proteins (MBDs) which mediate epigenetic regulation (see below) [6]. Single 5-methylcytosines in DNA that are not complexed by proteins are prone to hydrolysis to thymines, leading to a 5-methyl-C to A transition (Figure 8.3) [7]. This may occur spontaneously but is also catalyzed by DNA deaminases from the Aid/Apobec family [8]. This carries the risk of point mutation rates, but may be

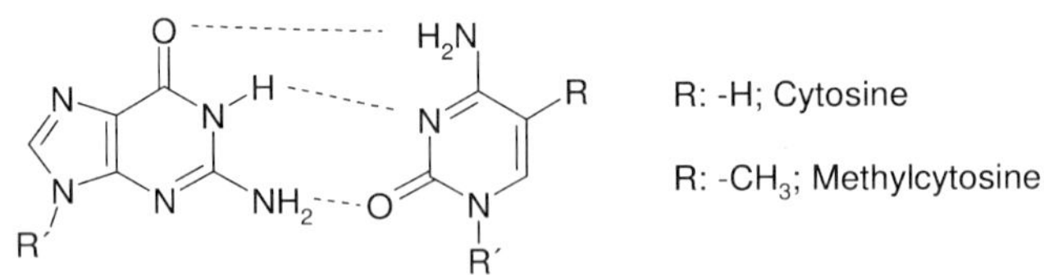

Figure 8.2 Base pairing of cytosine or methylcytosine with guanine in DNA. R′: Phosphodeoxyribose of the DNA backbone.

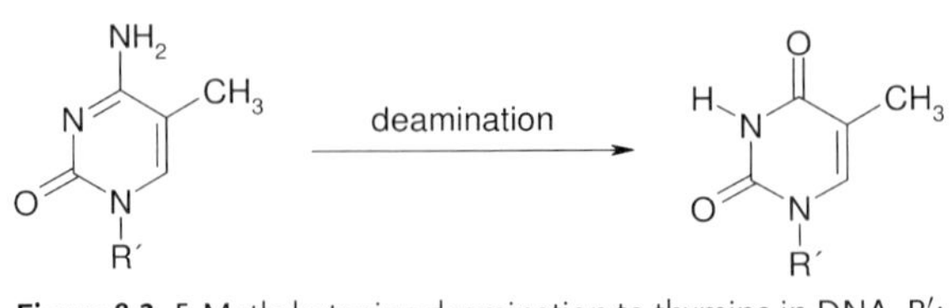

Figure 8.3 5-Methylcytosine deamination to thymine in DNA. R′: Phosphodesoxyribose of the DNA backbone.

beneficial. For example it plays a role in "hypermutations" of immunoglobulin loci which lead to an expansion of the armory of antigen receptors, hence strengthening the immune system [9].

Altogether about 70–80% of CpG sites are methylated [10–12]. CpG dinucleotides are found in short DNA regions with a length of about 0.5–4.0 kb, which are known as CpG islands and which are located in the proximal promoter regions of approximately half of the genes in our genome. These CpG islands represent about 1–2% of the total genome and contain more than half of the unmethylated CpG sites [10, 12–14]. High degrees of methylated sequences can be found in satellite DNA, repetitive elements, nonrepetitive intergenic DNA and exons of genes [15]. So far, no rigorous proof for an enzyme with 5-methylcytosine demethylating ability in humans has been obtained and the discussion continues whether such an activity exists [16], despite recent developments in the field [17, 18] (see also below).

8.3 DNA Methyltransferases

So far, four members of DNMTs are known in mammals: DNMT1, DNMT2, DNMT3A and the related DNMT3B [19–21]. The protein DNMT3L shows high sequence similarity with DNMT3A but it lacks a conserved segment in the C-terminal domain required for methyltransferase activity. Therefore, DNMT3L is not an active methyltransferase but has dual functions of binding the histone tail as well as activating DNMT3A. Due to homology it is therefore sometimes counted as a fifth DNMT protein in humans, belonging to the DNMT3 family [22]. DNMT3L was found to stabilize the conformation of the active-site loop of DNMT3A. Whereas DNA methylation in early embryogenesis is carried out by the *de novo* methylases DNMT3A and DNMT3B, the methylation level in differentiated cell is regulated by DNMT1. Therefore, DNMT1 is also called maintenance methyltransferase. DNMT1 was the first cytosine methyltransferase identified and is closely associated with the DNA replication process. It transfers the DNA methylation patterns from the parent strand to the newly synthesized strand. DNMT2 is a relative small protein (391 amino acids) and shows all the sequence and structural characteristics of the other DNMTs, except for the large N-terminal domain present in DNMT1 and DNMT3. Despite the sequence and structural similarity between DNMT2 and the other DNMTs, DNMT2 is not necessary for DNA methylation *in vivo*. It has been shown that genomic methylation level is not measurably altered in DNMT2-deficient mouse embryonic stem cells [19]. Recently, it was reported that human DNMT2 methylates cytosine 38 in the anticodon loop of aspartic acid transfer RNA [23].

Mammalian DNMTs (beside the enigmatic DNMT2) are built from two domains: the N-terminal regulatory domain and the C-terminal domain which bears the catalytic site. DNMTs possess ten conserved, characteristic sequence motifs; six of which are present in nearly all cytosine methyltransferases from bacteria through plants to mammals [24]. The different motifs are described regarding their function [25]: motifs I–III form the cofactor binding pocket, motif IV provides the cysteine that forms the thiolate initiating the methyl group transfer, motifs VI, VIII, X compose the substrate binding site and motifs V, VII form the target recognition domain.

The first methyltransferases that could be crystallized were prokaryotic enzymes (e.g. the bacterial cytosine methyltransferases M.HhaI, M.HaeIII) which are simpler in structure and less complex than the mammalian DNMT family members DNMT1 and DNMT3. Later, crystal structures were also reported for DNMT2 and DNMT3A, whereas no X-ray diffraction data have been derived so far for DNMT1 [26]. Three-dimensional structures are available for the PWWP domain of DNMT3B [27], intact DNMT3L in complex with a histone H3 amino-tail peptide [28] and a complex between the C-terminal domains of DNMT3A and DNMT3L [29]. Since all known DNA methyltransferases use SAM as the methyl donor, the active site shows high structural similarity; and it is suggested on the basis of a homology model of DNMT1 [30] that this enzyme has the same architecture of the binding site. The crystal structures of DNMT2, DNMT3 and the bacterial cytosine methyltransferases are essentially superimposable over the C-terminal domain including the catalytic site. The binding pockets show high structural conservation of residues interacting with deoxycytidine and the SAM cofactor (Figure 8.4(a)).

The crystal structure of the DNMT3A-DNMT3L complex contains two monomers of each protein (resulting in a tetramer) and was crystallized without bound DNA. In this complex DNMT3L stabilizes the conformation of the DNMT3A active site loop. Since the DNMT3A structure is similar to the bacterial methyltransferase M.HhaI (which was cocrystallized with DNA) the DNMT3A-DNMT3L-DNA complex could be modeled from the bacterial complex [29]. DNTM3A has a relatively small DNA binding domain (~50 base pairs) compared to the bacterial enzymes. However, in the tetramer two active sites come together closely which leads to doubling of the DNA binding surface. It was suggested that the DNA is bound to both binding sites, such that the two active sites are located in the major groove ~40 Angstroms apart, which corresponds to one DNA helical turn. In this modeled DNMT3a-DNA complex the cytosine is located between the nucleophile Cys706 and the cofactor SAM. Figure 8.4(b) shows the interaction of a stretch of DNA in which the inhibitor zebularine has been incorporated (from the crystal structure of M.HhaI) with the catalytic site of DNTM3A.

Since in differentiated cells DNMT1 is responsible for the transfer of the methylation patterns, it represents the more interesting target for experimental cancer therapies. Due to the lack of an experimental 3D structure for this enzyme, Lyko *et al.* [31] generated a homology model based on DNTM2 and bacterial enzymes. While this model demonstrated a significant conformational preservation of the catalytic site, it also revealed a number of unique structural features: His1459 of DNMT1 is substituted with alanine at the corresponding positions in the bacterial methyltransferases. In addition, the side-chains of Arg1310 and Arg1312 have different conformations compared to the corresponding side-chains in the two bacterial methylases. The authors stated that these differences influence the binding

(a)

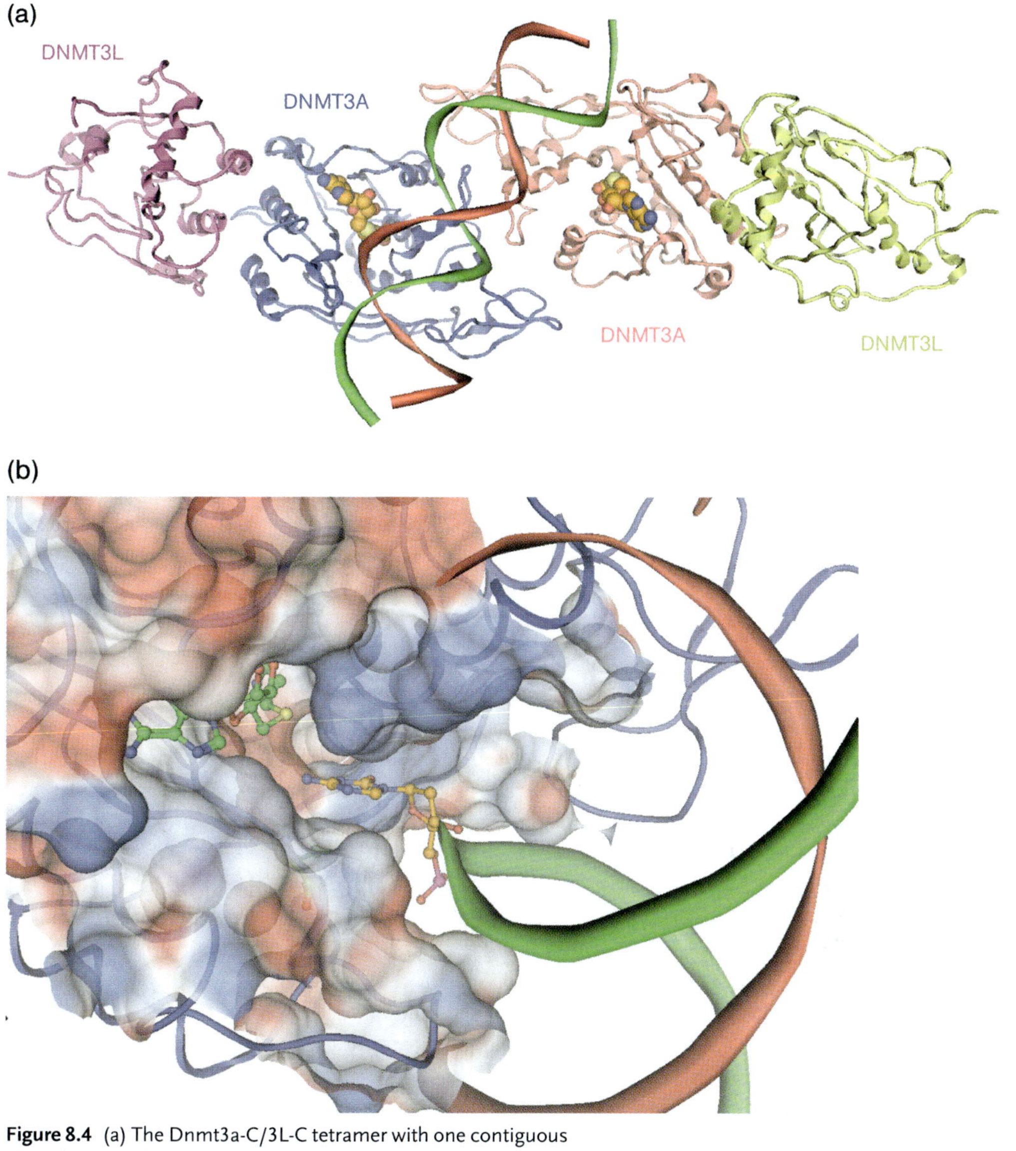

(b)

Figure 8.4 (a) The Dnmt3a-C/3L-C tetramer with one contiguous curved DNA molecule covering two active sites. The cofactor SAM is shown in orange. (b) Interaction of DNA-incorporated zebularine (colored orange, taken from the bacterial HhaI crystal structure) with the catalytic site of DNMT3A. The bound cofactor analog SAH is shown in green.

of the ribose ring in the cytosine ligand by creating a tighter cavity. Differences in DNMT1 were also observed for the number of charged residues neighboring the catalytic site. These differences could be used to design selective DNMT1 inhibitors. The quality of the homology model was demonstrated by a successful virtual

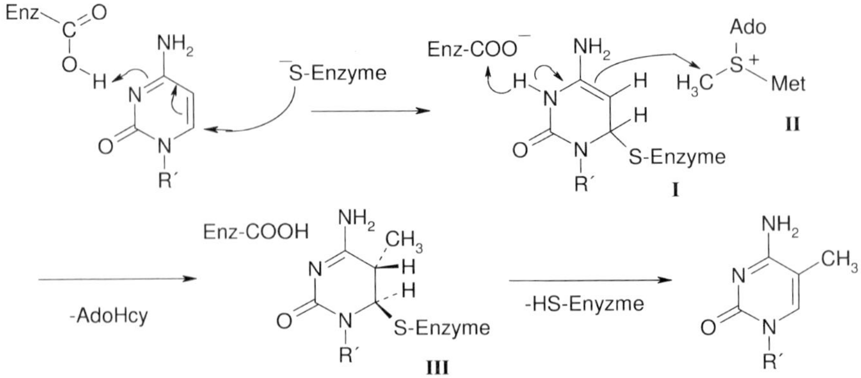

Figure 8.5 Mechanism of cytosine methylation. For a description see text. AdoHcy: S-Adenosylhomocysteine.

screening which let to two non-nucleoside DNMT1 inhibitors (for details see below) [30].

8.4 Biochemical Mechanism of DNA Methylation

The biochemical mechanism of cytosine methylation has been studied in detail [32, 33]. DNMT undergoes a complex with the DNA and the cytosine which will be methylated flips out of the DNA double helix [34]. The methyltransferase is then forming a covalent adduct (**I**) with the DNA by means of the conjugate addition of the thiol group of a cysteine residue in the active site to the double bond of the cytosine. This adduct (**I**) then reacts with the cosubstrate SAM (**II**) which is also present in the active site and a methylated adduct (**III**) is formed. A glutamate in the active site of the DNMT delivers the carboxylate that participates in the process. Finally, a retro-Michael-type elimination of the enzyme and an adjacent proton will liberate the enzyme from the DNA under formation of a 5-methylated cytosine base which finally flips back into its original position within the DNA double helix (Figure 8.5) [35]. This mechanism is the basis for the activity of the two inhibitors approved for human use and this knowledge can been exploited for further inhibitor design (see below). It has been proposed that from intermediate (**I**) in the absence of SAM a deamination to thymine occurs with subsequent base repair excision to cytosine [18]. This would be formally a demethylation reaction but not in a direct biochemical sense.

8.5 Physiological Role of DNA Methylation

DNA methylation is an essential function in normal mammalian cells. It is involved in genomic imprinting (restriction of the expression of a gene to only one of the two parental chromosomes) [36] which is important for development. It is also necessary for X chromosome inactivation [37], the mechanism of dosage compensation in female mammals.

DNA methylation may directly decrease the binding affinity of certain transcription factors to DNA [38]. Additionally, methylated CpG sites recruit MBD proteins, which in turn leads to transcriptional repression [39]. siRNA-mediated knockdown of MBD proteins leads to a re-expression of silenced tumor suppressor protein candidates [40]. DNA methylation and histone modification are dependent on each other [41, 42] and from this interplay a synergy in derepression (e.g. between histone deacetylase and DNMT inhibitors) can be observed [43–45] (see also below).

The importance of DNA methylation for normal genome function can also be shown by the finding that homozygous mutation of the DNMT gene results in embryonic lethality [46]. Thus, unwanted activation of certain genes by DNMT inhibitors may pose a risk, for example by derepression of proinvasive genes [47], which puts a caveat to those therapeutical approaches.

8.6 DNA Methylation and Disease

Epigenetics and hence also DNA methylation can be seen as a biochemical manifestation of environmental cues [48]. These epigenetic alterations may lead to an increased susceptibiliy to certain physical diseases, for example cancer [49, 50], but also psychiatric diseases [51, 52]. This increases over time, as was elegantly described in homozygotic twins who had the same gene set but became more and more different in terms of DNA methylation pattern with increasing age [53]. Genome-wide studies of epigenetic patterns will become increasingly important in order to correlate those patterns with human disease [54–56]. Ultimately, the goal will be to use those patterns as predictive markers for disease risk, disease progression and optimized treatment [57].

In cancer cells the hypermethylation of certain promoter regions is known as one of the most important epigenetic changes taking place in tumors, leading to transcriptional silencing of tumor suppressor genes [58–60]. This may be due to overexpression of the enzyme [61, 62], aberrant recruitment of the enzymatic proteins [63] or expression of truncated mutants [64]. A large variety of genes are aberrantly methylated in cancer cells, including genes that are involved in regulating DNA repair (e.g. BRCA1, MLH1), signal transduction (e.g. RASSF1), the cell cycle (e.g. $p16^{INK4a}$, $p15^{INK4b}$), metabolism of carcinogena (e.g. GSTP1), cell adherence phenomena (e.g. CDH1, CDH13), apoptosis (e.g. DAPK, TMS1) or angiogenesis (e.g. THBS1) [60, 65]. But besides the promotor regions of protein-coding genes also nonprotein-coding regions of the DNA can be affected and DNA methylation in the regulatory region has also an impact on microRNA expression [66]. An example is the suppression of the formation of miRNA-124a by DNA hypermethylation. This in turn leads to an activation of the oncogenic cyclin D kinase 6 [67].

8.7 DNMT Inhibitors

Whereas in the case of histone deacetylases one inhibitor is approved for human use, about 5–10 are in clinical trials and hundreds are known from preclinical research, which is almost opposite to the case of DNMT. Already two inhibitors are the active ingredient of a marketed drug but only a handful of mostly unselective and not very potent inhibitors are known beyond that. This is rather unusual for drug discovery research, but given the emergence of epigenetic research in the past 10 years, the development of novel preclinical entities with DNMT inhibitors is likely to emerge and selected candidates may approach the clinic as a second generation of inhibitors.

Generally, DNMT inhibitors can be divided in two big classes. One group consists of base analogs which are incorporated into DNA and act as suicide substrates for DNMT via a covalent adduct formation. The other group acts on the free enzyme in the same way as "classic" enzyme inhibitors do.

8.7.1 Covalent DNMT Inhibitors

This group contains the two marketed inhibitors, decitabine (Dacogen) and 5-azacytidine (AzaC, INN: azacitidine, Vidaza®) [68, 69]. Additionally, 5-fluorocytosine and zebularine also belong to the same group (Figure 8.6). These compounds act as prodrugs and show no activity during *in vitro* DNMT assays [70]; only after

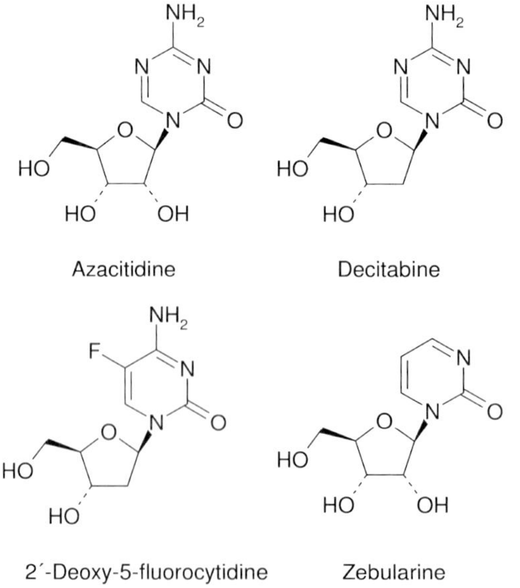

Figure 8.6 Nucleoside analogs as prodrugs for covalent inhibition of DNMT.

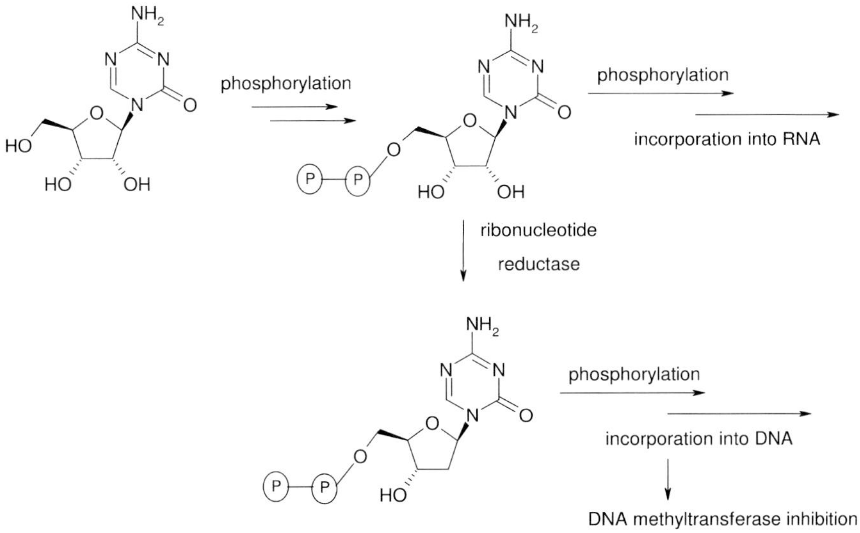

Figure 8.7 Metabolic activation of prodrug inhibitors.

incorporation into the DNA are they able to block DNMT. There is also an ester prodrug of decitabine available which is hence a prodrug of a prodrug [71]. While the deoxyriboside decitabine can be directly transformed into the triphosphate (by deoxycytidine kinase) which then serves as a building block for DNA polymerases, the riboside azacitidine needs to be deoxygenated in the sugar moiety before it is phosphorylated by cytidine–uridine kinase. This step is performed by ribonucleotide reductase on the level of the diphosphate. Then, the same triphosphate as from decitabine is formed and the false base is incorporated into DNA (Figure 8.7). Hence, the rate of DNA incorporation of azacitidine is much lower than for decitabine. Additionally, azacitidine as a riboside is incorporated into RNA [72] which might be a reason for additional side-effects. The activity of each inhibitors is in the low micromolar region [73].

Once the azacytosine analogs are incorporated into the DNA, they are also subject to a covalent addition of the thiol group of the DNMTand an adduct (**Ia**) similar to (**I**) in Figure 8.5 is formed. This adduct (**Ia**) in most cases also reacts with S-adenosyl methionine (**II**) to a methylated adduct (**IIIa**). But due to the absence of an α-proton the enzyme cannot be liberated by elimination and remains trapped to DNA (Figure 8.8).

In the case of 5-fluoro-deoxycytidine (FdC) an methylated adduct (**IIIb**) is also formed, from which (again due to substitution of the α-proton by the fluorine) no liberation of the enzyme by elimination is possible [74]. Zebularine is a riboside prodrug like azacitidine that is also incorporated in both RNA and DNA. It is somewhat different, though, as the covalent enzyme adduct (**Ib**) is formed but methylation does not occur and is not necessary for inhibition. Although elimination of the enzyme should be possible, a stable intermediate is formed [35] (Figure 8.9).

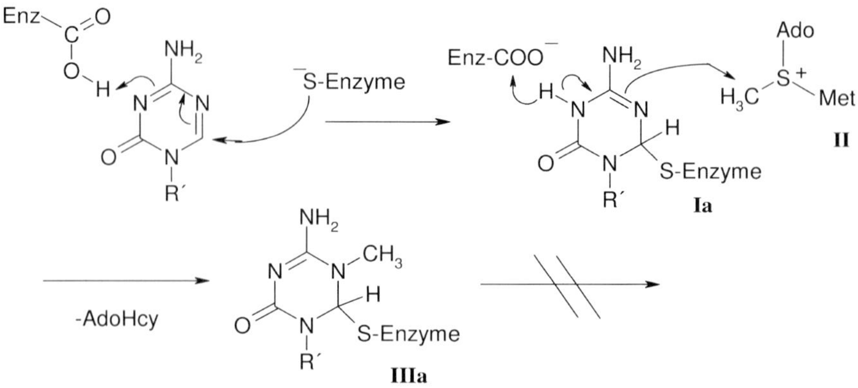

Figure 8.8 Mechanism of covalent DNMT inhibition for 5-azacytidine. For a description see text. AdoHcy: S-Adenosylhomocysteine.

The potency of zebularine is about 10-fold lower than for the azacytosines [73]. Zebularine also inhibits cytidine deaminase [75] which is involved in nucleoside catabolism and deactivates also for example azacitidine and its desoxy analog [76]. Thus, it increases the concentrations of nucleoside triphosphates for incorporation into DNA, the efficacy of DNA methylation and ultimately the anticancer activity of for example azacitidine [77, 78]. Zebularine is metabolized by aldehyde oxidase and it has been shown that its activity can be increases if an inhibitor of that enzyme, for example raloxifene is given in combination [79]. One big question about all epigenetic drugs is the origin of the observed selectivity towards cancer cells. For zebularine, it has been shown that much less activation towards triphosphate metabolites that can be incorporated into DNA occurs in normal muscle tissue as compared to cancer tissue [80].

The covalent trapping of the enzyme leads to a depletion of the cellular pool of DNMTs and subsequent DNA hypomethylation. This in turn results in activation with respect to the reactivation of silenced genes. Additionally, the covalently trapped DNMT may inhibit RNA and DNA polymerases, which leads to an inhibition of protein biosynthesis and DNA strand breaks. This may lead to apoptosis and hence cytotoxicity. Thus, it is not easy to dissect the reasons for the clinical efficacy of these inhibitors in terms of real epigenetic and plain cytotoxic effects [81].

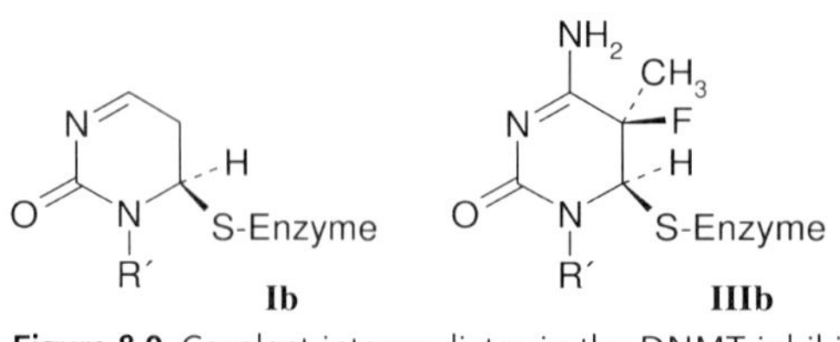

Figure 8.9 Covalent intermediates in the DNMT inhibition by zebularine (**Ib**) and 2′-deoxy-5-fluorocytidine (**IIIb**).

8.7.2 Noncovalent DNMT Inhibitors

These inhibitors act directly on the enzyme without the necessity for incorporation into the DNA. In theory, this should shift the dual activity of reactivation of silenced genes and cytotoxicity towards the epigenetic effects which may result in reduced side-effects. But the proof for that remains yet to be established.

Few reports are available for systematic approaches towards new selective inhibitors of DNMTs. The most prominent example is the tryptophan derivative RG108 (NSC401077) that was identified via a virtual screening approach [30, 82] and is active between 10 and 100 μM. In the same study, NSC 303530 was also identified as a somewhat weaker inhibitor (Figure 8.10). The analog of R108 that does not contain the carboxylic acid group was found to be inactive.

Hydralazine is a vasodilating drug and inhibition of DNA methyltransferases in the range of 10–20 μM have been reported *in vitro* [83]. In addition, hypomethylation in cell culture has also been shown [84]. Also the local anesthetic procaine [85] and its amide analog procainamide [84] have been identified as DNA methyltransferase inhibitors. Synthetic analogs of procaine have shown activity only around 500 μM [86] (Figure 8.10).

There are also some natural products that were identified as inhibitors of DNMTs [87]. Certain disulfide bromotyrosine derivatives, such as psammaplin

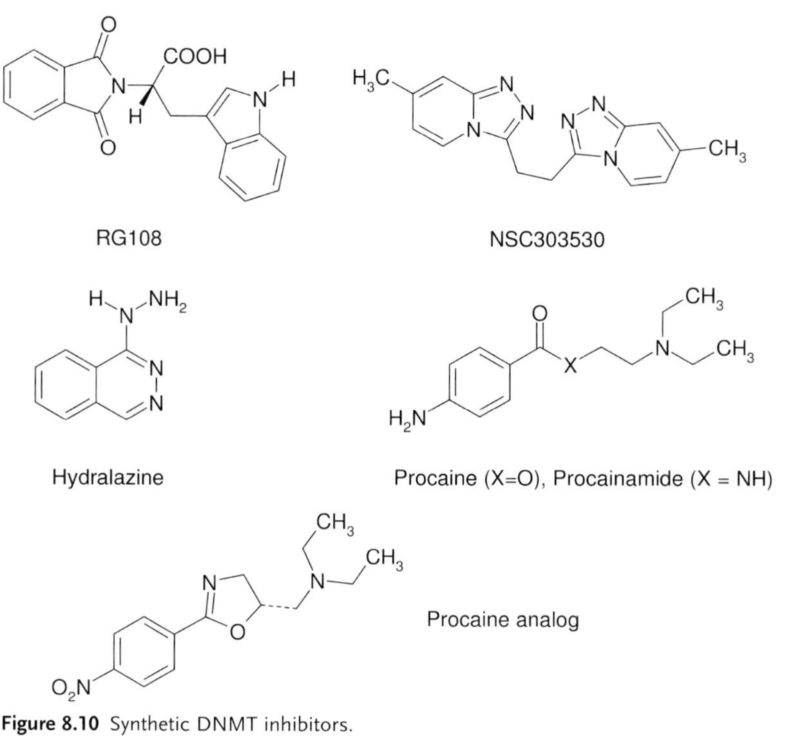

Figure 8.10 Synthetic DNMT inhibitors.

A, isolated from the sponge *Pseudoceratina purpurea*, were found to be potent inhibitors of both DNMT1 and also histone deacetylases [88] (see also the chapter on histone deacetylases). (−)-Epigallocatechin-3-gallate (EGCG), a major polyphenol from green tea leaves, inhibits DNA methyltransferases and is thereby able to reactivate silenced genes like *P16*^{INK4a} and *hMLH1* in tumor cells [89]. EGCG is a pleiotropic inhibitor that has received a lot of attention, especially for cancer chemoprevention, but with such inhibitors it remains to be determined which of its inhibitory or stimulatory activities are the most important for its net effect in biological systems [90]. Two polyphenols from coffee, caffeic acid and chlorogenic acid, have also been reported to inhibit DNMT1 in the low micromolar range [91] and polyphenols from apples have also been described to have a similar activity [92]. An isoflavone from soy beans, genistein, inhibits methylation of DNA and thus can lead to re-expression of methylation-silenced genes, such as *RAR*β, *p16*^{INK4} and *MGMT* in the esophageal squamous cell carcinoma cell line KYSE 510 [93] (Figure 8.11). As the histone acetylation status is also known to have an impact on the re-expression of these genes, the weak inhibition of histone deacetylase activity observed after treatment of the cells with genistein is also possibly contributing to the gene reactivation. Biochanin A and daidzein, two other isoflavones, are weaker inhibitors of DNMTs and as they also are less effective in reactivating the *RAR*β gene. Thus, a direct correlation between the inhibition of DNA methyltransferases and the re-activation of the silenced genes was assumed [93].

A further natural product inhibitor is mithramycin A, a structurally complex anticancer antibiotic. Mithramycin A is a member of a group of aureolic acid-type polyketides that are produced by the soil bacterium *Streptomyces argillaceus* [94].

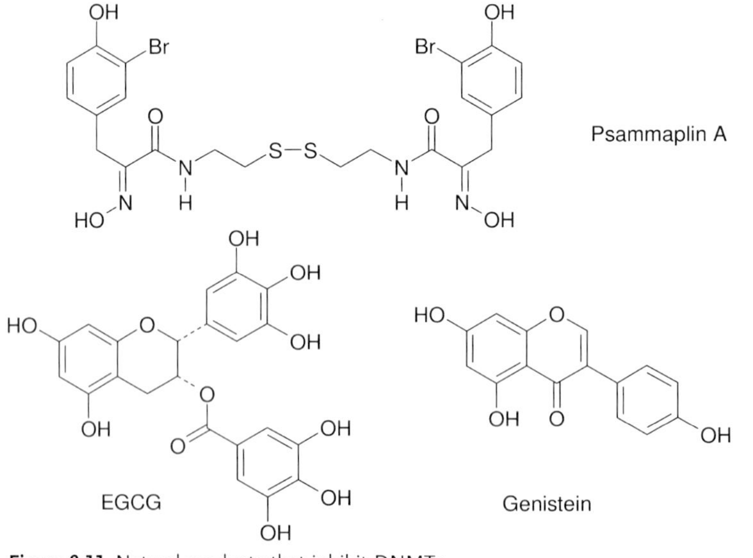

Figure 8.11 Natural products that inhibit DNMTs.

Mithramycin A binds to GC-rich or CG-rich DNA sequences and blocks DNMT methylation activity. Docking of mithramycin A into the DNMT1 catalytic domain indicates that the trisaccharide of the inhibitor can fit into the putative cytosine pocket and the aglycon core is bound between the two arms that fasten the hemimethylated DNA.

Novel approaches to therapeutically downregulate DNA methylation include the DNMT1 antisense compound MG98. However, clinical phase trials with the single drug showed no effect (partial or complete remission) or the effects could not be linked to DNMT inhibition [95–97].

8.8
Therapeutic Applications of DNMT Inhibitors

The inhibitors available for human use, azacitidine and decitabine, have been approved for the treatment of myelodysplastic syndrome (MDS) [98, 99]. MDS summarizes a set of different conditions that affect the maturation of blood cells. It is a group of bone marrow stem cell malignancies that have a pathogenetic overlap with acute myeloid leukemia, show peripheral blood cytopenias and, in more advanced subtypes, varied degrees of maturation arrest [100]. Both drugs are approved for all subtypes of MDS. Response rates are usually around 30%. The question whether the clinical benefit results more from epigenetic effects and re-activation of silenced maturation factors or more from cytotoxic effects on the immature hyperproliferative cells remains open.

Several studies have shown the ability of DNMT inhibitors to prevent cancer using different pathways [101–104]. Genistein demonstrated cancer chemopreventive activities in animal models [105]. It has been studied in different cancer cell lines and inhibition of cancer cell growth has been shown [106]. But several mechanisms, such as antihormonal effects, are discussed to explain this activity and the exact contribution of DNMT inhibition to in-vivo activity in cancer chemoprevention remains to be determined.

Many *in vitro* investigations have shown a cooperation of DNA methylation and histone deacetylation in the repression of transcription [107, 108]. Thus, it seems logical that the combination of DNMT and HDAC inhibition has been shown to induce differentiation, apoptosis and growth arrest in cancer cell lines [109]. The re-expression of hypermethylated genes such as MLH1, TIMP3, CDKN2B and CDKN2A was increased when HDAC inhibitors were combined with inhibitors of DNA methyltransferases. In contrast, HDAC inhibition alone was not able to reactivate transcription [110]. The silencing of the COX 2 gene, whose promoter was shown to be hypermethylated in gastric cancer, can be relieved with a synergistic treatment of DNMT and HDAC inhibitors [111]. More connections and hence potential for combined therapeutic approaches between inhibitors targeting histones and DNA methyltransferase inhibitors are becoming evident [112, 113].

8.9 Conclusion

DNA methylation is one cornerstone of epigenetic regulation. The mechanistic understanding of the biological implications of this modification is steadily increasing. Already, inhibitors of DNMTs are approved for human therapy. Many clinical studies with DNMT inhibitors both as single agents and in combination therapies for the treatment of cancer are currently under way. But there is clearly a lack of potent and selective inhibitors that do not act via incorporation into DNA. This next generation of DNMT inhibitors offers the promise of optimized epigenetic therapy with fewer side-effects.

Acknowledgements

We thank Frank Lyko, DKFZ Heidelberg, for critical reading of the manuscript and Victor Marquez, NCI, for valuable discussion.

References

1 Kouzarides, T. (2007) Chromatin modifications and their function. *Cell*, **128**, 693–705.
2 Bestor, T.H. (2000) The DNA methyltransferases of mammals. *Human Molecular Genetics*, **9**, 2395–2402.
3 Yoo, C.B., Valente, R., Congiatu, C., Gavazza, F., Angel, A., Siddiqui, M.A., Jones, P.A., McGuigan, C. and Marquez, V.E. (2008) Activation of p16 Gene Silenced by DNA Methylation in Cancer Cells by Phosphoramidate Derivatives of 2′-Deoxyzebularine. *Journal of Medicinal Chemistry* (in press).
4 Allis, C.D., Jenuwein, T. and Reinberg, D. (2007) Overview and concepts, *Epigenetics*, Cold Spring Harbor Laboratory Press, pp. 23–61.
5 Wolffe, A.P. and Matzke, M.A. (1999) Epigenetics: regulation through repression. *Science*, **286**, 481–486.
6 Lopez-Serra, L. and Esteller, M. (2008) Proteins that bind methylated DNA and human cancer: reading the wrong words. *British Journal of Cancer*, **98**, 1881–1885.
7 Schmutte, C. and Jones, P.A. (1998) Involvement of DNA methylation in human carcinogenesis. *Biological Chemistry*, **379**, 377–388.
8 Morgan, H.D., Dean, W., Coker, H.A., Reik, W. and Petersen-Mahrt, S.K. (2004) Activation-induced cytidine deaminase deaminates 5-methylcytosine in DNA and is expressed in pluripotent tissues: implications for epigenetic reprogramming. *The Journal of Biological Chemistry*, **279**, 52353–52360.
9 Petersen-Mahrt, S. (2005) DNA deamination in immunity. *Immunological Reviews*, **203**, 80–97.
10 Bird, A. (2002) DNA methylation patterns and epigenetic memory. *Genes and Development*, **16**, 6–21.
11 Ehrlich, M., Gama-Sosa, M.A., Huang, L.H., Midgett, R.M., Kuo, K.C., McCune, R.A. and Gehrke, C. (1982) Amount and distribution of 5-methylcytosine in human DNA from different types of tissues of cells. *Nucleic Acids Research*, **10**, 2709–2721.

12 McCabe, D.C. and Caudill, M.A. (2005) DNA methylation, genomic silencing, and links to nutrition and cancer. *Nutrition Reviews*, **63**, 183–195.

13 Gardiner-Garden, M. and Frommer, M. (1987) CpG islands in vertebrate genomes. *Journal of Molecular Biology*, **196**, 261–282.

14 Takai, D. and Jones, P.A. (2002) Comprehensive analysis of CpG islands in human chromosomes 21 and 22. *Proceedings of the National Academy of Sciences of the United States of America*, **99**, 3740–3745.

15 Dunn, B.K. (2003) Hypomethylation: one side of a larger picture. *Annals of the New York Academy of Sciences*, **983**, 28–42.

16 Ooi, S.K. and Bestor, T.H. (2008) The colorful history of active DNA demethylation. *Cell*, **133**, 1145–1148.

17 Kangaspeska, S., Stride, B., Metivier, R., Polycarpou-Schwarz, M., Ibberson, D., Carmouche, R.P., Benes, V., Gannon, F. and Reid, G. (2008) Transient cyclical methylation of promoter DNA. *Nature*, **452**, 112–115.

18 Metivier, R., Gallais, R., Tiffoche, C., Le Peron, C., Jurkowska, R.Z., Carmouche, R.P., Ibberson, D., Barath, P., Demay, F., Reid, G., Benes, V., Jeltsch, A., Gannon, F. and Salbert, G. (2008) Cyclical DNA methylation of a transcriptionally active promoter. *Nature*, **452**, 45–50.

19 Okano, M., Xie, S. and Li, E. (1998) Cloning and characterization of a family of novel mammalian DNA (cytosine-5) methyltransferases. *Nature Genetics*, **19**, 219–220.

20 Bestor, T., Laudano, A., Mattaliano, R. and Ingram, V. (1988) Cloning and sequencing of a cDNA encoding DNA methyltransferase of mouse cells. The carboxyl-terminal domain of the mammalian enzymes is related to bacterial restriction methyltransferases. *Journal of Molecular Biology*, **203**, 971–983.

21 Yoder, J.A. and Bestor, T.H. (1998) A candidate mammalian DNA methyltransferase related to pmt1p of fission yeast. *Human Molecular Genetics*, **7**, 279–284.

22 Goll, M.G. and Bestor, T.H. (2005) Eukaryotic cytosine methyltransferases. *Annual Review of Biochemistry*, **74**, 481–514.

23 Goll, M.G., Kirpekar, F., Maggert, K.A., Yoder, J.A., Hsieh, C.L., Zhang, X., Golic, K.G., Jacobsen, S.E. and Bestor, T.H. (2006) Methylation of tRNAAsp by the DNA methyltransferase homolog Dnmt2. *Science*, **311**, 395–398.

24 Posfai, J., Bhagwat, A.S., Posfai, G. and Roberts, R.J. (1989) Predictive motifs derived from cytosine methyltransferases. *Nucleic Acids Research*, **17**, 2421–2435.

25 Lauster, R., Trautner, T.A. and Noyer-Weidner, M. (1989) Cytosine-specific type II DNA methyltransferases. A conserved enzyme core with variable target-recognizing domains. *Journal of Molecular Biology*, **206**, 305–312.

26 Cheng, X. and Blumenthal, R.M. (2008) Mammalian DNA methyltransferases: a structural perspective. *Structure (London, England: 1993)*, **16**, 341–350.

27 Qiu, C., Sawada, K., Zhang, X. and Cheng, X. (2002) The PWWP domain of mammalian DNA methyltransferase Dnmt3b defines a new family of DNA-binding folds. *Nature Structural Biology*, **9**, 217–224.

28 Ooi, S.K., Qiu, C., Bernstein, E., Li, K., Jia, D., Yang, Z., Erdjument-Bromage, H., Tempst, P., Lin, S.P., Allis, C.D., Cheng, X. and Bestor, T.H. (2007) DNMT3L connects unmethylated lysine 4 of histone H3 to de novo methylation of DNA. *Nature*, **448**, 714–717.

29 Jia, D., Jurkowska, R.Z., Zhang, X., Jeltsch, A. and Cheng, X. (2007) Structure of Dnmt3a bound to Dnmt3L suggests a model for de novo DNA methylation. *Nature*, **449**, 248–251.

30 Siedlecki, P., Boy, R.G., Musch, T., Brueckner, B., Suhai, S., Lyko, F. and

Zielenkiewicz, P. (2006) Discovery of two novel, small-molecule inhibitors of DNA methylation. *Journal of Medicinal Chemistry*, **49**, 678–683.

31 Siedlecki, P., Boy, R.G., Comagic, S., Schirrmacher, R., Wiessler, M., Zielenkiewicz, P., Suhai, S. and Lyko, F. (2003) Establishment and functional validation of a structural homology model for human DNA methyltransferase 1. *Biochemical and Biophysical Research Communications*, **306**, 558–563.

32 Vilkaitis, G., Merkiene, E., Serva, S., Weinhold, E. and Klimasauskas, S. (2001) The mechanism of DNA cytosine-5 methylation. Kinetic and mutational dissection of Hhai methyltransferase. *The Journal of Biological Chemistry*, **276**, 20924–20934.

33 O'Gara, M., Klimasauskas, S., Roberts, R.J. and Cheng, X. (1996) Enzymatic C5-cytosine methylation of DNA: mechanistic implications of new crystal structures for HhaL methyltransferase-DNA-AdoHcy complexes. *Journal of Molecular Biology*, **261**, 634–645.

34 Klimasauskas, S., Kumar, S., Roberts, R.J. and Cheng, X. (1994) HhaI methyltransferase flips its target base out of the DNA helix. *Cell*, **76**, 357–369.

35 Zhou, L., Cheng, X., Connolly, B.A., Dickman, M.J., Hurd, P.J. and Hornby, D.P. (2002) Zebularine: a novel DNA methylation inhibitor that forms a covalent complex with DNA methyltransferases. *Journal of Molecular Biology*, **321**, 591–599.

36 Brannan, C.I. and Bartolomei, M.S. (1999) Mechanisms of genomic imprinting. *Current Opinion in Genetics & Development*, **9**, 164–170.

37 Hansen, R.S. (2003) X inactivation-specific methylation of LINE-1 elements by DNMT3B: implications for the Lyon repeat hypothesis. *Human Molecular Genetics*, **12**, 2559–2567.

38 Watt, F. and Molloy, P.L. (1988) Cytosine methylation prevents binding to DNA of a HeLa cell transcription factor required for optimal expression of the adenovirus major late promoter. *Genes and Development*, **2**, 1136–1143.

39 Wade, P.A. (2001) Methyl CpG binding proteins: coupling chromatin architecture to gene regulation. *Oncogene*, **20**, 3166–3173.

40 Lopez-Serra, L., Ballestar, E., Ropero, S., Setien, F., Billard, L.M., Fraga, M.F., Lopez-Nieva, P., Alaminos, M., Guerrero, D., Dante, R. and Esteller, M. (2008) Unmasking of epigenetically silenced candidate tumor suppressor genes by removal of methyl-CpG-binding domain proteins. *Oncogene*, **27**, 3556–3566.

41 Fahrner, J.A., Eguchi, S., Herman, J.G. and Baylin, S.B. (2002) Dependence of histone modifications and gene expression on DNA hypermethylation in cancer. *Cancer Research*, **62**, 7213–7218.

42 Kondo, Y., Shen, L. and Issa, J.P. (2003) Critical role of histone methylation in tumor suppressor gene silencing in colorectal cancer. *Molecular and Cellular Biology*, **23**, 206–215.

43 Venturelli, S., Armeanu, S., Pathil, A., Hsieh, C.J., Weiss, T.S., Vonthein, R., Wehrmann, M., Gregor, M., Lauer, U.M. and Bitzer, M. (2007) Epigenetic combination therapy as a tumor-selective treatment approach for hepatocellular carcinoma. *Cancer*, **109**, 2132–2141.

44 Griffiths, E.A. and Gore, S.D. (2008) DNA methyltransferase and histone deacetylase inhibitors in the treatment of myelodysplastic syndromes. *Seminars in Hematology*, **45**, 23–30.

45 Walton, T.J., Li, G., Seth, R., McArdle, S.E., Bishop, M.C. and Rees, R.C. (2008) DNA demethylation and histone deacetylation inhibition co-operate to re-express estrogen receptor beta and induce apoptosis in prostate cancer cell-lines. *Prostate*, **68**, 210–222.

46 Li, E., Bestor, T.H. and Jaenisch, R. (1992) Targeted mutation of the DNA methyltransferase gene results in embryonic lethality. *Cell*, **69**, 915–926.

47 Ateeq, B., Unterberger, A., Szyf, M. and Rabbani, S.A. (2008) Pharmacological inhibition of DNA methylation induces proinvasive and prometastatic genes in vitro and in vivo. *Neoplasia (New York, NY)*, **10**, 266–278.

48 Choi, J.K. and Kim, S.C. (2007) Environmental effects on gene expression phenotype have regional biases in the human genome. *Genetics*, **175**, 1607–1613.

49 Weidman, J.R., Dolinoy, D.C., Murphy, S.K. and Jirtle, R.L. (2007) Cancer susceptibility: Epigenetic manifestation of environmental exposures. *Cancer Journal (Sudbury, Mass)*, **13**, 9–16.

50 Jones, P.A. and Baylin, S.B. (2007) The epigenomics of cancer. *Cell*, **128**, 683–692.

51 Kuratomi, G., Iwamoto, K., Bundo, M., Kusumi, I., Kato, N., Iwata, N., Ozaki, N. and Kato, T. (2008) Aberrant DNA methylation associated with bipolar disorder identified from discordant monozygotic twins. *Molecular Psychiatry*, **13**, 429–441.

52 Kaminsky, Z., Petronis, A., Wang, S.C., Levine, B., Ghaffar, O., Floden, D. and Feinstein, A. (2008) Epigenetics of personality traits: An illustrative study of identical twins discordant for risk-taking behavior. *Twin Research and Human Genetics*, **11**, 1–11.

53 Fraga, M.F., Ballestar, E., Paz, M.F., Ropero, S., Setien, F., Ballestart, M.L., Heine-Suner, D., Cigudosa, J.C., Urioste, M., Benitez, J., Boix-Chornet, M., Sanchez-Aguilera, A., Ling, C., Carlsson, E., Poulsen, P., Vaag, A., Stephan, Z., Spector, T.D., Wu, Y.Z., Plass, C. and Esteller, M. (2005) Epigenetic differences arise during the lifetime of monozygotic twins. *Proceedings of the National Academy of Sciences of the United States of America*, **102**, 10604–10609.

54 Esteller, M. (2006) The necessity of a human epigenome project. *Carcinogenesis*, **27**, 1121–1125.

55 Wang, S.S., Smiraglia, D.J., Wu, Y.Z., Ghosh, S., Rader, J.S., Cho, K.R., Bonfiglio, T.A., Nayar, R., Plass, C. and Sherman, M.E. (2008) Identification of novel methylation markers in cervical cancer using restriction landmark genomic scanning. *Cancer Research*, **68**, 2489–2497.

56 Yu, L., Liu, C., Vandeusen, J., Becknell, B., Dai, Z., Wu, Y.Z., Raval, A., Liu, T.H., Ding, W., Mao, C., Liu, S., Smith, L.T., Lee, S., Rassenti, L., Marcucci, G., Byrd, J., Caligiuri, M.A. and Plass, C. (2005) Global assessment of promoter methylation in a mouse model of cancer identifies ID4 as a putative tumor-suppressor gene in human leukemia. *Nature Genetics*, **37**, 265–274.

57 Mulero-Navarro, S. and Esteller, M. (2008) Epigenetic biomarkers for human cancer: The time is now. *Critical Reviews in Oncology/Hematology*, **68**, 1–11.

58 Baylin, S.B. and Herman, J.G. (2000) DNA hypermethylation in tumorigenesis: epigenetics joins genetics. *Trends in Genetics*, **16**, 168–174.

59 Costello, J.F. and Plass, C. (2001) Methylation matters. *Journal of Medical Genetics*, **38**, 285–303.

60 Esteller, M. (2002) CpG island hypermethylation and tumor suppressor genes: a booming present, a brighter future. *Oncogene*, **21**, 5427–5440.

61 Butcher, D.T. and Rodenhiser, D.I. (2007) Epigenetic inactivation of BRCA1 is associated with aberrant expression of CTCF and DNA methyltransferase (DNMT3B) in some sporadic breast tumours. *European Journal of Cancer (Oxford, England: 1990)*, **43**, 210–219.

62 Lin, R.K., Hsu, H.S., Chang, J.W., Chen, C.Y., Chen, J.T. and Wang, Y.C. (2007) Alteration of DNA methyltransferases contributes to 5′CpG methylation and poor prognosis in lung cancer. *Lung Cancer (Amsterdam, Netherlands)*, **55**, 205–213.

63 Liu, S., Shen, T., Huynh, L., Klisovic, M.I., Rush, L.J., Ford, J.L., Yu, J., Becknell, B.,

Li, Y., Liu, C., Vukosavljevic, T., Whitman, S.P., Chang, K.S., Byrd, J.C., Perrotti, D., Plass, C. and Marcucci, G. (2005) Interplay of RUNX1/MTG8 and DNA methyltransferase 1 in acute myeloid leukemia. *Cancer Research*, **65**, 1277–1284.

64 Ostler, K.R., Davis, E.M., Payne, S.L., Gosalia, B.B., Exposito-Cespedes, J., Le Beau, M.M. and Godley, L.A. (2007) Cancer cells express aberrant DNMT3B transcripts encoding truncated proteins. *Oncogene*, **26**, 5553–5563.

65 Costello, J.F. and Plass, C. (2001) Methylation matters. *Journal of Medical Genetics*, **38**, 285–303.

66 Esteller, M. (2008) Epigenetics in cancer. *The New England Journal of Medicine*, **358**, 1148–1159.

67 Lujambio, A., Ropero, S., Ballestar, E., Fraga, M.F., Cerrato, C., Setien, F., Casado, S., Suarez-Gauthier, A., Sanchez-Cespedes, M., Git, A., Spiteri, I., Das, P.P., Caldas, C., Miska, E. and Esteller, M. (2007) Genetic unmasking of an epigenetically silenced microRNA in human cancer cells. *Cancer Research*, **67**, 1424–1429.

68 Jones, P.A. and Taylor, S.M. (1980) Cellular differentiation, cytidine analogs and DNA methylation. *Cell*, **20**, 85–93.

69 Christman, J.K. (2002) 5-Azacytidine and 5-aza-2′-deoxycytidine as inhibitors of DNA methylation: mechanistic studies and their implications for cancer therapy. *Oncogene*, **21**, 5483–5495.

70 Stresemann, C., Brueckner, B., Musch, T., Stopper, H. and Lyko, F. (2006) Functional diversity of DNA methyltransferase inhibitors in human cancer cell lines. *Cancer Research*, **66**, 2794–2800.

71 Byun, H.M., Choi, S.H., Laird, P.W., Trinh, B., Siddiqui, M.A., Marquez, V.E. and Yang, A.S. (2008) 2′-Deoxy-N4-[2-(4-nitrophenyl)ethoxycarbonyl]-5-azacytidine: a novel inhibitor of DNA methyltransferase that requires activation by human carboxylesterase 1. *Cancer Letters*, **266**, 238–248.

72 Plagemann, P.G., Behrens, M. and Abraham, D. (1978) Metabolism and cytotoxicity of 5-azacytidine in cultured Novikoff rat hepatoma and P388 mouse leukemia cells and their enhancement by preincubation with pyrazofurin. *Cancer Research*, **38**, 2458–2466.

73 Brueckner, B., Kuck, D. and Lyko, F. (2007) DNA methyltransferase inhibitors for cancer therapy. *Cancer Journal (Sudbury, Mass)*, **13**, 17–22.

74 Santi, D.V., Garrett, C.E. and Barr, P.J. (1983) On the mechanism of inhibition of DNA-cytosine methyltransferases by cytosine analogs. *Cell*, **33**, 9–10.

75 Xiang, S.B., Short, S.A., Wolfenden, R. and Carter, C.W. (1995) Transition-state selectivity for a single hydroxyl group during catalysis by cytidine deaminase. *Biochemistry*, **34**, 4516–4523.

76 Laliberte, J., Marquez, V.E. and Momparler, R.L. (1992) Potent inhibitors for the deamination of cytosine arabinoside and 5-aza-2′-deoxycytidine by human cytidine deaminase. *Cancer Chemotherapy and Pharmacology*, **30**, 7–11.

77 Lemaire, M., Momparler, L.F., Bernstein, M.L., Marquez, V.E. and Momparler, R.L. (2005) Enhancement of antineoplastic action of 5-aza-2′-deoxycytidine by zebularine on L1210 leukemia. *Anti-Cancer Drugs*, **16**, 301–308.

78 Lemaire, M., Momparler, L.F., Raynal, N.J., Bernstein, M.L. and Momparler, R.L. (2009) Inhibition of cytidine deaminase by zebularine enhances the antineoplastic action of 5-aza-2′-deoxycytidine. *Cancer Chemotherapy and Pharmacology*, **63**, 411–416.

79 Klecker, R.W., Cysyk, R.L. and Collins, J.M. (2006) Zebularine metabolism by aldehyde oxidase in hepatic cytosol from humans, monkeys, dogs, rats, and mice: influence of sex and inhibitors. *Bioorganic and Medicinal Chemistry*, **14**, 62–66.

80 Ben-Kasus, T., Ben-Zvi, Z., Marquez, V.E., Kelley, J.A. and Agbaria, R. (2005) Metabolic activation of zebularine, a novel DNA methylation inhibitor, in human

bladder carcinoma cells. *Biochemical Pharmacology*, **70**, 121–133.

81 Stresemann, C. and Lyko, F. (2008) Modes of action of the DNA methyltransferase inhibitors azacytidine and decitabine. *International Journal of Cancer*, **123**, 8–13.

82 Brueckner, B., Boy, R.G., Siedlecki, P., Musch, T., Kliem, H.C., Zielenkiewicz, P., Suhai, S., Wiessler, M. and Lyko, F. (2005) Epigenetic reactivation of tumor suppressor genes by a novel small-molecule inhibitor of human DNA methyltransferases. *Cancer Research*, **65**, 6305–6311.

83 Arce, C., Segura-Pacheco, B., Perez-Cardenas, E., Taja-Chayeb, L., Candelaria, M. and Duennas-Gonzalez, A. (2006) Hydralazine target: from blood vessels to the epigenome. *Journal of Translational Medicine*, **4**, 10.

84 Segura-Pacheco, B., Trejo-Becerril, C., Perez-Cardenas, E., Taja-Chayeb, L., Mariscal, I., Chavez, A., Acuna, C., Salazar, A.M., Lizano, M. and Duenas-Gonzalez, A. (2003) Reactivation of tumor suppressor genes by the cardiovascular drugs hydralazine and procainamide and their potential use in cancer therapy. *Clinical Cancer Research*, **9**, 1596–1603.

85 Villar-Garea, A., Fraga, M.F., Espada, J. and Esteller, M. (2003) Procaine is a DNA-demethylating agent with growth-inhibitory effects in human cancer cells. *Cancer Research*, **63**, 4984–4989.

86 Castellano, S., Kuck, D., Sala, M., Novellino, E., Lyko, F. and Sbardella, G. (2008) Constrained analogues of procaine as novel small molecule inhibitors of DNA methyltransferase-1. *Journal of Medicinal Chemistry*, **51**, 2321–2325.

87 Hauser, A.-T. and Jung, M. (2008) Targeting Epigenetic Mechanisms: Potential of Natural Products in Cancer Chemoprevention. *Planta Medica* (in press).

88 Pina, I.C., Gautschi, J.T., Wang, G.Y., Sanders, M.L., Schmitz, F.J., France, D., Cornell-Kennon, S., Sambucetti, L.C., Remiszewski, S.W., Perez, L.B., Bair, K.W. and Crews, P. (2003) Psammaplins from the sponge Pseudoceratina purpurea: inhibition of both histone deacetylase and DNA methyltransferase. *The Journal of Organic Chemistry*, **68**, 3866–3873.

89 Fang, M.Z., Wang, Y., Ai, N., Hou, Z., Sun, Y., Lu, H., Welsh, W. and Yang, C.S. (2003) Tea polyphenol (−)-epigallocatechin-3-gallate inhibits DNA methyltransferase and reactivates methylation-silenced genes in cancer cell lines. *Cancer Research*, **63**, 7563–7570.

90 Narayanan, B.A. (2006) Chemopreventive agents alters global gene expression pattern: predicting their mode of action and targets. *Current Cancer Drug Targets*, **6**, 711–727.

91 Lee, W.J. and Zhu, B.T. (2006) Inhibition of DNA methylation by caffeic acid and chlorogenic acid, two common catechol-containing coffee polyphenols. *Carcinogenesis*, **27**, 269–277.

92 Fini, L., Selgrad, M., Fogliano, V., Graziani, G., Romano, M., Hotchkiss, E., Daoud, Y.A., De Vol, E.B., Boland, C.R. and Ricciardiello, L. (2007) Annurca apple polyphenols have potent demethylating activity and can reactivate silenced tumor suppressor genes in colorectal cancer cells. *The Journal of Nutrition*, **137**, 2622–2628.

93 Fang, M.Z., Chen, D., Sun, Y., Jin, Z., Christman, J.K. and Yang, C.S. (2005) Reversal of hypermethylation and reactivation of p16INK4a, RARbeta, and MGMT genes by genistein and other isoflavones from soy. *Clinical Cancer Research*, **11**, 7033–7041.

94 Lin, R.K., Hsu, C.H. and Wang, Y.C. (2007) Mithramycin A inhibits DNA methyltransferase and metastasis potential of lung cancer cells. *Anti-Cancer Drugs*, **18**, 1157–1164.

95 Davis, A.J., Gelmon, K.A., Siu, L.L., Moore, M.J., Britten, C.D., Mistry, N., Klamut, H., D'Aloisio, S., MacLean, M., Wainman, N., Ayers, D., Firby, P., Besterman, J.M., Reid, G.K. and Eisenhauer, E.A. (2003) Phase I and pharmacologic study of the human

DNA methyltransferase antisense oligodeoxynucleotide MG98 given as a 21-day continuous infusion every 4 weeks. *Investigational New Drugs*, **21**, 85–97.

96 Winquist, E., Knox, J., Ayoub, J.P., Wood, L., Wainman, N., Reid, G.K., Pearce, L., Shah, A. and Eisenhauer, E. (2006) Phase II trial of DNA methyltransferase 1 inhibition with the antisense oligonucleotide MG98 in patients with metastatic renal carcinoma: a National Cancer Institute of Canada Clinical Trials Group investigational new drug study. *Investigational New Drugs*, **24**, 159–167.

97 Klisovic, R.B., Stock, W., Cataland, S., Klisovic, M.I., Liu, S., Blum, W., Green, M., Odenike, O., Godley, L., Burgt, J.V., Van Laar, E., Cullen, M., Macleod, A.R., Besterman, J.M., Reid, G.K., Byrd, J.C. and Marcucci, G. (2008) A phase I biological study of MG98, an oligodeoxynucleotide antisense to DNA methyltransferase 1, in patients with high-risk myelodysplasia and acute myeloid leukemia. *Clinical Cancer Research*, **14**, 2444–2449.

98 Issa, J.P. (2007) DNA methylation as a therapeutic target in cancer. *Clinical Cancer Research*, **13**, 1634–1637.

99 Melchert, M. and List, A. (2008) Targeted therapies in myelodysplastic syndrome. *Seminars in Hematology*, **45**, 31–38.

100 Sekeres, M.A. (2007) The myelodysplastic syndromes. *Expert Opinion on Biological Therapy*, **7**, 369–377.

101 Laird, P.W., Jackson-Grusby, L., Fazeli, A., Dickinson, S.L., Jung, W.E., Li, E., Weinberg, R.A. and Jaenisch, R. (1995) Suppression of intestinal neoplasia by DNA hypomethylation. *Cell*, **81**, 197–205.

102 Davis, C.D. and Uthus, E.O. (2002) Dietary selenite and azadeoxycytidine treatments affect dimethylhydrazine-induced aberrant crypt formation in rat colon and DNA methylation in HT-29 cells. *The Journal of Nutrition*, **132**, 292–297.

103 Lantry, L.E., Zhang, Z., Crist, K.A., Wang, Y., Kelloff, G.J., Lubet, R.A. and You, M. (1999) 5-Aza-2′-deoxycytidine is chemopreventive in a 4-(methyl-nitrosamino)-1-(3-pyridyl)-1-butanone-induced primary mouse lung tumor model. *Carcinogenesis*, **20**, 343–346.

104 McGregor, F., Muntoni, A., Fleming, J., Brown, J., Felix, D.H., MacDonald, D.G., Parkinson, E.K. and Harrison, P.R. (2002) Molecular changes associated with oral dysplasia progression and acquisition of immortality: potential for its reversal by 5-azacytidine. *Cancer Research*, **62**, 4757–4766.

105 Dixon, R.A. and Ferreira, D. (2002) Genistein. *Phytochemistry*, **60**, 205–211.

106 Dean, N.M., Kanemitsu, M. and Boynton, A.L. (1989) Effects of the tyrosine-kinase inhibitor genistein on DNA synthesis and phospholipid-derived second messenger generation in mouse 10T1/2 fibroblasts and rat liver T51B cells. *Biochemical and Biophysical Research Communications*, **165**, 795–801.

107 Jones, P.L., Veenstra, G.J., Wade, P.A., Vermaak, D., Kass, S.U., Landsberger, N., Strouboulis, J. and Wolffe, A.P. (1998) Methylated DNA and MeCP2 recruit histone deacetylase to repress transcription. *Nature Genetics*, **19**, 187–191.

108 Nan, X., Ng, H.H., Johnson, C.A., Laherty, C.D., Turner, B.M., Eisenman, R.N. and Bird, A. (1998) Transcriptional repression by the methyl-CpG-binding protein MeCP2 involves a histone deacetylase complex. *Nature*, **393**, 386–389.

109 Zhu, W.G. and Otterson, G.A. (2003) The interaction of histone deacetylase inhibitors and DNA methyltransferase inhibitors in the treatment of human cancer cells. *Current Medicinal Chemistry Anticancer Agents*, **3**, 187–199.

110 Cameron, E.E., Bachman, K.E., Myohanen, S., Herman, J.G. and Baylin, S.B. (1999) Synergy of demethylation and histone deacetylase inhibition in the re-expression of genes silenced in cancer. *Nature Genetics*, **21**, 103–107.

111 Kikuchi, T., Itoh, F., Toyota, M., Suzuki, H., Yamamoto, H., Fujita, M., Hosokawa, M. and Imai, K. (2002) Aberrant methylation and histone deacetylation of cyclooxygenase 2 in gastric cancer. *International Journal of Cancer*, **97**, 272–277.

112 Jones, P.A. and Baylin, S.B. (2002) The fundamental role of epigenetic events in cancer. *Nature Reviews. Genetics*, **3**, 415–428.

113 Yoo, C.B. and Jones, P.A. (2006) Epigenetic therapy of cancer: past, present and future. *Nature Reviews. Drug Discovery*, **5**, 37–50.

9
Histone Deacetylase Inhibitors

Philip Jones

9.1
Introduction

For decades it has been known that nucleosomes, made up of DNA wrapped around a core of eight histones, form the key structural units of chromatin that are essential for the packaging of eukaryotic DNA. Equally, it has been thoroughly described that the long *N*-terminal extensions of these histones undergo a plethora of posttranslational modifications such as: acetylation, methylation and phosphorylation, as well as ubiquitinylation, sumoylation and ADP-ribosylation [1]. Despite speculation more that 40 years ago by Vincent Alfrey *et al.* that these modifications could have a functional role in modulating transcription efficiency, it is only now in the past decade or so that the scientific community has established the role of posttranslational modifications in the epigenetic regulation of DNA; and for novel pharmacological agents targeting chromatin remodeling to undergo development. Indeed, it was a serendipitous observation 30 years ago that dimethyl sulfoxide (DMSO), and several other agents, caused the terminal differentiation of murine erythroleukemia cells that unbeknowingly triggered the development of the first chromatin remodeling agents, such as butyric acid. Moving ahead two decades, it took until the 1990s for the first of the enzymes responsible for the deacetylation of histone tails of chromatin to be identified – histone deacetylase 1 (HDAC 1) [2]. Subsequently, there has been an explosion of research in this area, culminating with the FDA approval in October 2006 of the first HDAC inhibitor (HDACi), vorinostat, for the treatment of cutaneous T-cell lymphoma (CTCL) [3].

Histone deacetylases (HDACs) and their counterparts the histone acetyl transferases (HATs) are two opposing enzyme families responsible for controlling the acetylation status of chromatin; thereby playing a crucial role in chromatin remodeling and in the regulation of gene transcription [1, 4, 5]. Whilst the HATs add acetyl (Ac-) groups onto lysine residues on histone tails, the HDACs are responsible for their removal. Acetylation of the ε-amino group of lysine residues on the histone tails neutralizes their positive charge and thereby prevents the histone tails interacting

Epigenetic Targets in Drug Discovery. Edited by Wolfgang Sippl and Manfred Jung

ISBN: 978-3-527-32355-5

with the negatively charged DNA, thereby giving rise to a relaxed chromatin structure, allowing transcriptional activation. In contrast, deacetylation by the HDACs acts as a method of transcription repression, by removing the Ac-groups and condensing the chromatin. The HDACis therefore act to selectively alter gene transcription by chromatin remodeling. HDACs also function on a range of nonhistone substrates, thereby affecting protein stability, protein–protein interactions, protein localization and DNA binding.

In humans, 18 HDACs have been identified and classified according to their homology to yeast HDACs [6]. Class I, II and IV HDACs are zinc-dependent enzymes, whereas the third class (sirtuins) are NAD^+-dependent enzymes and are covered elsewhere in this book. Class I (HDACs 1, 2, 3, 8) are closely related to yeast Rpd3; class IIa (HDACs 4, 5, 7, 9) and class IIb (HDACs 6, 10) are related to yeast Hda1 and this latter subclass contains two catalytic sites. Finally, class IV HDACs contain just one member (HDAC 11). Whilst classes I and IV HDACs are mainly found in the nucleus of cells, class II HDACs are free to shuttle between the nucleus and the cytoplasm. The exact physiological role of each of the individual HDAC isoforms in cells is far from fully understood, yet it is known that these enzymes act on many other nonhistone substrates. They also often function as part of larger multiprotein complexes and are frequently associated with other HDAC isoforms and/or require the presence of several coregulators.

HDACis have emerged as interesting drug candidates, in particular antineoplastic, and a number of agents are being explored in the clinic in both solid and hematological tumors, where they reverse the aberrant epigenetic state associated with cancer, thereby regulating: cell differentiation, proliferation and/or apoptosis and angiogenesis, as well as immune response [4, 7]. Imbalance of histone and nonhistone protein acetylation is common in human cancer and is related to HDAC overexpression and aberrant recruitment by oncoproteins, or mutation in malignant cells. Also several mutations affecting HATs have also been described in tumors. However, the full physiological role of HDACs and their inhibitors is not fully understood and continues to be investigated [5]. HDACis are also being investigated for the treatment of neurodegenerative and psychiatric disorders [8] and inflammation.

9.2
Mechanism and X-Ray Crystal Structure

The understanding of the mechanism of action and the rational design of HDACis is greatly facilitated by the availability of structural information and several X-ray crystal structures of HDACs are available. The first of these was of HDAC-like protein (HDLP) bound by two inhibitors [9]. Two independent groups have also published crystal structures of HDAC8 [10, 11]. The architecture of these structures is very similar, with the residues within and in the immediate vicinity of the active site being conserved between HDLP and HDAC8 (Figure 9.1a). Also, based on sequence homology these are likely to be common to all Zn-dependent HDACs. However, the organization of the loop and distal helices make the active site of HDAC8 more open

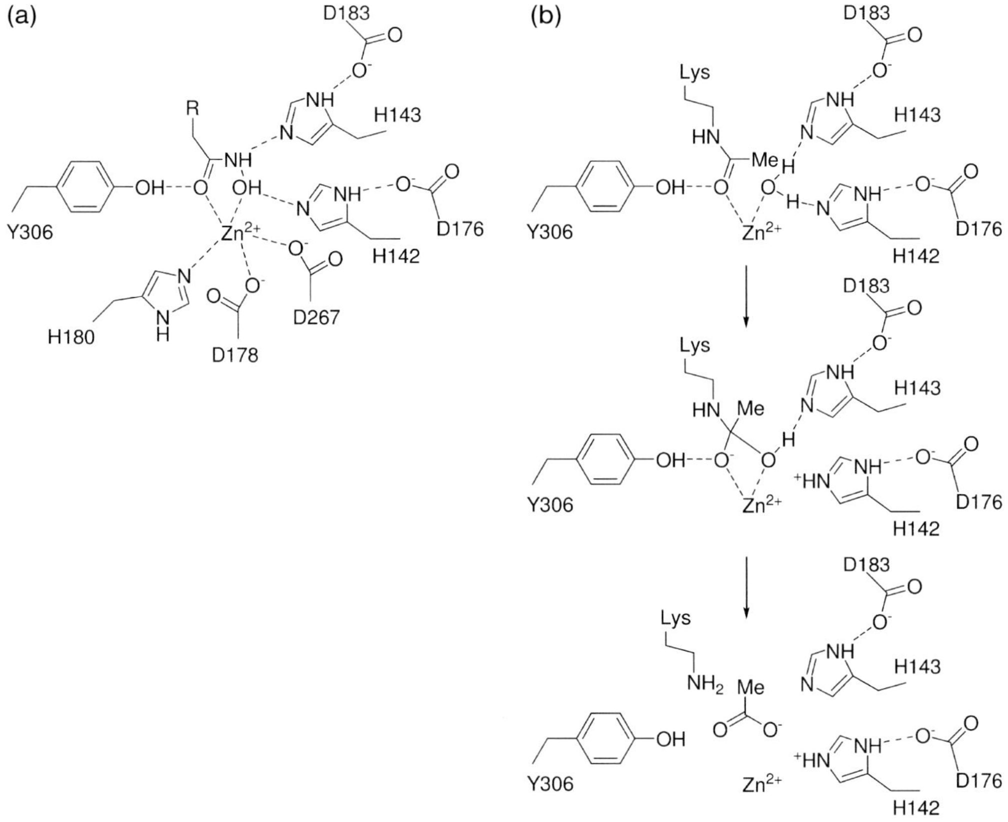

Figure 9.1 (a) Representation of crucial binding interactions of hydroxamic acid inhibitor in the HDAC active site (HDAC8 numbering). (b) Proposed catalytic mechanism.

and accessible compared to HDLP. The deacetylase active site is an approximately 12 Å tunnel, containing the catalytic zinc at one end. The zinc ion is pentacoordinated by two aspartic acids and one histidine residue; the remaining two sites are occupied by a bound inhibitor. Immediately above this are a critical tyrosine residue (histidine in some class II HDACs) and two histidine–aspartic acid charge relay systems, that both play a key role in the deacetylation reaction. The remainder of the tunnel is made up of lipophilic amino acids which are highly conserved across the isoforms; notable are two phenylalanine side chains which restrict the width of the tunnel. At the top of this binding cavity is a rim leading to the surface of the HDAC, which is made from several loop regions that differ between subtypes. The binding mode of the inhibitors are very similar between crystal structures, with the hydroxamic acid acting as a bidentate chelator of the zinc ion. This functional group also makes a number of other key contacts within the active site, with the conserved tyrosine residue forming a hydrogen bond to the carbonyl oxygen and making interactions with the two charge relay systems. The central portion of the inhibitor then threads its way through the long narrow binding cavity, making a number of lipophilic binding interactions, whilst the remote terminus of the inhibitor is correctly positioned to interact with the rim of the HDAC. Interestingly, the structure of a catalytically inactive HDAC 8 mutant bound to an Ac-lysine substrate reveals that an essential conserved aspartic acid located at the mouth of the binding cavity makes two hydrogen bonds to the substrate [10b]. Very recently, small molecule HDACis bound to the catalytic domain of HDAC 4 have also been described [12].

The binding mode of these inhibitors gives an insight into the mechanism of the deacetylation reaction based on the hypothesis that the bound hydroxamic acids act as substrate analogs [9]. It is proposed that the Ac-lysine residue binds to both the active site zinc and the tyrosine residue, these two interactions acting to polarize the C=O to attack (Figure 9.1b). The nucleophile in the deacetylation reaction is a water molecule whose nucleophilicity is increased through coordination to both the zinc ion, and to the Asp-His charge relay system. Upon attack, the resulting tetrahedral intermediate is then stabilized through two zinc–oxygen interactions, plus binding to the active site tyrosine. Collapse of this intermediate then liberates the deacetylated lysine residue.

9.3 Histone Deacetylase Inhibitors

To date there are seven distinct classes of HDAC inhibitors that are discussed in this review: short-chain fatty acids like valproic acid (**1**), hydroxamic acids such as vorinostat (**2**), aminoanilines exemplified by SNDX-275 (**3**), natural cyclic peptides like romidepsin (**4**) and apicidin (**5**), electrophilic ketones like **6**, small molecule inhibitors derived from natural products, and thiols (Figure 9.2). All classes of HDACis contain three key structural elements to their pharmacophore: (i) a zinc-binding group which coordinates the zinc ion at the bottom of the long narrow active site cavity, (ii) a capping group which interacts both with the amino acids on the rim of the binding cavity and the protein surface and (iii) a linker domain whose role is to ensure the correct positioning of the two former groups and to interact with the lipophilic binding tunnel.

9.3.1 Short-Chain Fatty Acids

The simplest class of HDACis in terms of structure are the short-chain fatty acids, exemplified by butyric acid (BA; **7**) and valproic acid (**1**; Figure 9.3). Unsurprisingly given their low molecular weight, lipophilicity and lack of functionality, these agents are the least potent of the various classes of HDACis, with IC_{50} values in the millimolar range. However in 1975 BA was shown to induce the differentiation in Friend leukemia cells [13]; and then three years later to cause a dramatic and reversible increase in histone acetylation [14]. These findings together with growth arrest seen in many cell lines caused BA to be evaluated in the clinic. Despite very

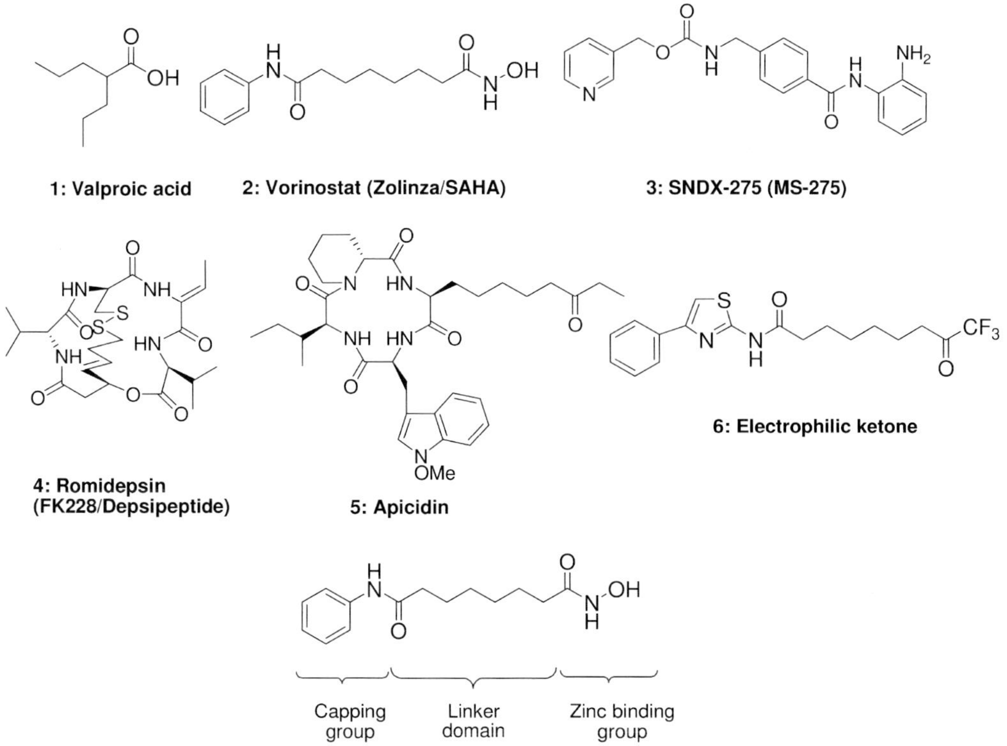

Figure 9.2 Representative HDACis and proposed HDAC inhibitor pharmacophore.

encouraging results seen in the first patients, more extensive clinical trials failed to reproduce these findings, probably due to its short half life and low plasma levels achievable. In an effort to obtain higher plasma levels several prodrugs of BA have been developed [15], the most studied of these was AN9/Pivanex (**8**), which progressed as far as phase II clinical trials. Other aliphatic acids, like valproic acid (**1**), have also been demonstrated to be modestly active HDACis (HDAC2 $IC_{50} = 0.54$ mM), relieving HDAC-dependent transcriptional repression and causing histone hyperacetylation both in cell culture and *in vivo* [16]. Moreover, reduced tumor growth and metastasis formation have been observed in a rat breast cancer model following twice daily i.p. dosing.

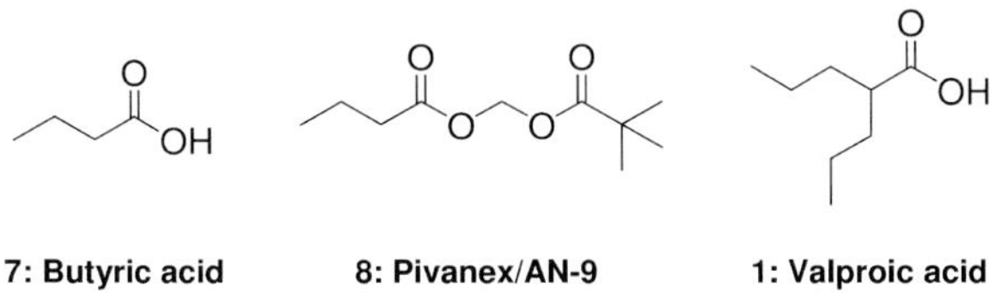

Figure 9.3 Short-chain fatty acid HDACis.

9.3.2
Hydroxamic Acids

The hydroxamic acid class is probably the most widely explored class of HDACis and indeed, since the discovery of Trichostatin A (**9**), significant progress has been made culminating with the approval of vorinostat (**2**) for the treatment cutaneous manifestations of advanced CTCL that has relapsed or progressed on or following two or more systemic therapies. Multiple other compounds from this class are now being explored in man. The following section tries to capture all the key developments of this class of HDACi, nevertheless several excellent reviews can be consulted for further details [17].

Trichostatin A (TSA; **9**) [18] was the first hydroxamic acid HDACi to be discovered, being isolated from the fungus *Streptomyces hydroscopicus* (Figure 9.4). This compound has subsequently become one of the main research tools for probing the function of histone acetylation. Like butyric acid, interest in this natural product arouse due to the demonstration that it was able to cause induction of Friend leukemia cell differentiation, as well as G_1 and G_2/M cell cycle arrest. In 1990 TSA was identified to be a potent HDACi, giving rise to a marked accumulation of acetylated histones in a variety of mammalian cells. Subsequently it was shown that doses as low as 6.7 nM were sufficient to cause an accumulation of acetylated histone H4 in cells. Using partially purified HDACs from mouse FM3A cells it was demonstrated that TSA strongly inhibits HDAC with $K_i = 3.4$ nM [19]. Interestingly, the *S*-enantiomer of the natural product is devoid of activity. Unfortunately poor pharmacokinetics precluded further development, but stimulated researchers to development related HDACis with improved properties.

Following TSA, probably the most widely studied HDACi is vorinostat (**2**; SAHA/ Zolinza). Interestingly, the discovery of this compound arose by chance, as the groups of P. Marks, R. Breslow and R. Rifkind were working to understand the mechanism

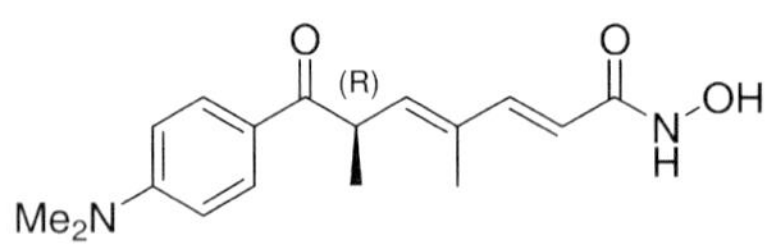

9: Trichostatin A

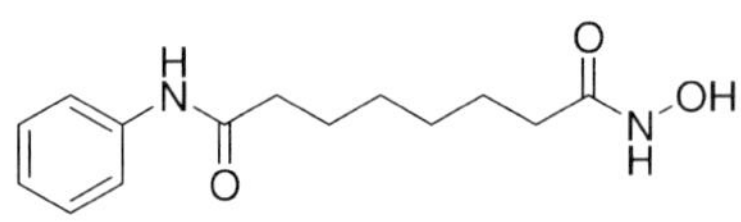

2: Vorinostat (Zolinza/SAHA)

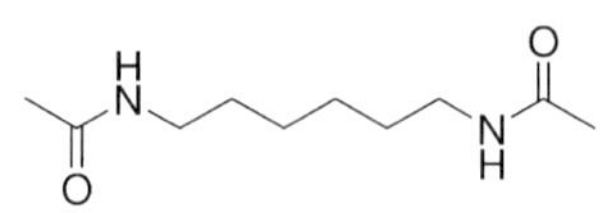

11: Hexamethylene bisacetamide (HMBA)

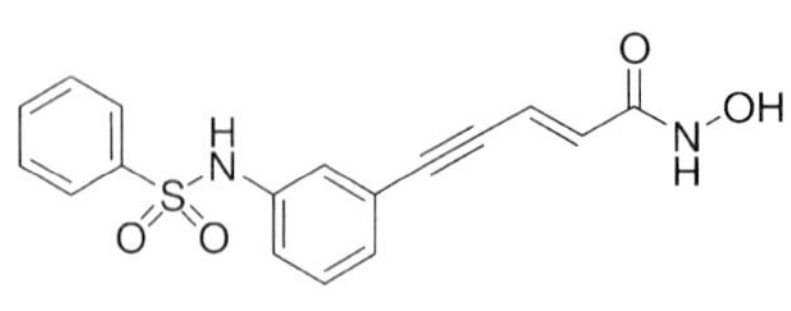

10: Oxamflatin

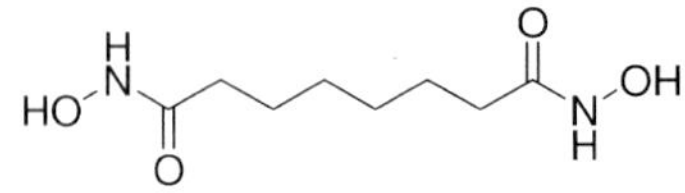

12: Suberoyl bishydroxamic acid (SBHA)

Figure 9.4 The first examples of hydroxamic acid HDACis.

by which DMSO was able to arrest the growth and induce terminal differentiation of transformed cells [20]. They identified that hexamethylene bisacetamide (HMBA; **11**; optimum concentration 5 mM) was a more potent differentiating agent [21] and although this compound caused minor and partial remissions in myelodysplastic syndrome (MDS) and acute myelogenous leukemia (AML) in the clinic, these remissions were only transient and a more potent derivative was sought. Hypothesizing that a stronger binding group was required they prepared suberoyl bishydroxamic acid (SBHA; **12**) which was two orders of magnitude more potent than **11**, optimum concentration 30 μM [22]. They also rationalized that two hydroxamic acid groups were probably not required so replaced the second of these with a lipophilic anilide moiety giving rise to suberoylanilide hydroxamic acid (vorinostat/SAHA; **2**) which was itself sixfold more active than **12**. This compound is capable of inducing differentiation of murine erythroleukemia cells, causing increased levels of p21 and G_1 cell cycle block. Subsequently, V. Richon recognized the similarities to TSA and thereafter was able to reveal that this agent was capable of inhibiting HDAC, with $IC_{50} = 10$ and 20 nM on HDACs 1 and 3 respectively. Vorinostat has been shown to induce differentiation, cell growth arrest and/or apoptosis in a wide variety of cell lines at low micromolar concentrations and to have antiproliferative effects against a range of cultured transformed cells. These findings are the subject of several other recent reviews [23, 24]. *In vivo* vorinostat inhibits tumor growth with little toxicity in a wide range of animal models of solid tumors (e.g. breast, prostate, lung, gastric cancer) and hematological malignancies. In a phase IIb study for advanced, refractory CTCL the overall response rate was 29.7% following a daily oral dose of 400 mg [3, 25]. Clinical studies have also been initiated against a wide range of solid and hematological malignancies, both as single agent and in combination. Ongoing studies include: mesothelioma, renal cell, bladder, prostate and breast carcinomas, as well as glioblastoma, melanoma, non-Hodgkin's lymphoma, MDS and AML. Phase II/III clinical studies are also underway in nonsmall cell lung cancer in combination with carboplatin and paclitaxel.

Another related hydroxamic acid HDACi is oxamflatin (**10**), an unsaturated hydroxamic acid prepared as part of a chemical library designed to identify compounds capable to cause morphological revision of ras transformed NIH3T3 cells [26]. Oxamflatin has been profiled in a wide range of cancer cell lines and demonstrated to cause growth inhibition at concentrations in the range of 0.02–0.72 μg/mL. Subsequent work revealed that this inhibitor is capable of inducing morphologic change of HeLa cells in a similar manner to TSA and follow up revealed that it caused hyperacetylation. Thereafter, it was demonstrated that this agent directly inhibits partial purified mouse HDACs with an $IC_{50} = 15.7$ nM. Interestingly, in a mouse B16 leukemia model oxamflatin administered every other day at 8–50 mg/kg i.p. was able to cause a dose-dependent increase in lifespan, with doses of 20 and 50 mg/kg resulting in 30 and 67% increases.

As already mentioned, the field of hydroxamic acid HDACis is extensive, therefore the next paragraphs are divided into sections depending on the nature of the group attached to the hydroxamic acid, including: aliphatic, cinnamic, phenyl and heterocyclic hydroxamic acids.

9.3.2.1 Aliphatic Hydroxamic Acids

One of the first papers to describe synthetic HDACis described the development of hybrid derivatives of TSA and the cyclic peptides. The group of Jung recognized that both classes of compounds contained a zinc-binding group, a linker domain and a capping region, therefore they hypothesized to combine various elements of the two classes (Figure 9.5). The most effective unification of these classes was to link the hydroxamic acid to a 6-aminohexanoic acid capped off with methyl phenylalanine which inhibited maize HD2 76% at 30 μM. Similarly, the *para*-dimethylaminobenzoic acid derivative of 6-aminohexanoic acid (**13d**) inhibited 94% at 30 μM [27]. Further exploration of this latter compound investigated the influence of the chain length on HDAC activity [28]. A five- or six-carbon chain between the hydroxamic acid and the amide group was found to be optimal, with **13c** and **13e** displaying $IC_{50} = 100$ nM. Further extension to a heptanyl spacer was tolerated but less potent ($IC_{50} = 300$ nM). In contrast, a shorter butyl spacer was 20-fold less active, with $IC_{50} = 2$ μM. The inclusion of a benzyl linker was also studied, and whereas when the phenyl ring was linked to the hydroxamic acid (**13h**) a 180 nM inhibitor was obtained, in contrast the isomer **13g** with the methylene adjacent to the hydroxamic acid was devoid of activity at 40 μM. All these derivatives were significantly less active than TSA ($IC_{50} = 3$ nM).

Related investigation of the structure–activity relationship (SAR) of HDAC inhibition, including cellular activity, was undertaken by the groups of Novartis and Methylgene [29]. The former group described an extensive investigation of vorinostat and TSA analogs, and focusing on analogs of the former, they were able to demonstrate that 2-aminopyridine analog (**14a**) was equipotent to vorinostat (HDAC $IC_{50} = 248$ and 194 nM respectively) and maintained cellular activity (HCT116 $IC_{50} = 2.0$ and 1.9 μM respectively). The other pyridyl isomers despite displaying similar enzymatic activity were less active in cells. In parallel, simplified analogs of TSA were described, this time the inhibitors being tested on human HDAC nuclear extracts (NE) with rank order of potency $6 > 7 > 5 \gg 4$. The **13d** displayed antiproliferative activity against HCT116 cells ($IC_{50} = 210$ nM) and also on a broad panel of cancer cell lines including colon SW620, lung A549, breast MDA-MB-435 and lung H1299 cells ($IC_{50} = 0.7$–3.9 μM). Interestingly, alkylation of the amide resulted in a twofold loss of activity. Almost simultaneously, the group at Methylgene reported the investigation of analogs of TSA (**16a–d**) and tested them against human HDAC1 [29b]. They too found that the optimal spacer between the hydroxamic acid and the capping group was six methylenes, with potencies in the order of $6 > 7 > 5 \gg 4$ atom spacer.

Meanwhile, the researchers at Abbott were also designing other potent HDACis which they hoped could be subtype-selective by the incorporation of a macrocyclic capping group on the 6-aminohexanoic hydroxamic acid framework [30]. Although the targeted compound proved to be a relatively weak HDACi ($IC_{50} = 2.1$ μM), the group identified **19** as a potent byproduct ($IC_{50} = 38$ nM), with antiproliferative activity in the range of hundreds of nanomoles. Subsequent SAR work on these succinimide derivatives gave little overall improvement in terms of activity, but did result in simplified structures such as **20**. Key SAR findings included that both carbonyl groups are required for activity and the addition of a second alkyl group on

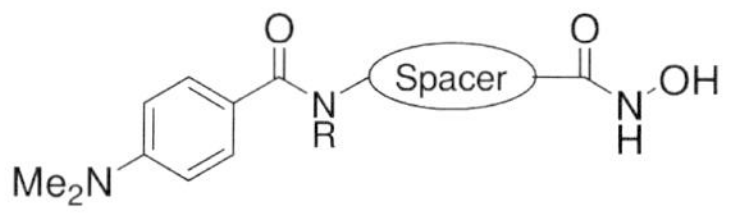

	Spacer	R	Maize HD2 IC50 (nM)	HDAC NE IC50 (nM)	HCT116 IC50 (μM)
13a	3 x CH_2	H	NA at 40 μM		
13b	4 x CH_2	H	2000	>10000	
13c	5 x CH_2	H	100	244	
13d	6 x CH_2	H	100	46	0.21
13e	7 x CH_2	H	300	145	0.5
13f	5 x CH_2	Me	ND	443	
13g	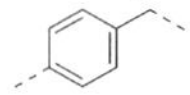		NA at 40 μM		
13h	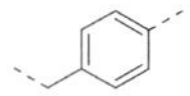		180		

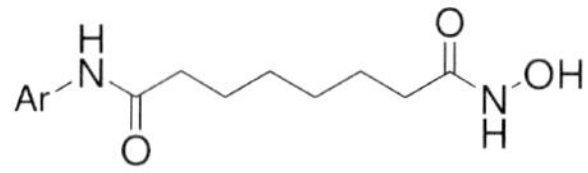

	Ar	HDAC NE IC50 (nM)	HCT116 IC50 (μM)
2	Ph	194	1.9
14a	2-Pyridyl	248	2.0
14b	3-Pyridyl	200	6.5
14c	4-Pyridyl	306	5.4

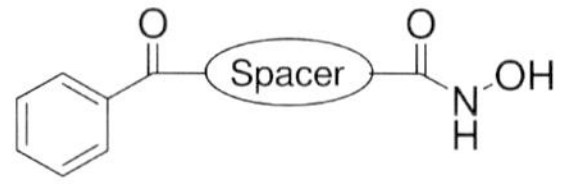

	Spacer	HDAC 1 IC50 (nM)
16a	4 x CH_2	1500
16b	5 x CH_2	500
16c	6 x CH_2	65
16d	7 x CH_2	135

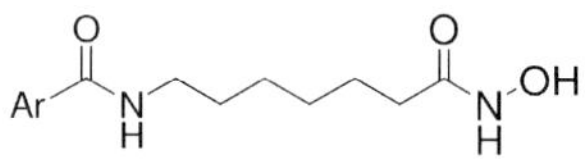

	Ar	HDAC NE IC50 (nM)	HT1080 IC50 (μM)	MDA435 IC50 (μM)
2	SAHA	143	2.4	1.9
15a	Ph (reverse SAHA)	1006		
15b	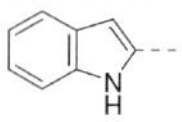	14.6	0.14	0.15
15c	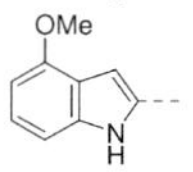	3.1	0.12	0.13

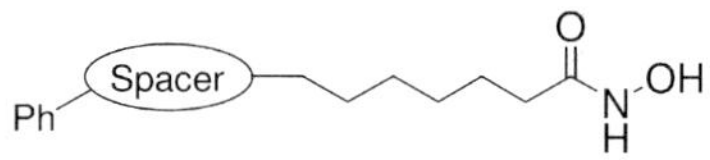

	Ar	HDAC NE IC50 (nM)	HT1080 IC50 (μM)	MDA435 IC50 (μM)
18a	CH_2	560		
18b	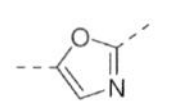	9.8	8.4	2.2
18c	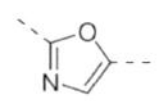	13	23%inh at 50 μM	6%inh at 50 μM
18d	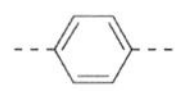	58		

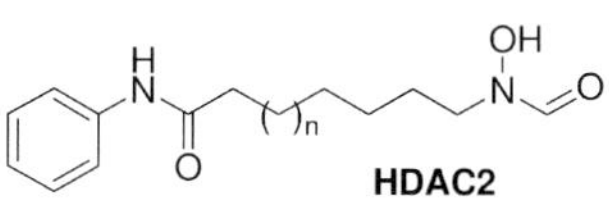

	n	HDAC2 IC50 (nM)
17a	0	19000
17b	1	11000
17c	2	7800

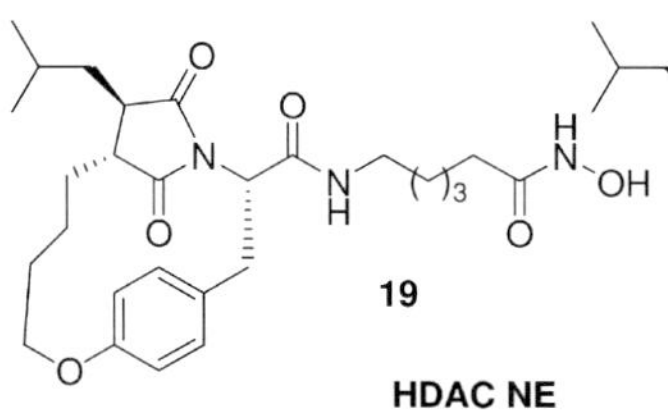

19

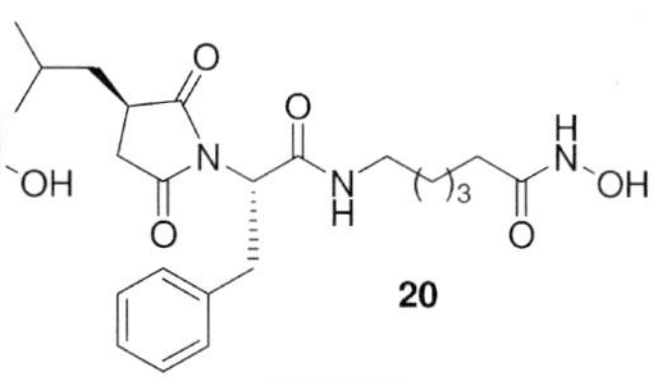

20

	HDAC NE IC50 (nM)	MDA435 IC50 (μM)
19	38	0.15
2	120	1.9
20	99	0.67

Figure 9.5 SAR exploration of aliphatic hydroxamic acid HDACis.

the succinimide results in an improvement of activity and finally that a five-methylene chain was optimal.

Further work by the same group resulted in the identification of indole amides as an alternative capping group for aliphatic hydroxamic acids [31]. Starting from a reverse amide version of SAHA (**15a**) which displays only micromolar HDAC inhibitory activity, they were able to show that replacement of the phenyl group with an indol-2-yl group results in a 60-fold improvement in activity. This gain in activity was also seen in cells with **15b** displaying $IC_{50} = 0.14$ and 0.15 μM in HT1080 and MDA435 cells respectively. Further improvements in activity could be achieved by substitution of the indole ring (e.g. **15c**). The unsubstituted derivative was tested in a HT1080 fibrosarcoma xenograft model and was shown to cause 36 and 39% tumor growth inhibition (TGI) when dosed every other day at 30 and 100 mg/kg.

The Abbott group also investigated different linkers between the aliphatic chains of these hydroxamic acids and the capping group; and in an effort to enlarge the number of connecting units they explored 'conformation restricted' heterocyclic moieties [32]. Using SAHA and reverse SAHA as benchmarks ($IC_{50} = 140$ and 1010 nM) this group made a number of heterocycles as alternative connection motifs and demonstrated that the isomeric oxazoles **18b** and **18c** are potent HDACis ($IC_{50} = 9.8$ and 13 nM), showing the N–H bond is not essential. They also showed that simple phenyl (**18d**) or methylene (**18a**) groups are much less active, with $IC_{50} = 58$ and 560 nM respectively. Unfortunately **18b** showed only weak cellular activity with $IC_{50} = 8.4$ μM against HT1080 cells, but further improvements in potency and cellular activity could be achieved by the incorporation of substituents on the phenyl ring.

A limited amount of work was also conducted by the group of Schultz to investigate the potential of *N*-formyl hydroxylamine head group to inhibit HDAC. This bidentate chelating moiety was used successfully in inhibitors of angiotensin converting enzyme and neural endopeptidase, however, in the case of HDAC a 50-fold loss in activity was observed with this group (**17a–c**) [33].

9.3.2.2 Cinnamic Hydroxamic Acids

Following the aliphatic hydroxamic acids, the second most widely investigated class of hydroxamate HDACi are those of the cinnamic acid derivatives (Figure 9.6), alternatively known as *N*-hydroxyphenyl-2-propeneamides. Indeed, several compounds from this class have advanced into the clinic, including: panobinostat (**24**) and belinostat (**26a**). Interest in this class of inhibitors arose from the finding that *m*-carboxycinnamic acid bishydroxamide (CBHA) was a potent differentiating agent (optimum concentration 4 μM) [21, 22] and was only twofold less active than SAHA. Furthermore, comparing these structures to TSA and oxamflatin it can be imagined how the remote double bond in TSA, or the alkyne in oxamflatin could readily be substituted for an aromatic ring.

Researchers at Novartis identified NVP-LAK974 during an HTS campaign, however despite this compound being a potent HDACi it had only poor efficacy in a HCT116 colon cancer xenograft [34]. Efforts were then made to alter the structure in the hope of improving the *in vivo* activity, concentrating primarily on the amine substituents. In the secondary amine series, no clear SAR trend was observed, but promising compounds like the fluoroindole **22a** and indole **22b** were identified as being relatively potent HDACis with good antiproliferative activity. However, the tertiary amines were generally more potent, with small aliphatic, nonpolar substituents giving a significant boost in activity. For instance, adding an *iso*-propyl (**22c**)

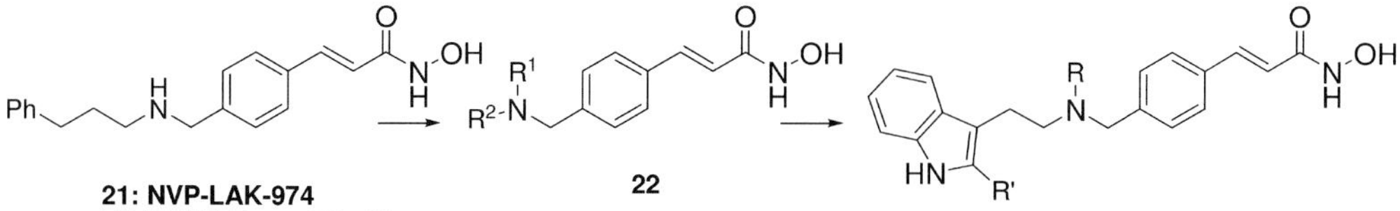

21: NVP-LAK-974
HDAC NE IC_{50} = 150 nM
HCT116 IC_{50} = 50 nM
H1299 IC_{50} = 800 nM

22

23: NVP-LAQ824 R = $(CH_2)_2OH$, R' = H
24: Panobinostat (LBH-589) R = H, R' = Me

Number	R^1	R^2	HDAC NE IC_{50} (nM)	HCT116 IC_{50} (µM)	H1299 IC_{50} (µM)	in vivo MTD (mg/kg)	Xenograft dose (mg/kg)	Efficacy %T/C
22a	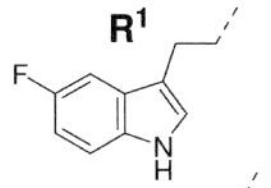	H	14	30	310	100	100	16
22b	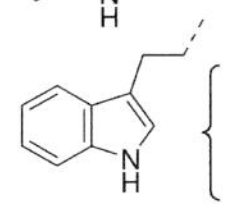	H	63	30	400	100	100	17
22c		^iPr	23	6	30	25	25	29
23		CH_2CH_2OH	32	10	150	>200	100	12

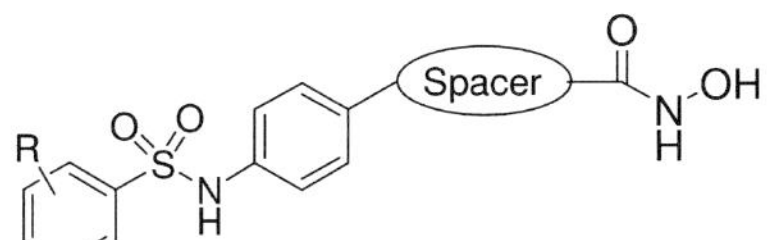

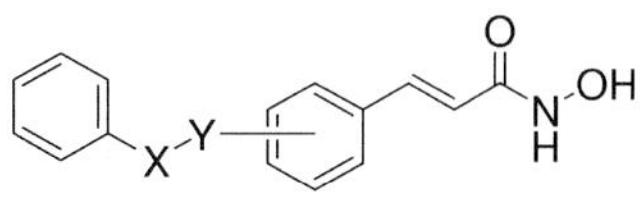

Number	R	R	HDAC1 IC_{50} (µM)	HCT116 IC_{50} (µM)
25a	bond	H	0.9	2
25b	CH_2	H	1	22
25c	$(CH_2)_2$	H	0.1	2
25d	$(CH_2)_3$	H	1	8
25e	CH=CH	H	0.2	3
25f	CH=CMe	H	2	15
25g	CH=CH	4-Cl	0.075	1
25h	CH=CH	4-MeO	0.060	0.4
25i	CH=CH	3,4-di-MeO	0.090	0.2

Number	Substitution	-X-Y-	HDAC1 IC_{50} (nM)	WST-1 IC_{50} (µM)
26a: Belinostat (PXD-101)	*meta*	$-NH-SO_2-$	28	1.27
26b	*meta*	$-SO_2-NH-$	188	8.85
26c	*para*	$-NH-SO_2-$	29	1.13
25e	*para*	$-SO_2-NH-$	59	3.75
26d	*meta*	$-NMe-SO_2-$	476	7.29

Figure 9.6 SAR exploration of cinnamyl hydroxamic acid HDACis.

or hydroxyethyl (**24**) chain results in a three- to 13-fold increase in activity. The most promising compounds from this series were then studied *in vivo* to determine both their maximum tolerated doses (MTDs) and their *in vivo* efficacy in a HCT116 xenograft. Although most of these compounds showed good tumor growth inhibition (TGI) this was occasionally compromised by body weight loss and/or efficacy was seen only close to the MTD. NVP-LAQ824 (**23**) was identified as the most promising compound due to the fact that good efficacy (55–20% T/C between 10–100 mg/kg) was seen, with no changes in body weight. Also these efficacious doses were significantly below the MTD of 200 mg/kg. Similarly, in an A549 lung xenograft model statistically significant tumor growth inhibition was observed, with T/C of 7–32%. NVP-LAQ824 entered the clinical trials as a treatment for hematological malignancies, but no recent development has been reported for this agent. However, Novartis are developing panobinostat (**24**), a structurally related HDACi which is currently in phase II/III clinical trials for chronic myeloid leukemia (CML), refractory CTCL, MDS and multiple myeloma (MM). In a phase I study in patients with refractory hematological malignancies a reduction in peripheral blasts was seen in eight out of 11 patients during the 7-day treatment period and increases in histone H3 acetylation were detected [35]. Little preclinical data for panobinostat is available but the compound is reported to be a potent HDACi ($IC_{50} = 37\,nM$) and shows activity in a p21 promoter assay ($EC_{50} = 69\,nM$) [36].

A related series of cinnamyl hydroxamic acids bearing sulfonamides was developed by the groups at Methylgene [37] and TopoTarget [38, 39]. The researchers at Methylgene identified a series of compounds (**25a–i**) whereby the hydroxamic acid moiety was linked to a phenyl sulfonamide by distinct spacer groups. Initial work focused on the identification of the optimal linker between the two groups; and it was established that a two-carbon linker gave the most potent compounds, being fivefold more active than a simple bond, or a one- or three-carbon linker. Interestingly, substitution of this two-carbon linker was detrimental for activity. Despite there being little difference in activities between the saturated (**25c**) and unsaturated (**25e**) linkers, the group in Montreal decided to focus entirely on the cinnamyl series and to investigate the role of the capping group. They determined that electron-withdrawing groups were not tolerated on the phenyl ring. Instead, simple 4-chloro, 4-methoxy and 3,4-dimethoxy groups were beneficial for activity. The 3,4-dimethoxy analog (**25i**) was studied in a lung A549 xenograft model and daily doses of 20, 40 and 50 mg/kg i.p. resulted in 41–57% TGI.

The group at TopoTarget concentrated on designing a novel HDACi scaffold based on the structures of known HDACis and concentrated on motifs that they considered to be compatible with drug development; in this way they evolved a series of related sulfonamide HDACis (**26a–d**). Most of their work revolved around cinnamyl hydroxamic acids with 'forward' or 'reverse' sulfonamides in the *meta* or *para* positions of the phenyl ring (sulfonamide *N* or *S* attached respectively) where highly potent inhibitors were identified. In the *meta* series they showed that reverse sulfonamides were always more potent and culminated in the identification of belinostat (formerly PXD-101; **26a**). In the *para* series no clear trend emerged and both forward and reverse compounds are tolerated. In contrast, substituents at the *ortho* position are devoid of activity. With regard to the aromatic head group a wide range of substituents are tolerated irrespectively of their electronic properties, while interestingly *N*-substitution of the sulfonamide results in a 17-fold loss of activity. With regard to SAR of the cinnamyl double bond, saturation of the alkene results in an order of magnitude loss of activity, while replacement with an ether gives an inactive compound. Belinostat (**26a**) is expected to be studied in an initial regulatory study as monotherapy to treat peripheral T-cell lymphoma (PTCL) in the second half of 2008 following i.v. administration and is under going phase II trials in solid tumors (ovarian, hepatocarcinoma, mesothelioma) and hematological malignancies (B- and T-cell lymphomas, MDS, AML, MM), as well as several combination and phase I studies. Belinostat is a potent HDACi ($IC_{50} = 27\,nM$) and shows cytotoxicity against a wide panel of tumor cell lines with IC_{50} values in the range of 0.2–3.4 μM [39]. These cytotoxic effects correlate with histone H4 acetylation. Similarly, induction of apoptosis was observed following treatment with belinostat, as was induction of p21. In preclinical xenograft studies the compound was shown to cause a dose-dependent growth delay of both ovarian A2780 and colon HCT116 xenografts at doses of 10–40 mg/kg daily i.p., with no obvious signs of toxicity.

9.3.2.3 Phenyl Hydroxamic Acids

Turning attention to the phenyl hydroxamic acids, these are a relatively sparsely explored series of HDACi, probably due to the fact that simple analogs are somewhat less potent HDACis compared to alkyl or cinnamyl linkers. Nevertheless, the group at Celera Genomics was able to identify the phenyl hydroxamic acid **27a**, $IC_{50} = 43$ nM, as a promising lead (Figure 9.7) [40a]. Through SAR studies they were able to increase the activity sevenfold by replacement of the phenyl with a naphthyl group. Substitution by a benzofuran further improved potency and addition of a dimethylaminomethyl group at the 3-position gave PCI-24781 (formerly CRA-24781; **27d**). PCI-24781 is a potent HDAC 1 inhibitor ($K_i = 7$ nM) and also inhibits many other HDAC isoforms, with $K_i = 19, 8, 17, 280, 24$ nM, respectively, on HDACs 2, 3, 6, 8, 10. In pre-clinical studies, the compound was demonstrated to give rise to an increase in both histone and tubulin acetylation in many tumor cell lines, resulting in inhibition of growth and induction of apoptosis (e.g. HCT116 $GI_{50} = 200$ nM). In a HCT116 xenograft study a reduction in tumor growth was seen when administered i.v. 4 days/week with 57, 82 and 80% TGI at 40, 80 and 160 mg/kg respectively. Currently PCI-24781 is being evaluated in phase I/II clinical trials for solid tumors. The group at Pharmacyclics developed a related phenyl hydroxamic acid HDACi, PCI-34051 (**27e**) and demonstrated this to display greater than 200-fold selectivity for HDAC8 ($IC_{50} = 10$ nM) over the other HDAC isoforms [40b]. Interestingly, this compound induced caspase-dependent apoptosis in T-cell lymphomas and leukemias at low micromolar concentrations, but not in other hematopoietic or solid tumor cell lines. Furthermore, PCI-34051 does not cause detectable tubulin or histone acetylation.

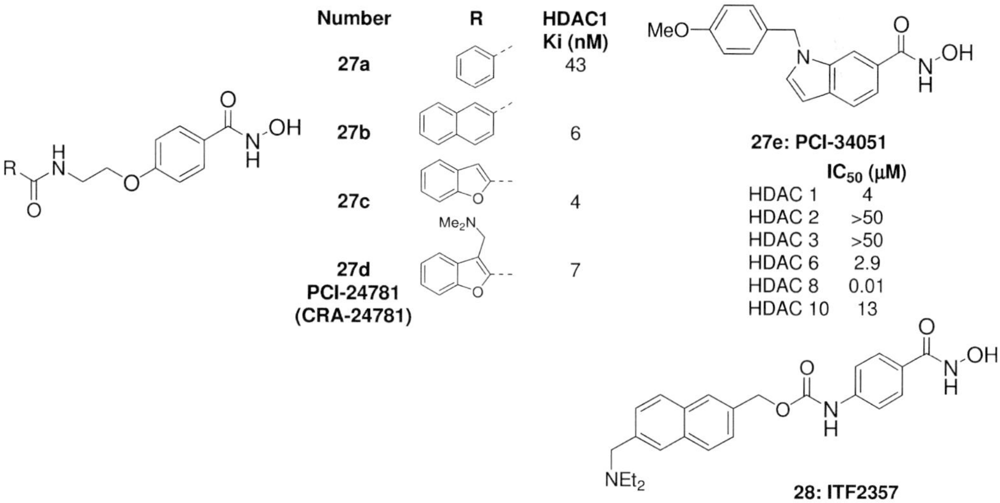

Figure 9.7 SAR exploration of phenyl hydroxamic acid HDACis.

A related *N*-hydroxybenzylamide that has advanced into phase II clinical studies is ITF2357 (**28**), developed by Italfarmaco [41]. This compound was demonstrated to inhibit class I and II HDACs, and to inhibit the proliferation of 9 MM and 7 AML cell lines, with mean IC_{50}'s = 0.17 μM and 0.23 μM respectively. In a mouse model of AML, injected cells home in on the blood, spleen, bone marrow and liver, usually resulting in death in 35–40 days. Daily administration of ITF2357 at 10 or 100 mg/kg resulted in an increase of survival of 6 and 10 days respectively.

9.3.2.4 Heterocycle Hydroxamic Acids

In place of the aryl ring a number of groups investigated the possibility of linking a heteroaromatic ring to the hydroxamic acid (Figure 9.8). Arguably the most successful of these was the group at Johnson and Johnson, who identified the pyrimidine hydroxamic acid R306465 (formerly JNJ-16241199; **29**), which is undergoing phase I trials as an oral agent. In preclinical models R306465 was demonstrated to be a potent HDACi (IC_{50} = 3.3 nM) and induced histone H3 and H4 acetylation in human A2780 ovarian cancer cells [42]. Against a broad panel of human cancer cell lines antiproliferation was observed, with IC_{50} = 15–486 nM. This compound also showed efficacy in a range of xenograft studies, including A2780 ovarian, H460 lung and HCT116 colon carcinoma models, when dosed once a day at 10–40 mg/kg.

Another related series of compounds was developed by the group at Argenta, who developed a series of thiophen-2-yl hydroxamic acids [43]. This series arose from a virtual screen on a virtual library comprised of 644 potential hydroxamic acids, derived *in silico* from all the carboxylic acids available to Argenta. The results of the virtual screen encouraged the company to synthesize 75 compounds, from which ADS100380 (**30**) was identified as a moderately active HDACi (IC_{50} = 750 nM), displaying antiproliferative activity against MDA-MD-231 cells (IC_{50} = 11.4 μM). Other closely related analogs (**31a–e**) with substituents off the pyrazole *N*-atoms were then designed to make additional interactions at the mouth of the active cavity. This resulted in substantial improvements in potency and cellular activity. One of the preferred substitutions was the introduction of a four-atom tether to an additional aromatic ring, especially including a nitrogen atom as the third atom. Further investigation into the aromatic ring demonstrated that a range of heteroaromatic groups were tolerated, including indoles (**31d**) and benzodioxoles (**31e**). The latter was studied in a human HCT116 xenograft and daily dosing of 50 mg/kg i.p. resulted in 33% TGI. Unfortunately, this compound was a potent CYP3A4 inhibitor and was also only sparingly orally bioavailable in rats. In an effort to improve these properties a search for replacements to pyrazole moiety was undertaken, which resulted in the identification of heterocycles bearing a heteroatom in the 2-position as moderately active HDACis. The 2-pyridyl (**32b**) and the 2-pyrimidinyl (**32e**) analogs were fivefold more active than the corresponding phenyl analog. Further SAR work in the 2-pyridyl series and the addition of a benzylamino-methyl group in the 5- or 6-postion of the pyridine gave potent compounds, with the 5-position being preferred. In fact, **32f** had 10-fold weaker CYP inhibition liabilities and also enhanced permeability, with F = 50% in rats, although it suffered from high clearance in mice.

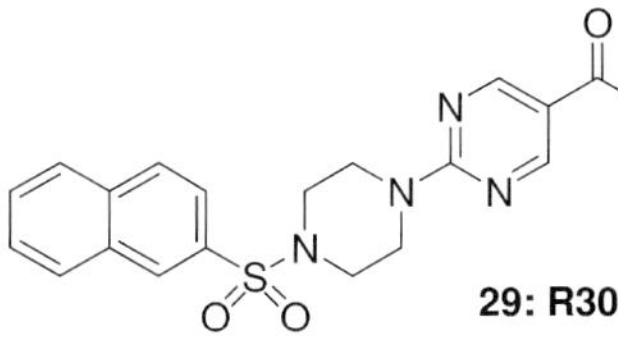

29: R306465 (JNJ-1624119)

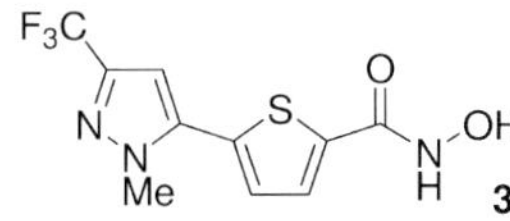

30: ADS100380
HDAC IC_{50} = 750 nM
MCF7 IC_{50} = 11.4 μM

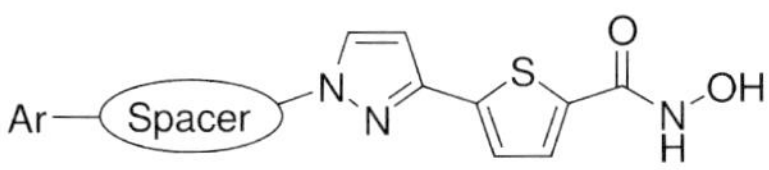

Number	Spacer	Ar	HDAC1 IC_{50} (nM)	MCF7 IC_{50} (μM)
31a	CH_2	Ph	153	2.06
31b	$(CH_2)_3$	Ph	34	0.52
31c	$CH_2NH(CH_2)_2$	Ph	33	0.46
31d	$CH_2NH(CH_2)_2$	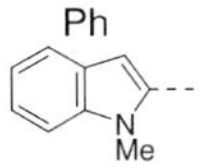	6	0.17
31e **ADS102550**	$CH_2NH(CH_2)_2$	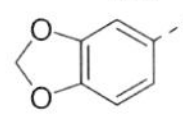	29	0.30

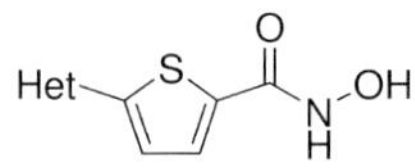

Number	Ar	HDAC1 IC_{50} (nM)	MCF7 IC_{50} (μM)
32a	Ph	900	31
32b	2-Pyridyl	243	2.25
32c	3-Pyridyl	1130	
32d	4-Pyridyl	1260	
32e	2-Pyrimidinyl	186	2.12
32f	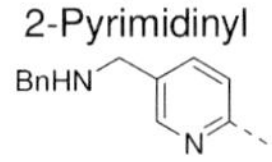	16	0.08

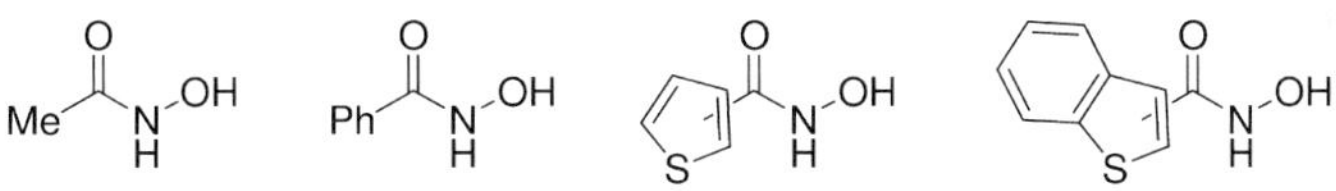

	33a	**33b**	**33c**: C-2	**33d**: C-3	**33e**: C-2	**33f**: C-3
HDAC IC_{50} (μM)	625	20	6.6	9.7	0.67	38%inh at 10 μM

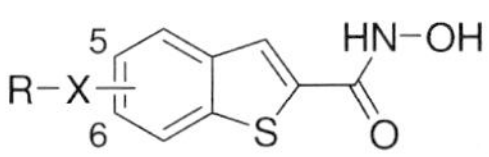

Number	Substitution	Spacer	HDAC1 IC_{50} (nM)	SC9 IC_{50} (nM)
34a	5	PhNHCO-	600	6135
34b	6	"	615	2775
34c	5	BnNHCO-	75	1705
34d	6	"	55	1105
34e	5	BnCONH-	30	1165
34f	6	"	10	220
34g	5	$BnNHCH_2$-	145	475
34h	6	"	50	160
34i	6	$PhCONHCH_2$-	10	190

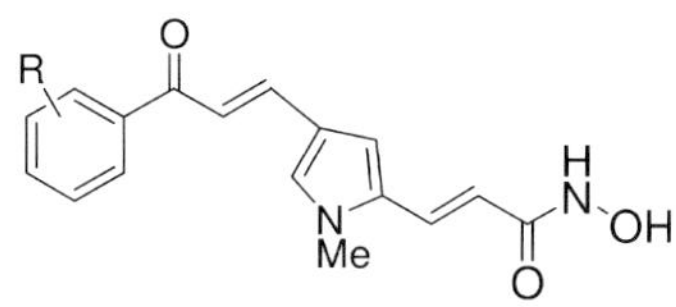

Number	R	HD1-B IC_{50} (μM)	HD1-A IC_{50} (μM)
TSA (9)		0.0004	0.0008
35a	2-Cl	1.6	0.05
35b	3-Cl	31.4	0.44
35c	3-F	38.8	0.22
35d	2-Me	0.39	0.06
35e	2-MeO	0.17	0.16

Figure 9.8 SAR exploration of heterocyclic hydroxamic acid HDACis.

Researchers at Merck developed a series of benzothiophen-2-yl hydroxamic acids as HDACis [44] which can be considered a hybrid of the cinnamyl and thiophenyl hydroxamic acids. Starting from simple acetyl hydroxamic acid (**33a**; $IC_{50} = 625\,\mu M$), they showed that incremental boost in activity could be achieved introducing first a phenyl ring ($IC_{50} = 20\,\mu M$), then replacing this with a thiophene ($IC_{50} = 6.6\,\mu M$).

Finally, the fusion of a benzo-ring resulted in benzothiophene **33e** with HDAC $IC_{50} = 670$ nM. Further improvements in potency were accomplished by the introduction of groups at the 5- and 6- positions of the benzothiophene. Optimal activity could be achieved by the incorporation of an aromatic ring at the end of a three-atom spacer, giving double-digit nanomolar HDACis. The most active compounds from this series were phenylacetylamino (**34f**; HDAC $IC_{50} = 10$ nM, SC9 $IC_{50} = 220$ nM) and benzoylaminomethyl (**34i**; HDAC $IC_{50} = 10$ nM, SC9 $IC_{50} = 190$ nM).

The group of Mai conducted an in-depth investigation of a series of pyrrole containing analogs (**35a–e**) of TSA. His group found that, by replacing the remote double bond of the natural product with this heterocycle, they could generate potent HDACis [45]. Extensive SAR investigations were conducted in order to determine: the optimal linker between the hydroxamic acid and the pyrrole, the desired substitution pattern and the preferred capping groups. Furthermore, docking models were developed to assist with the rational design of these inhibitors. Through this comprehensive work the group was able to evolve compounds with distinct HDAC selectivity profiles, identifying compounds that are selective for maize HD1-A over maize HD1-B, the homologs of mammalian class IIa HDACs (HDACs 4, 5, 7, 9) and class 1 HDACs respectively. For instance, although prototypical HDACis like TSA show essentially no selectivity between HD1-A and HD1-B, through the introduction of substituents on the terminal aryl ring, Mai and coworkers were able to develop potent dual HD1-A/HD1-B inhibitors like the *o*-methyl or *o*-methoxy analogs **35d** and **35e**. The introduction of groups in the *meta* position gave selective HD1-A inhibitors like **35c** with 176-fold selectivity over HD1-B. Yet, when this compound was tested against human HDACs 1 and 4, no activity was seen at 5 μM against HDAC1, whereas 55% of HDAC 4 activity was inhibited at the same concentration. Completing the SAR study, substituents were also introduced in the *para* position of the aromatic ring but these were substantially less active.

9.3.3 Aminoanilines

Besides aliphatic carboxylic acids and hydroxamic acids, another class of HDACis receiving extensive attention is that of the aminoaniline class (Figure 9.9), exemplified by CI-994 (**36**), SNDX-275 (**3**) and MGCD0103 (**38**). The latter two of these are still undergoing clinical investigation. The mechanism of action of these compounds is a controversial subject of extensive debate, although one yet to be proven hypothesis is that the *ortho*-amino aniline acts as a zinc-binding group.

CI-994 (**36**) was the first member of this class to be identified and arose from the serendipitous observation that dinaline, a potential anticonvulsant and the des-acetyl derivative of CI-994, caused bone marrow suppression. Furthermore, in preclinical models it showed good antitumor activity [46] and it was revealed that dinaline undergoes rapid acetylation *in vivo*, with CI-994 as the active species. After extensive preclinical work CI-994 was evaluated in the clinic, but development has been terminated. It was more recently shown that the antitumor activity is the result of

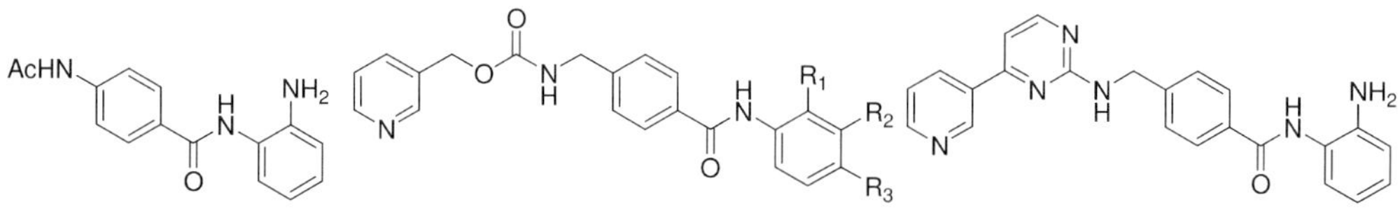

36: CI-994

Number	Spacer	HDAC1 IC_{50} (μM)
3: SNDX-275 (MS-275)	$R_1 = NH_2$	4.8
37a	R_1 = OH	2.2
37b	R_1 = NHAc	>100
37c	$R_2 = NH_2$	>100
37d	$R_3 = NH_2$	>100

38: MGCD0103

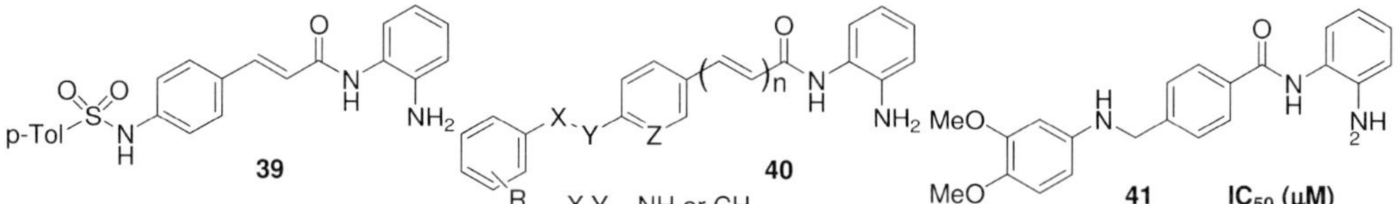

39

40

X,Y = NH or CH_2
Z = N or CH
n = 0, 1

41	IC_{50} (μM)
HDAC 1	2
HCT116	2

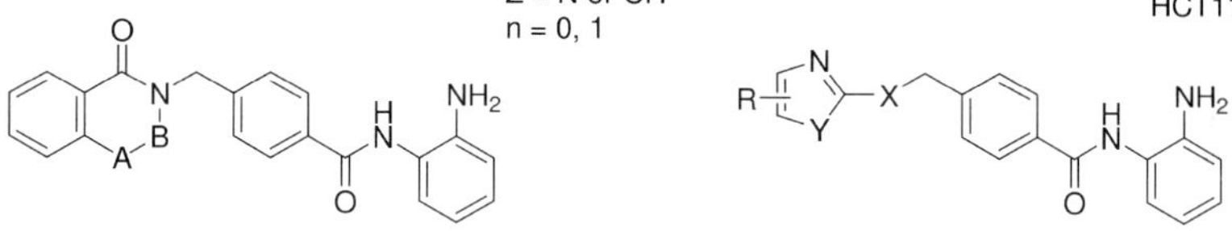

Number	Aromatic	HDAC1 IC_{50} (μM)	HCT116 IC_{50} (μM)
42a	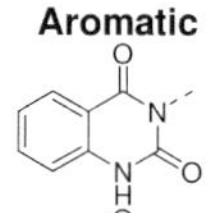	0.06	0.8
42b	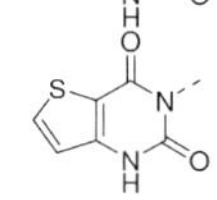	0.06	0.4

Number	Aromatic	HDAC1 IC_{50} (μM)	HCT116 IC_{50} (μM)
43a	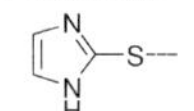	0.5	5
43b	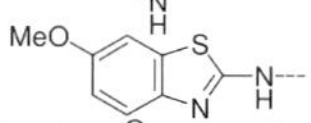	0.03	0.2
43c	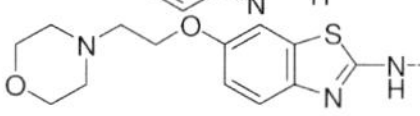	0.06	0.2

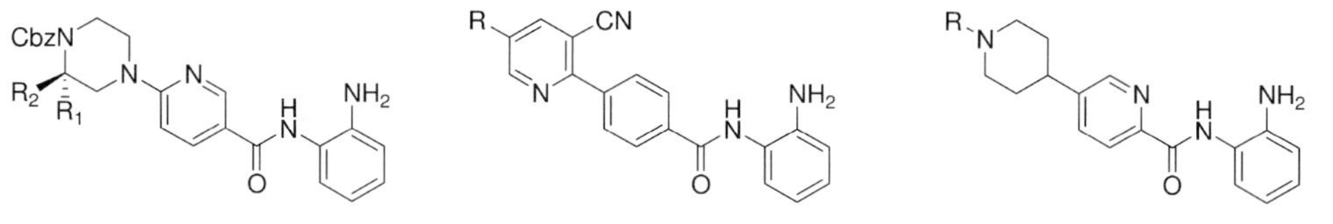

Number	R_1	R_2	HDAC1 IC_{50} (nM)	HCT116 IC_{50} (nM)
44a	H	H	168	
44b	Me	H	73	81
44c	H	Me	40	495

Number	R	HDAC1 pIC_{50}	HCT116 pIC_{50}
45a	H	7.91	6.54
45b	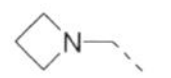	8.01	6.86

Number	R	HDAC1 pIC_{50}	HCT116 pIC_{50}
46a	Me	6.86	6.08
46b	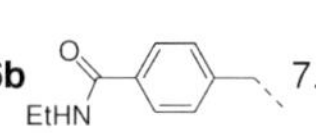	7.46	6.44

Figure 9.9 SAR exploration of aminoanilines HDACis.

HDAC inhibition [47], as growth of HCT-8 colon carcinoma cells is inhibited by CI-994 ($IC_{50} = 4.7\,\mu M$), with simultaneous dose-dependent increases in histone hyperacetylation. *In vitro* work also demonstrated that HDAC could be inhibited 50% at 25–50 μM.

Following in the footsteps of CI-994 is SNDX-275 (formerly MS-275; **3**), which is being developed by Syndax, who acquired worldwide rights from Bayer Schering Pharma. This compound is currently in phase I/II development for non-small cell lung cancer in combination with erlotinib or azacitidine; and it is also being studied in hematological malignancies (MDS, CML or AML), with or without azacitidine or growth factors. The compound is also being profiled as a monotherapy in solid tumors and has a relatively long half life, allowing weekly or biweekly administration [48]. Preclinically, SNDX-275 was shown to inhibit HDACs with $IC_{50} = 2.0\,\mu M$ and was demonstrated to cause hyperacetylation of histone H4, induce $p21^{WAF1/CIP}$ and cause G_1 cell cycle arrest [49, 50]. The *ortho*-amino group or *ortho*-hydroxy group (**37a**; $IC_{50} = 2.2\,\mu M$) are crucial for activity, as the corresponding *meta*- and *para*- isomers are devoid of HDAC activity. The SAR of these compounds is also limited by the fact that further substituents are only tolerated in the position *para* to the NH_2 group. Antiproliferative activities on a wide panel of cancer cell lines range over 0.042–4.7 µM and activity has been demonstrated in a broad set of xenograft models at nontoxic doses. Further details of both the clinical and preclinical development of this agent were recently described [51].

The other pioneers in the development of aminoanilines are the group at Methylgene, which culminated in the discovery and development of MGCD0103 (**38**) [52, 53], now undergoing phase II trials in hematological cancers, including: AML, MDS, CML, Hodgkin's lymphoma, chronic lymphocytic leukemia and B-cell lymphomas. Furthermore, studies in solid tumors are underway, as well as combination studies with azacitidine and gemzar.

This group in an effort to develop HDACi with more desirable pharmaceutical properties than hydroxamic acids focused on combining known HDACi scaffolds with the aminoaniline group present in CI-994 and SNDX-275 [54, 55]. Using their knowledge, they rapidly evolved compounds like **39** equipotent to SNDX-275, which showed low micromolar antiproliferative activities across a range of cancer cell lines; and in a HCT116 xenograft model at 20 mg/kg i.p. gave 54% TGI.

By moving away from sulfonamide linkers, these researchers were able to improve the antitumor activity of this class of compounds, both *in vitro* and *in vivo* [56]. They developed a series of cinnamides with the generic structure of **40**, with a two-atom linker to a terminal aryl ring. Through an extensive SAR study interchanging NH and CH_2 groups on the linker and by the introduction of mono-, di- and tri- methoxy groups on the aryl ring, they developed potent compounds, exemplified by **41**. These compounds show low micromolar antiproliferative activity, cause histone hyperacetylation in cancer cells from 1 µM upwards and show higher %TGI than SNDX-275 in xenograft models. Other developments include the incorporation of 4-(heteroarylmethyl) capping groups, resulting in inhibitors like **42a** and **42b** [57]. These compounds are potent HDAC1 inhibitors with $IC_{50} < 0.1\,\mu M$, displaying antiproliferative activities in the 400–800 nM range against HCT116 cells. While **42a** shows good *in vivo* activity flowing i.p. administration (59% TGI at 40 mg/kg), **42b** also shows efficacy following oral administration at 80 mg/kg, with 55 and 67% TGI in NSCLC A549 and prostate DU145 xenografts. Other potent analogs have been developed by the scientists in Montreal with a series of 4-(heteroarylaminomethyl) derivatives [58]. Starting from modestly active imidazole sulfide **43a** ($IC_{50} = 0.5\,\mu M$), this group was able to improve the enzymatic activity more than 15-fold to give a 2-aminobenzothiazole analog **43b** ($IC_{50} = 30\,nM$). Through subsequent manipulations they were able to engineer the molecules to give **43c** (HDAC1 $IC_{50} = 60\,nM$), with good antiproliferative activity (HCT116 $IC_{50} = 0.2\,\mu M$), but moreover good *in vivo* efficacy. This compound showed activity in four xenograft models (62–74% TGI) following either administration at 20 mg/kg i.p., or oral administration at 90 mg/kg.

However, the most advanced compound developed by Methylgene is MGCD0103 (**38**), which is a selective inhibitor of HDACs 1, 2, 3, 11 with $IC_{50} = 0.15$, 0.29, 1.66, 0.59 μM, respectively. In contrast to hydroxamic acid HDACis, MGCD0103 does not inhibit the other isoforms at 10 μM [52, 53]. This isoform selectivity is maintained in cells, while NVP-LAQ824 inhibits almost all deacetylase activity in cells, MGCD0103 inhibits only 75–85% of HDAC activity. The compound shows good antiproliferative activities on a broad range of cell lines, both solid tumors and hematological malignancies, with IC_{50} values in the range 0.2–1.45 μM. Furthermore, histone hyperacetylation is observed, as well as the induction of both cell cycle block and apoptosis. This compound is orally bioavailable in preclinical species, with a modest half-life, $t_{1/2} = 0.6–1.3\,h$. In tumor-bearing animals dose-dependent tumor growth inhibition was observed in multiple xenograft models following daily oral doses of 60–120 mg/kg.

Other related series of compounds have been designed by the groups at Merck and AstraZeneca.

The former group evolved their series of compounds from *N*-(2-aminophenyl) nicotinamide, a 12.4 μM screening hit [59]. The group rationalized that the 6-position of the pyridine could easily be functionalized and set about a rapid SAR exploration. This primary effort culminated in the identification of **44a**, having almost a 100-fold improvement in enzymatic activity ($IC_{50} = 168\,nM$). A more extensive SAR exploration was then carried out on the piperazine ring, introducing substituents at every position. Small alkyl groups proved beneficial for potency, with the two enantiomeric 3-methyl derivatives being particularly interesting. Although the *S*-enantiomer (**44b**) was a weaker HDAC1 inhibitor ($IC_{50} = 73$ vs 40 nM), the reduced cellular shift made this *S*-enantiomer more potent in cells. In fact, this compound is a selective class I HDACi with $IC_{50} = 73$, 272, 939, >50 000, 16 720 nM against HDACs 1, 2, 3, 6, 8 respectively. This compound also displayed acceptable PK in preclinical species with good oral bioavailability, acceptable clearance and half-lives. The compound is also active in a HCT116 xenograft model at 100 and 150 mg/kg.

The latter group evolved a series of related pyridine-containing aminoanilines [60, 61]. Compound **45a** was identified as a potent, low molecular weight lead and was subjected to optimization efforts. Consequently, a range of more soluble analogs were made with different C-3 substituents, as well as a range of amines in the 5-position of the pyridine. One compound (**45b**) was of particular interest, with HDAC 1 $pIC_{50} = 8.01$ and good antiproliferative activity, HCT116 $pIC_{50} = 6.86$. Furthermore, this compound was demonstrated to show low clearance and good oral exposure in rats. A second related series developed by this group focused on a series of compounds with a piperidine-4-yl group appended [61]. The group started from *N*-(2-aminophenyl)pyridine-2-carboxamide and identified piperidine-4-yl as an optimal substituent. A further round of SAR culminated with the identification of **46b**, that was a potent HDACi with $pIC_{50} = 7.46$, displayed $pIC_{50} = 6.44$ against HCT116 cells and gave an excellent dose response profile in an A549 xenograft model following five doses per week.

9.3.3.1 HDAC1 and 2 Selective Aminoanilines

More recently, two groups simultaneously reported the development of a series of selective HDAC 1 and 2 inhibitors (Figure 9.10) [62]. The roles of HDACs 1 and 2 are well supported in regulating cell proliferation; furthermore both HDAC isoforms have been shown to be over expressed in certain types of cancer; and RNA interference to knockdown HDAC 1 and 2 results in inhibition of proliferation and the induction of apoptosis. Through the introduction of an aromatic group in the *para* position to the amino group in the previous series of compounds, the groups at Merck and Methylgene claim they are able to exploit additional binding interactions in the internal cavity of these two HDAC isoforms, thereby engineering HDAC 1 and 2 selective inhibitors. The corresponding analog **47** of SNDX-275 bearing a 2-thienyl group was prepared and this resulted in 27- and fivefold improvements in HDAC 1 and 2 activities ($IC_{50} = 20$ and 100 nM respectively), while abolishing HDAC 3 activity. Similarly, the NH_2 group could be replaced by a hydroxyl group (**48c**), invoking a similar selectivity profile. The 2-thienyl group could be replaced by phenyl (**48d**) and furyl (**48e**) groups, although bulkier groups were not tolerated. Several derivatives were also tested in cellular assays and antiproliferative activities in the range of hundreds of nanomoles were obtained. Related work by the Merck group identified the biaryl phenol **49** as an HTS hit. This compound displayed greater than 10-fold selectivity for HDAC 1 over 3, so the group decided to add substituents off the thiophene ring in a hope of improving activity. This work lead them to the *para*-phenyl analog of SNDX-275 (**50**), which like **47** was a selective HDAC 1 and 2 inhibitor ($IC_{50} = 10, 72, 6180$ nM against HDACs 1, 2, 3 respectively) and displayed no activity on HDACs 4–8 at 20 μM. Further exploration of the SAR, replacing 3-pyridyl group with amide and carbamates resulted in the identification of compounds, such as **51**, which were potent HDAC1 inhibitors ($IC_{50} = 6$ nM) and displayed growth inhibition of HCT116 cells at 100 nM. This compound proved to be well tolerated and efficacious in a HCT116 xenograft in a dose-dependent manner. Further work on another HTS hit **52a** investigated in detail the structural requirements for good affinity. Focusing on the carboxylic acid fragment of this inhibitor it was revealed that many (hetero)aryl rings were tolerated including phenyl, 3- and 4- substituted pyridines. In contrast, pyrid-2-yl, as well as 2- and 3-aminophenyl groups resulted in a loss of affinity. Fortunately, an amino group could be accommodated in the *para* position and functionalized to make analogs of CI-994, including compound **53e** which displayed $IC_{50} = 7$ and 49 nM on HDACs 1 and 2, with no activity on the other HDACs isoforms at 10 μM. This compound too proved to be efficacious *in vivo*, causing 52% TGI in a HCT116 xenograft at 30 mg/kg i.p.. SAR investigation was also conducted on the biaryl fragment, where it was demonstrated that phenyl and 2- or

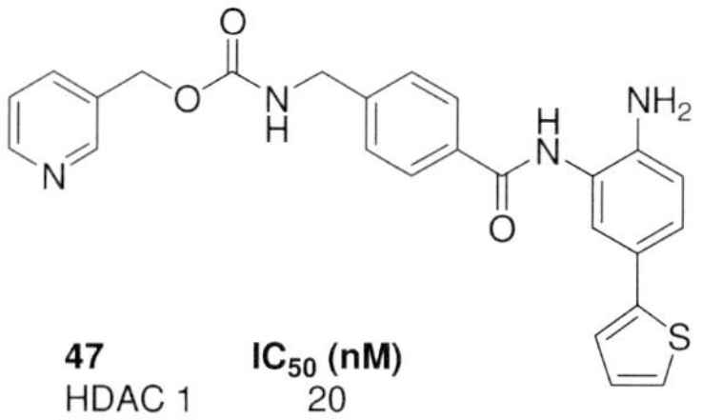

47	IC_{50} (nM)
HDAC 1	20
HDAC 2	100
HDAC 3	Not active

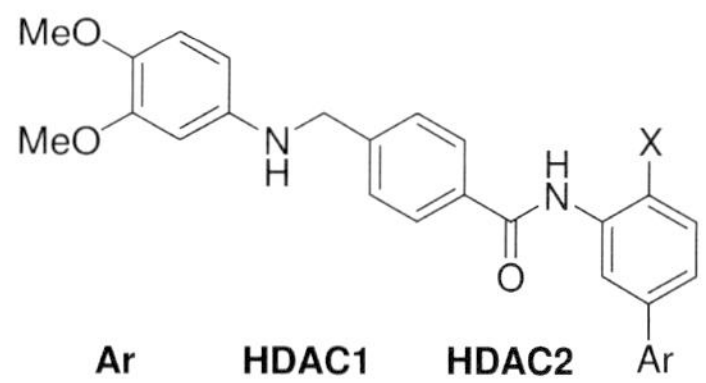

Number	X	Ar	HDAC1 IC_{50} (nM)	HDAC2 IC_{50} (nM)
48a	NH_2	H	440	500
48b	NH_2	2-Thienyl	50	80
48c	OH	2-Thienyl	40	60
48d	NH_2	Phenyl	60	100
48e	NH_2	3-Furyl	50	70

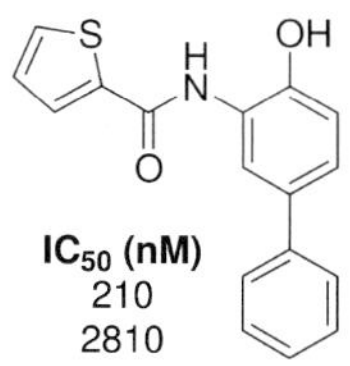

49	IC_{50} (nM)
HDAC 1	210
HDAC 3	2810

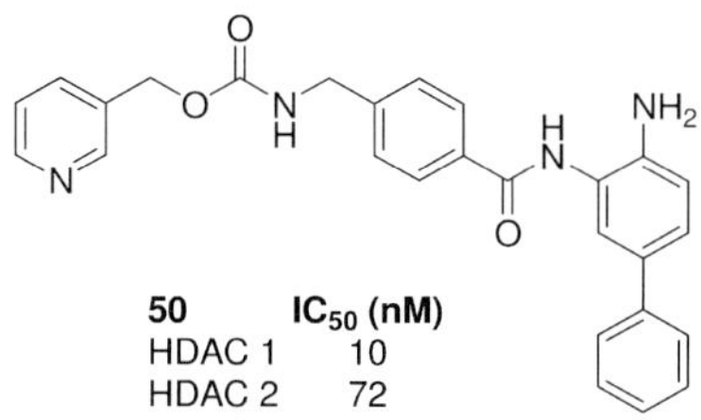

50	IC_{50} (nM)
HDAC 1	10
HDAC 2	72
HDAC 3	6180
HCT116	225

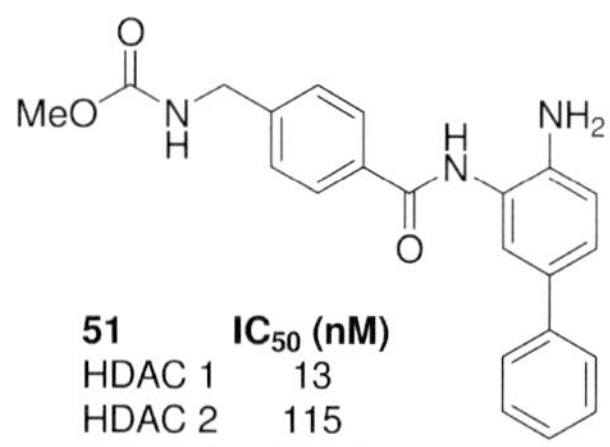

51	IC_{50} (nM)
HDAC 1	13
HDAC 2	115
HDAC 3	22450
HCT116	230

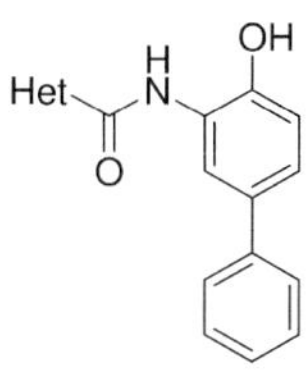

Number	Ar	HDAC1 IC_{50} (nM)
52a	Phenyl	58
52b	2-Pyridyl	310
52c	3-Pyridyl	68
52d	4-Pyridyl	75
52e	2-Aminophenyl	1800
52f	3-Aminophenyl	440
52g	4-Aminophenyl	40

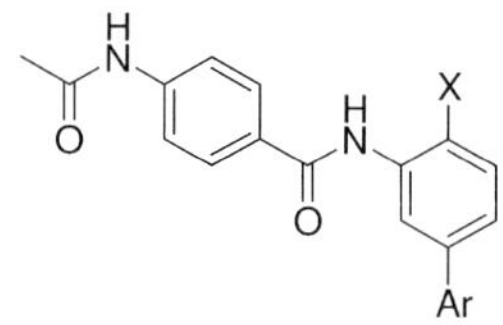

Number	X	Ar	HDAC1 IC_{50} (nM)	HDAC2 IC_{50} (nM)
CI-994 (36)	NH_2	H	570	
53a	OH	Phenyl	18	
53b	NH_2	Phenyl	28	
53c	NH_2	2-Thienyl	7	49
53d	NH_2	3-Thienyl	7	

Figure 9.10 SAR exploration of HDAC1 and 2 selective aminoaniline HDACis.

3-thienyl groups were optimal and polar groups were not tolerated. When non-aromatic substituents were introduced, all with the exception of pyrrolidine were only micromolar HDACis.

In some elegant work Schreiber designed a library of more than 7000 carboxylic and hydroxamic acids, and aminoanilines capable of inhibiting deacetylases [63]. The group used high-throughput, cell-based assays to screen for the induction of α-tubulin and histone acetylation, from which they were able to identify molecules capable of inhibiting one or both of these deacetylases. Interestingly, none of the aminoanilines showed any induction of α-tubulin acetylation, suggesting this class

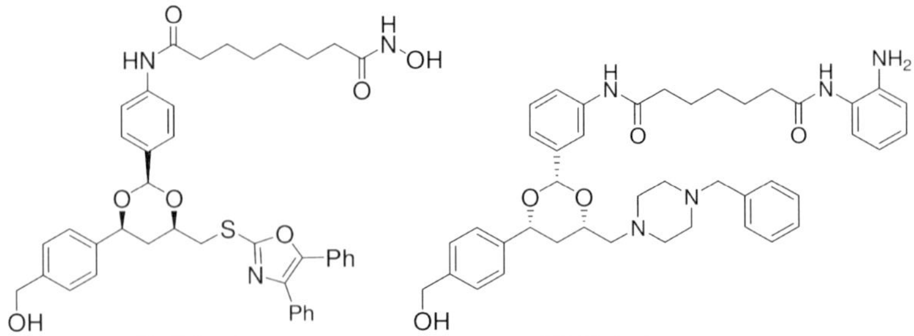

54: Tubacin **55: Histacin**

Figure 9.11 Selective tubulin and histone deacetylase inhibitors developed by Schreiber.

of inhibitors is inactive against HDAC 6 (the α-tubulin deacetylase). From this work they identified a selective, reversible inhibitor of α-tubulin deacetylation, tubacin (**54**; Figure 9.11), which was shown to induce α-tubulin acetylation threefold at 10 μM (EC_{50} = 2.5 μM), while causing no changes to histone acetylation. They also identified a selective inducer of histone acetylation – histacin (**55**).

9.3.4
Electrophilic Ketones

In an attempt to move away from the hydroxamic acid zinc binding group, which is known to causes poor pharmacokinetics as a result of hydrolysis or glucuronidation, the group at Abbott searched for alternative zinc chelators culminating in the development of a series of electrophilic ketone HDACis (Figure 9.12) [64–66]. Subsequently, a group at IRBM developed a related series of thiophene trifluoromethyl ketones and showed these to be selective class II HDACis [12].

Given that electrophilic ketones have been shown to be hydrated and able to inhibit other zinc dependent enzymes, several activated ketones were prepared and tested for HDAC inhibition. The trifluoromethyl ketone analog of SAHA (**56**) was synthesized and shown to display weak but measurable HDAC inhibitory activity, IC_{50} = 6.7 μM. Subsequently, these trifluoromethyl ketones were further optimized with changes to the lipophilic tether and the capping groups in order to develop more potent analogs, such as **6** which was shown to be a modestly active HDACi (IC_{50} = 310 nM) but unfortunately displayed only weak cellular activity (IC_{50} = 4.2 μM against HT1080 fibrosarcoma cells) [64]. The electrophilic carbonyl group is required as the corresponding methyl ketones are inactive. Unfortunately these compounds suffer from poor pharmacokinetics *in vivo*, being readily reduced to the inactive alcohol. A related series of heterocyclic ketones was also explored; and oxazoles exemplified by **57** proved to be potent HDACis, IC_{50} = 30 nM. These too suffered due to rapid reduction of the ketone group, even in MDA435 cells, and consequently displayed only modest antiproliferative activities [65]. More promising however were a series of α-ketoamides, which ultimately were shown to be efficacious *in vivo* [66]. The researchers at Abbott found *N*-methyl α-keto amides were

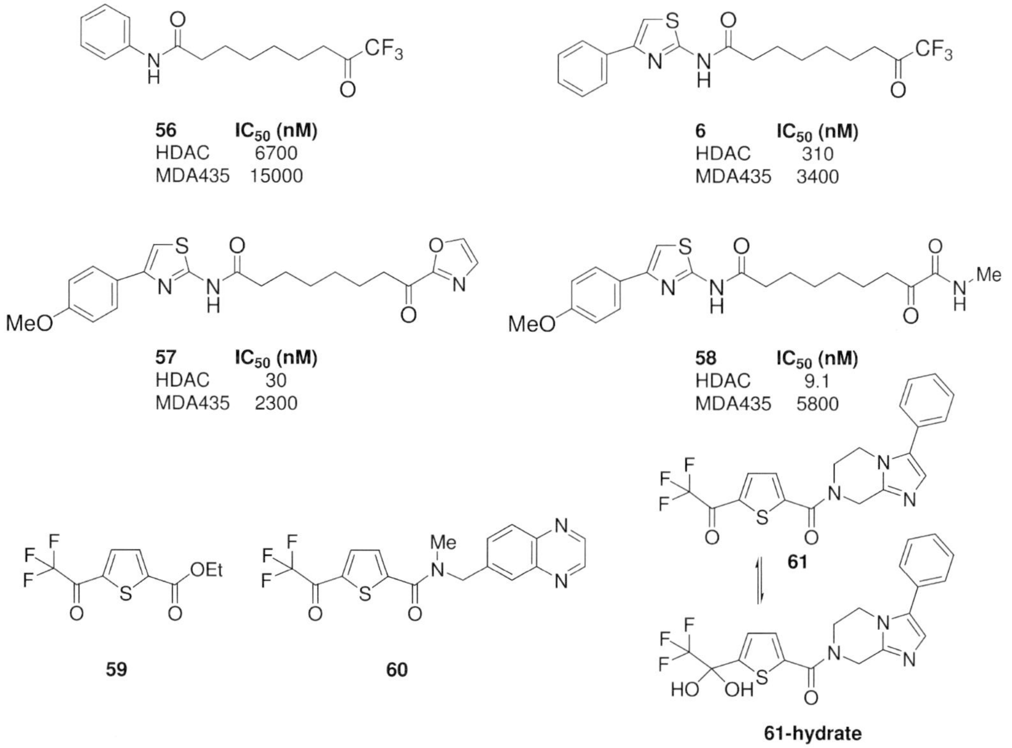

Figure 9.12 SAR exploration of electron deficient ketone HDACis, including selective class II HDACis.

potent HDACis and that the *N*-methyl amides were optimal. The corresponding carboxylic acids, as well as the primary, dimethyl and *N*-ethyl amides, were significantly less active. Whilst maintaining a simple alkyl chain, investigation of the capping groups identified *bis*-(hetero)aryl groups as optimal for potency and cellular activity, with substituted aryl thiazoles being especially promising. For instance, **58** inhibited HDAC with $IC_{50} = 9$ nM and displayed low micromolar antiproliferation activities against HT1080 and breast MDA435 cancer cells. This compound gave rise to tumor growth inhibition in a HT1080 xenograft model when dosed every other day at 30 or 100 mg/kg i.p.

During work to identify second-generation HDACis, the group at IRBM became interested in exploring selective class II inhibitors. It is widely debated whether class IIa HDACs (HDACs 4, 5, 7) have catalytic deacetylase activity, yet this group was able to demonstrate that HDAC4 can be prepared and isolated cleanly from *Escherichia coli*; and these bacteria preparations have weak but measurable deacetylase activity [67]. Furthermore, they were able to show that the low enzymatic efficiency can be restored either by: mutation of an active site histidine to tyrosine, or by the use of a non-acetylated lysine substrate, allowing the development of two HDAC 4 assays (4GOF 'gain of function', 4WT). With these assays to hand, a novel series of class II HDACis were developed [12]. A focused screen of both in-house and commercial compounds containing known zinc-binding groups was initially carried out on both HDAC4 assays, identifying **59** to be a potent inhibitor of class II HDACs, showing $IC_{50} = 350$ and 320 nM on HDAC 4GOF and 4WT assays respectively. This compound also inhibited HDAC6 ($IC_{50} = 550$ nM) and was shown to be modestly selective over the class I isoforms ($IC_{50} = 5.7$ and 3.5 μM against HDACs 1 and 3). ^{1}H NMR data showed that the trifluoromethyl ketone was readily hydrated, suggesting these may bind as the hydrate. Interestingly, the importance of the thiophene moiety was demonstrated by the fact that the corresponding furan derivative was 10-fold less potent, while most other (hetero)aryl replacements were inactive. Studies into the zinc binding group showed that electron withdrawing groups were essential for activity as the simple methyl ketone was inactive and also that there was a steric constraint as homologation to the pentafluoroethyl ketone was not tolerated. Ultimately, the series was further optimized to give potent and selective class II HDACis displaying around 10-fold selectivity over class I HDACs. A representative being **60** which displays modest selectivity for class II HDACs ($IC_{50} = 87$, 98, and 89 on HDAC 4GOF, 4WT and 6; $IC_{50} = 580$ and 670 nM on HDACs 1 and 3). Interestingly, this compound inhibits tubulin deacetylation with $IC_{50} = 12$ μM in HCT116 cells, whereas only 40% inhibition of histone H3 deacetylation was seen at 50 μM, thereby demonstrating that these compounds are selective class II HDACis in cells. Recently it became possible to obtain X-ray crystal structures of one of these inhibitors **61** bound to the catalytic domain of both HDAC 4GOF and 4WT; and this demonstrated these inhibitors are active site binders, with the hydrated ketone (**61-hydrate**) chelating the active site zinc in a bidentate manner.

9.3.5
Natural Products

As well as hydroxamic acids like TSA, nature also delivers a wealth of cyclic tetrapeptides that have been demonstrated to display excellent levels of HDAC inhibition. Probably the best known of these is romidepsin (**4**; formerly known as FK228/FR-901228/depsipeptide) which is currently in late-stage clinical trials. However, 30 years or so of screening natural products for antiproliferative activity and in phytochemical assays led to the discovery of multiple HDACis, including: HC-toxin (**62**), chlamydocin (**63**), trapoxin A (**64a**) and apicidin (**5**; Figure 9.13). The vast majority of these structures contain some common features, including: hydrophobic capping groups, at least one amino acid whose stereocentre in a *R*-configuration and a nonproteinogenic long aliphatic amino acid (often *L*-Aoe or *L*-Aoda) that may act as an Ac-lysine substrate analog. Furthermore, these natural products often, but not always, contain a proline or pipecolinic acid residue. This field of natural product HDACis has been recently reviewed [17c].

Romidepsin (**4**) is a natural product produced by *Chromobacterium violaceum* and was shown to display potent antitumor activity both *in vitro* ($IC_{50} = 0.55$–4.4 nM), and *in vivo* where growth of mouse and human tumors in mice was inhibited [68].

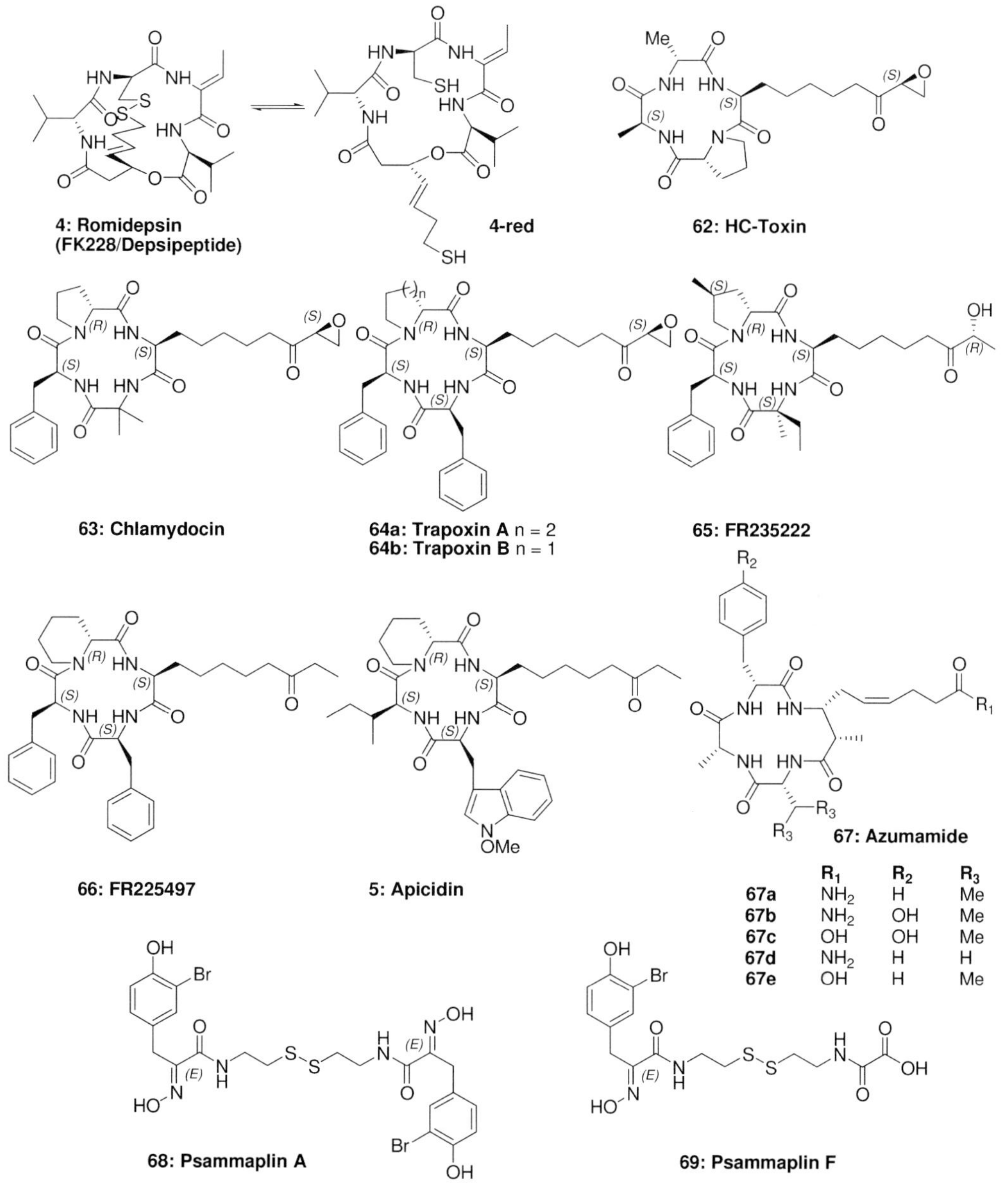

Figure 9.13 Cyclic peptide HDACis.

Initially its mechanism of action was unknown but, after showing similar pharmacology to TSA, it was revealed that romidepsin induced histone hyperacetylation in cells [69]; and subsequently it was shown to inhibit purified HDACs ($IC_{50} = 1.1$ nM). Romidepsin is actually a natural prodrug and is activated by cellular reduction to a dithiol (**4-red**; Figure 9.13) [70] and these thiols act as zinc-binding groups.

Romidepsin has been shown to be a selective class I HDACi, with activities on HDACs 1, 2, 4 and 6 of $IC_{50} = 36, 47, 510$ and 14 000 nM respectively. A single-arm registration trial of romidepsin in CTCL has been completed and an NDA submission for romidepsin in CTCL is anticipated in 2008. Data from this phase 2b study were presented at the International Investigative Dermatology meeting in May 2008 [71]; and the results reported included 72 evaluable patients with CTCL and an overall response rate of 40%: five complete responses (7%) and 24 partial responses (33%). A separate registration trial in peripheral T-cell lymphoma (PTCL) is underway and other trials are ongoing in additional indications, including MM. Related natural products to romidepsin are spiruchostatin A and B [17c].

HC-toxin (**62**) was one of the first HDACi natural products to be identified back in the 1970s. The compound is produced by the fungus *Cochliobolus carbonum* and is responsible for causing northern corn leaf disease, which affects maize [72]. The cyclic tetrapeptide is comprised of two alanine resides and a proline moiety, together with a *L*-Aoe group (2-amino-9,10-epoxy-8-oxodecanoic acid). It was only in the mid-1990s that the compound was revealed to indeed be an HDACi [73]. Contemporaneously, chlamydocin (**63**) was isolated as a cytostatic compound from the soil fungus *Diheterospora chlamydosporia* and was revealed to contain the same epoxy ketone side-chain, together with *D*-proline, *L*-phenylalanine and α-aminoisobutyric acid groups [74]. The compound demonstrated high cytotoxic activity against mastocytoma cells, with $ED_{50} = 0.8$ nM. Interestingly a derivative lacking the key epoxy ketone group proved to be inactive. Like the other members of this family, chlamydocin was shown to be a potent HDACi, with $IC_{50} = 1.3$ nM, causing histone hyperacetylation in A2780 ovarian cancer cells and simultaneously arresting cells in G_2/M phase [75]. Moreover, the compound was demonstrated to exhibit nanomolar antiproliferative activities against a broad panel of cancer cell lines. Two other related natural products, trapoxin A and B (**64a**, **64b**) were isolated from *Helicoma ambiens* RF-1023 [76]. They both contain two *L*-phenyl alanine moieties together with an *L*-Aoe side chain and differ from each other only by the presence of a *D*-pipecolinic acid or *D*-proline group respectively. Yoshida demonstrated that trapoxin A causes histone hyperacetylation in cells in a similar manner to TSA and is able to inhibit HDAC at low nanomolar concentrations [77]. In mechanistic studies, it was shown that this compound appeared to be a slow and irreversible HDACi, as HDACs treated with trapoxin no longer recovered their activity, even following dialysis for 18 h. These findings suggest that the epoxide may be alkylating a residue in the active site of the HDAC. The critical importance of the epoxy ketone group was also revealed, as the reduced derivative was devoid of HDAC activity at 100 nM. Trapoxin has also yielded some elegant reagents; and Schreiber developed a K-Trap, enabling him to purify trapoxin's target to homogeneity, thereby enabling the identification of HDAC 1. Also, a radiolabeled version of the natural product was synthesized, which enabled the demonstration that trapoxin and TSA bind in the same active site [2, 78]. Interestingly, preparation of a ^{125}I-labeled derivative of the natural products provided some suggestion that these epoxy ketones may not be irreversible inhibitors.

Probably the most recently discovered natural product of this class is FR235 222 (**65**) [79], a potent HDACi with $IC_{50} = 17$ nM. This compound differs from some of the other members of the class due to the isovaline and methyl proline moieties, although more markedly contains a α-hydoxyketone *L*-Ahoda amino acid as a zinc-chelating moiety.

Despite Yoshida demonstrating that the epoxy ketone seems essential for activity, several other related compounds lack this functionality and yet maintain HDAC inhibitory activity. For instance, FR225497 (**66**; desepoxy trapoxin A) was isolated from *Helicoma ambiens* and nevertheless inhibited HDACs (67% inhibition at 100 nM). FR225497 was shown to display both immunosuppressive and anticancer activities, for example colon HT-29 cells, $IC_{50} = 270$ nM [80]. Another class of these natural products that lack the 9,10-epoxy group is apicidin (**5**), and its derivatives, which were isolated from *Fusarium pallidoroseum* [81, 82]. Despite the absence of the epoxy ketone, these fungal metabolites were demonstrated to have potent, broad spectrum, antiprotozoal activity in the range 6–200 nM. In mouse malaria studies it was shown that apicidin administered orally twice daily at 25 or 50 mg/kg was able to substantially reduce the percentage of infected erythrocytes. Subsequently, it was elucidated that its antiprotozoal activity was a result of HDAC inhibition ($IC_{50} = 0.7$ nM). Interestingly, despite these compounds lacking the epoxide they are 30-fold more potent than HC-toxin, revealing the contribution of the cyclic tetrapeptide core on affinity. More recently, it has been illustrated that apicidin displays broad-spectrum antiproliferation activity against a wide panel of cancer cell lines, with $IC_{50} = 0.21$–3.8 μM; and this occurs with G_1 cell cycle arrest, accumulation of hyperacetylated histone H4 and changes in cell morphology.

Beside epoxyketone and ketone natural products, cyclic peptides bearing carboxylic acids and primary amides were recently isolated and demonstrated to be HDACis, the azumamides A–E; (**67a–e**). These were isolated from the marine sponge *Mycale izuensis* [83] and shown to be made up of three *D*-amino acids, plus a unique (*Z*,2*S*,3*R*)-3-amino-2-methyl-5-nonenedioic acid for azumamides C and E, or the corresponding amide for azumamides A, B and D. These compounds display HDAC inhibitory activity in the range 0.045–1.3 μM; and azumamide A was shown to display modest growth inhibitory activity on colon cancer WiDr and leukemia K562 cells ($CC_{50} = 5.8$ and 4.5 μM, respectively).

Another related class of natural product HDACis are those of the psammaplin family, isolated from the marine sponge *Pseudoceratina purpurea* [84]. These are highly functionalized bromotyrosine derivatives containing a disulfide bond. It is hypothesized that these are natural prodrugs. Psammaplin A (**68**) was initially identified; and further isolation work enlarged the family to ten members, plus the structurally related bisaprasin. Profiling of these derivatives confirmed some compounds to be very potent HDACis, with psammaplins A (**68**) and F (**69**) displaying $IC_{50} = 4.2$ and 8.6 nM respectively. The other family members were also confirmed to be HDACis, although with weaker activity ($IC_{50} = 14$–330 nM). Psammaplin A was also tested in antiproliferation assays and shown to inhibit growth of several human cancer cell lines, including lung A549 tumor cells with $IC_{50} = 1.3$ μM, and caused tumor growth inhibition in an A549 xenograft model.

9.3.6
Hybrid Cyclic Tetrapeptides

A number of groups have taken the approach of combining the cyclic tetrapeptide scaffolds which typically contain *L*-Aoe epoxy ketone zinc-binding groups with more potent zinc-binding groups found in other HDACis, for instance hydroxamic acids or thiol groups (Figure 9.14). One of the first examples of this was the evolution of the cyclic hydroxamic acid-containing peptides (CHAPs), which combined the scaffolds found in compounds such as trapoxin B and introduced a hydroxamic acid containing *L*-Asu(NHOH) chain [85]. These synthetic derivatives were potent reversible HDACis with the trapoxin B analog CHAP1 (**70**), showing $IC_{50} = 1.9$ nM,

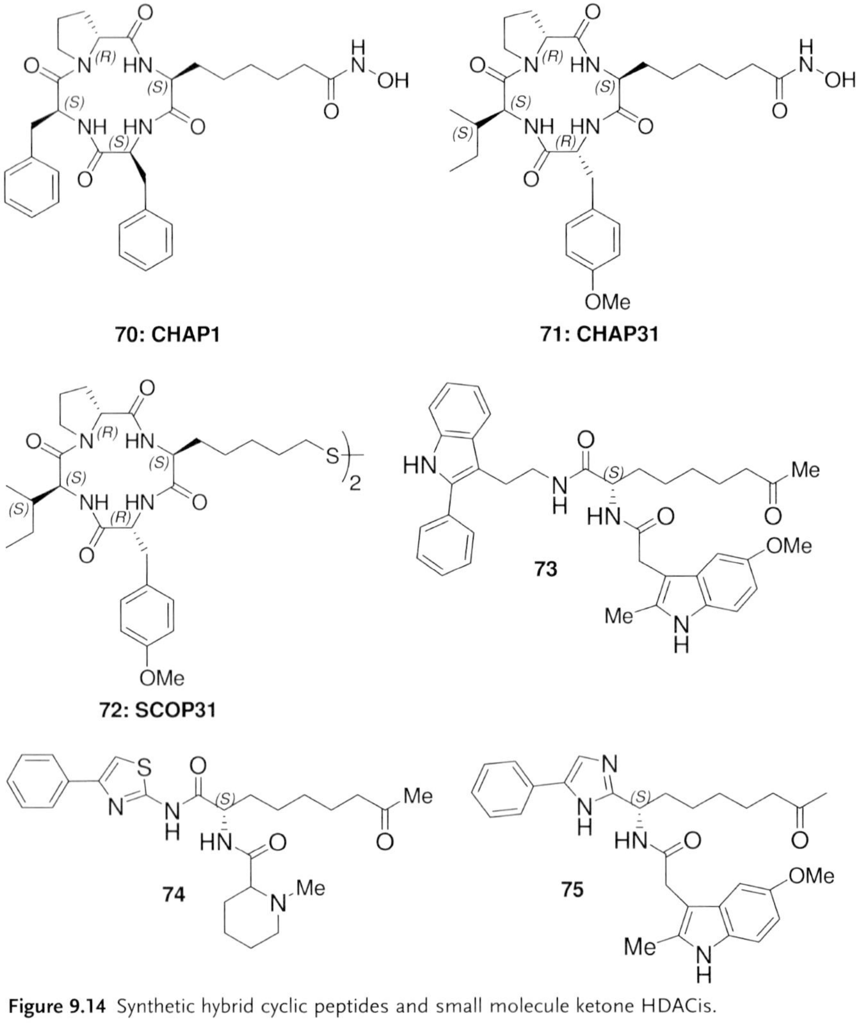

Figure 9.14 Synthetic hybrid cyclic peptides and small molecule ketone HDACis.

compared to 0.11 nM for the natural product. The potential of these synthetic derivatives was revealed when CHAP31 (**71**), the analog of Cyl-1, was prepared. Despite having only nanomolar potency, $IC_{50} = 3.3$ nM, it caused growth inhibition in B16/BL6 melanoma cells ($IC_{50} = 5.4$ nM), induced histone acetylation at 10 nM and moreover proved to have *in vivo* efficacy [86]. CHAP31 displayed tumor growth inhibition in multiple xenograft models at daily doses of 1–10 mg/kg i.v.. A related series of compounds are the sulfur-containing cyclic peptides (SCOPs), where the *L*-Aoe group of the natural products has been replaced by *L*-2-amino-7-mercapto-heptanoic acid. These too have been shown to be potent HDACis, with SCOP31 (**72**) displaying HDAC $IC_{50} = 4.6$ nM [87].

9.3.7
Aliphatic Ketones

Recently, the researchers at IRBM used apicidin as a starting point for a drug discovery program and evolved a series of potent, low molecular weight, nonhydroxamic acid HDACis (Figure 9.14) [88, 89]. Rationalizing that apicidin (**5**) presented potential issues in terms of chemical tractability and pharmacokinetic liabilities, they sought a new lead and identified acyclic *bis*-indole **73**, containing the key *L*-Aoda aliphatic side-chain. Despite a 10-fold loss in terms of enzymatic activity, $IC_{50} = 590$ nM (compared to 44 nM for **5**), submicromolar cellular activity was maintained in, cervical HeLa cancer cells $IC_{50} = 730$ nM. Interestingly, the *R*-enantiomer is inactive. SAR to replace both the amino and carboxy terminal capping groups was undertaken, identifying analogs exemplified by **74** as potent, selective HDACs 1, 2, 3, 6 inhibitor $IC_{50} = 55$, 170, 14, 13 nM, respectively. Furthermore, **74** showed submicromolar activity on a broad panel of cancer cell lines. Unfortunately, the anilide bond was unstable in rodent plasma [89] and efforts were undertaken to replace this bond by noncleavable bioisosteric groups. Indeed, imidazole **75** proved to be plasma stable and moreover maintained good HDAC inhibition with $IC_{50} = 59$, 110, 120 nM against HDACs 1, 2, 3. The compound showed modest activity on HDAC 6 ($IC_{50} = 340$ nM), but no activity on HDACs 4, 5, 7. This compound showed good antiproliferative activity against a wide range of cancer cell lines, for instance HeLa $IC_{50} = 880$ nM. When dosed at their MTDs, **75** displayed tumor growth inhibition comparable to the benchmark HDACis vorinostat and SNDX-275 in a HCT116 xenograft model. This is the first example of a synthetic small molecule aliphatic ketone HDACi showing efficacy in an *in vivo* model.

9.3.8
Thiols and Related HDAC Inhibitors

Related to the natural product thiol-containing HDAC inhibitors like romidepsin and the psammaplin family, a number of research groups explored the use of thiol-containing compounds as HDACis (Figure 9.15). One of the first people to do so was Suzuki, who recognized that: (i) thiols are used as inhibitors of zinc-dependent enzymes such as angiotensin-converting enzyme and matrix metalloproteinases and

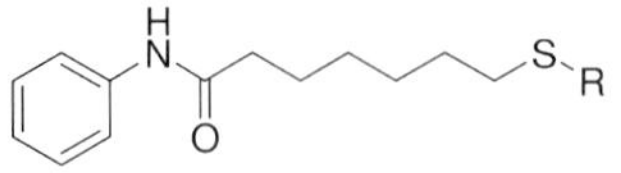

Number	R	HDAC NE IC_{50} (μM)	NCI-H460 cells IC_{50} (μM)
76a	H	0.21	34% inh. at 50 μM
76b	Ac	7.1	36
76c	Me	>100	NT
76d	CO^iPr	NT	20

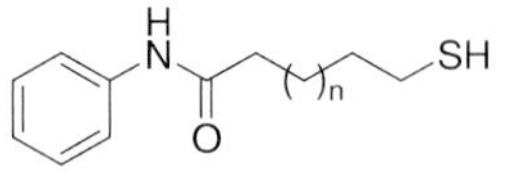

Number	n	HDAC NE IC_{50} (μM)
76e	1	6.2
76f	2	0.37
76a	3	0.21
76g	4	1.5

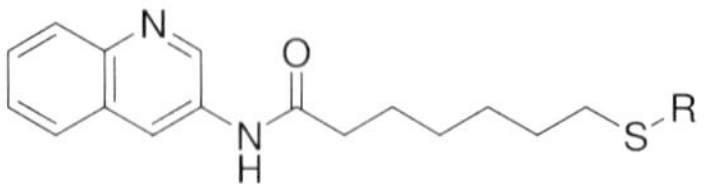

77a R = H, HDAC NE IC_{50} = 72 nM
77b R = -CO^iPr, NCI-H460 IC_{50} = 8 μM

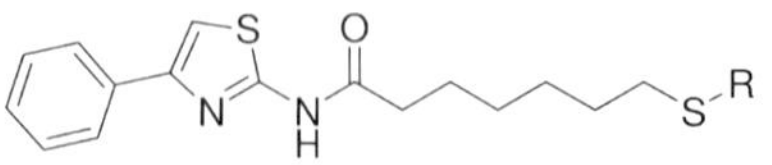

78a R = H, HDAC NE IC_{50} = 170 nM
78b R = -CO^iPr, NCI-H460 IC_{50} = 2.1 μM

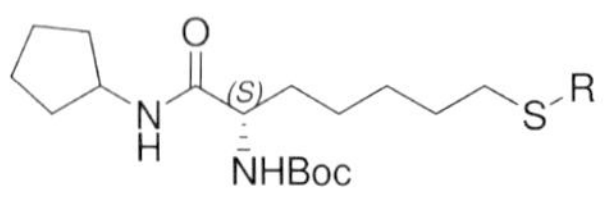

79a R = H
HDAC1 IC_{50} = 1210 nM
HDAC4 IC_{50} = 1030 nM
HDAC6 IC_{50} = 29 nM

79b R = -CO^iPr
His H4-Ac EC_{50} > 32 μM
Tub-Ac EC_{50} = 0.23 μM

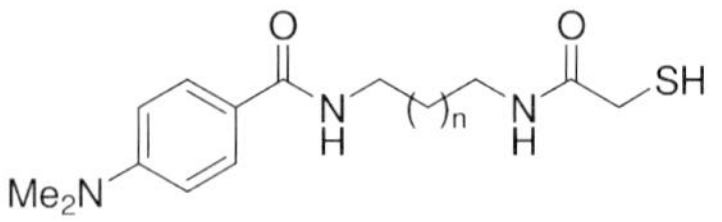

Number	n	HDAC NE IC_{50} (μM)
80a	1	0.8
80b	2	4.7
80c	3	0.2
80d	4	0.45

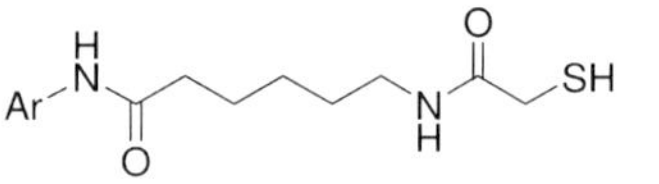

Number	n	HDAC NE IC_{50} (nM)
81a	Quinolin-8-yl	44
81b	Quinolin-3-yl	48
81c	Phenyl	300

81a:	**IC_{50} (nM)**
HDAC 1	3220
HDAC 2	7380
HDAC 6	95
HDAC 8	6120
HDAC 10	10700

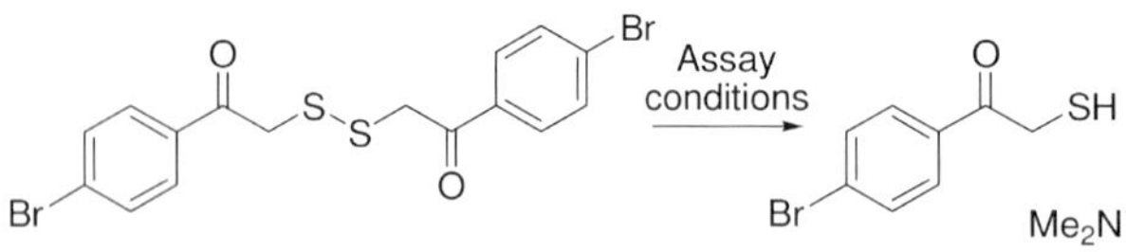

82	**IC_{50} (nM)**
HDAC NE	135

83

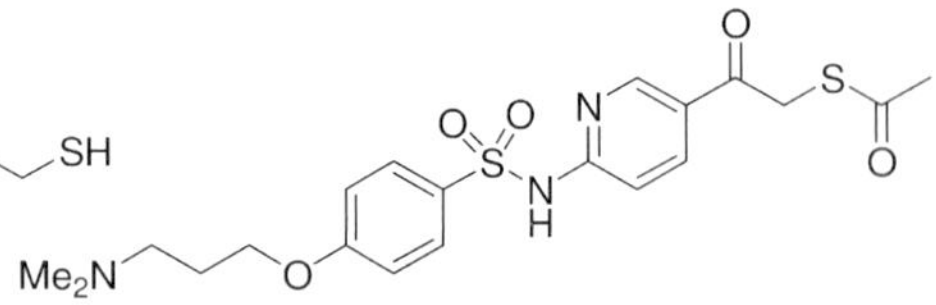

84: KD5170	**IC_{50} (nM)**
HDAC NE	45
HDAC 1	20
HDAC 2	2060
HDAC 3	75
HDAC 4	26
HDAC 5	950
HDAC 6	14
HDAC 7	85
HDAC 8	2500
HDAC 9	150
HDAC 10	18

Figure 9.15 SAR exploration of thiol and related HDACis.

(ii) the zinc ion is highly thiophilic. Therefore his group set about replacing the hydroxamic acid present in HDACis like vorinostat. Surprisingly, although the inhibitory ability of a monodentate zinc-binding group like a thiol was expected to be less effective than that of a bidentate zinc chelator like a hydroxamic acid, the analog of vorinostat (**76a**) was a potent HDACi with $IC_{50} = 210$ nM [90]. The corresponding thioacetate (**76b**) and methyl sulfide (**76c**) were substantially less active, demonstrating the critical importance of the free thiol group. Similarly, the corresponding sulfonamide and sulfone were also inactive. In order to explore the SAR the effect of chain length was investigated (**76e–g**) and it was revealed that, similarly to the hydroxamic acids, the optimal length was five or six methylene units. The same group carried out an optimization of the aromatic capping group and it was demonstrated that quinoline-3-yl (**77a**) and 4-phenylthiazol-2-yl (**78a**) groups were able to improve HDAC activity. When **76a** was tested in human NCI-H460 lung cancer cells, it showed only weak activity despite the high enzymatic activity. It was assumed this was due to poor membrane permeability and therefore the corresponding disulfide was explored as a potential prodrug, but it too failed to show growth inhibition. However, the acetyl (**76b**) and isobutyryl (**76d**) derivatives proved to be good prodrugs, with growth inhibitory $IC_{50} = 36$ and 20 μM respectively. The corresponding isobutyryl derivatives were made of **77a** and **78a**, and were shown to demonstrate strong growth inhibition of NCI-H460 cells, with $IC_{50} = 8$ and 2.1 μM for **77b** and **78b** respectively. The latter was explored on a panel of nine other cancer cell lines and was shown to have a mean $IC_{50} = 3.8$ μM, compared to 3.7 μM for vorinostat. Subsequently this class of HDACis was developed into a series of highly potent and selective HDAC 6 inhibitors, developed from a HDAC 6 selective substrate [91]. A series of *N*-Boc substrate mimetics were developed like **79b**, whilst maintaining the *S*-isobutyryl prodrug portion. These compounds were evaluated in cells for their ability to cause accumulation of acetylated α-tubulin and histone H4 in HCT116 cells. Interestingly, although the phenylthiazole and other aromatic derivatives were shown to offer poor selectivity, simple aliphatic derivatives caused dose-dependent increases in α-tubulin acetylation, without major increases in histone H4 acetylation. For example the cyclopentyl derivative **79b** showed $EC_{50} = 0.23$ μM and >32 μM respectively. The corresponding thiol (**79a**) was prepared and was evaluated in enzyme assays, whereby it was demonstrated to be a potent and selective HDAC 6 inhibitor with $IC_{50} = 29$ nM, with greater than 35-fold selectivity over HDACs 1 and 4.

Simultanously, Kozikowski and his group developed a series of mercaptoacetamides as potential HDACis [92, 93]. This functional group was designed as a bidentate zinc-chelating motif; and analogs of TSA (**80a–d**) with diverse chain lengths were demonstrated to be weak HDACis with IC_{50} values in the range of hundreds of nanomoles. More potent derivatives were developed by inverting the terminal amide group and replacing the *para*-dimethylbenzamide portion by 8-aminoquinoline (**81a**), 3-aminoquinoline (**81b**) or aniline (**81c**) with $IC_{50} = 44$, 48, 300 nM, respectively. Unfortunately, these compounds proved to have antiproliferation activities only in the range of tens of micromoles. However, more recently it was demonstrated that these compounds are in fact potent and selective HDAC

6 inhibitors [93], where **81a** inhibits HDAC 6 with $IC_{50} = 95$ nM and the other HDAC isoforms only in the micromolar range.

Related mercaptoketones were developed by the group at Kalypsys [94]. This group sought nonhydroxamate HDACis, and after a uHTS screen of 600 000 compounds, they identified disulfide **82** as a hit, $IC_{50} = 135$ nM. This compound is actually a prodrug, and during their enzyme assay, in the presence of reducing agent DTT, the disulfide was reduced to the α-mercaptoketone **83**. This series of compounds was optimized to KD5170 (**84**), which is a prodrug with $IC_{50} = 45$ nM on HDACs extracted from HeLa cells. This compound causes histone hyperacetylation in HeLa cells with $EC_{50} = 25$ nM and induces α-tubulin acetylation with $EC_{50} = 325$ nM. The thioester group serves to protect the thiol group from oxidative dimerization and in serum undergoes facile hydrolysis by serum esterases. KD5170 shows significant antiproliferative activity across a broad panel of cancer cells lines and in the NCI-60 human tumor cell line panel shows $IC_{50} = 0.1$–7.7 μM, with a mean $IC_{50} = 1.6$ μM. This compound was also demonstrated to cause significant tumor growth inhibition *in vivo* when dosed orally in colon HCT-116, prostate PC-3 and non-small cell lung NCI-H460 xenograft models.

9.4
Conclusions

HDAC inhibitors are exciting new epigenetic therapeutic agents; and the field has come a long way from the observation that the first agents caused terminal differentiation of mouse erythroleukemia cells. HDACis offer a diverse range of potential therapeutic applications, most notably in the arena of anticancer therapy. Following the successful approval of vorinostat for the treatment of cutaneous T-cell lymphoma, a multitude of other clinical applications, together with more than a dozen other structurally diverse HDACis, are currently being explored in man, both as monotherapy and also in combination. Although the first-generation HDACis target a broad selection of HDAC isoforms, medicinal chemists have shown it is possible to design inhibitors targeting a more restricted set of HDAC subtypes. Furthermore, as the molecular processes regulated by each of the individual isoforms become elucidated, this will provide the stimulus for further development of selective inhibitors. It will also allow patient stratification in the clinic, allowing the full potential of these epigenetic therapies to be exploited. Ultimately, there is hope these agents will be used therapeutically for the treatment of human diseases other than cancer.

References

1 Yoo, C.B. and Jones, P.A. (2006) Epigenetic therapy of cancer: past, present and future. *Nature Reviews Drug Discovery*, **5**, 37–50.

2 Taunton, J., Hassig, C.A. and Schreiber, S.L. (1996) A Mammalian Histone Deacetylase Related to the Yeast

Transcriptional Regulator Rpd3p. *Science*, **272**, 408–411.

3 Grant, S., Easley, C. and Kirkpatrick, P. (2007) Vorinostat. *Nature Reviews Drug Discovery*, **6**, 21–22.

4 Bolden, J.E., Peart, M.J. and Johnstone, R.W. (2006) Anticancer activities of histone deacetylase inhibitors. *Nature Reviews Drug Discovery*, **5**, 769–784.

5 Minucci, S. and Pelicci, P.G. (2006) Histone deacetylase inhibitors and the promise of epigenetic (and more) treatments for cancer. *Nature Reviews Cancer*, **6**, 38–51.

6 de Ruijter, A.J.M., van Gennip, A.H., Caron, H.N., Kemp, S. and van Kuilenburg, A.B.P. (2003) Histone deacetylases (HDACs): characterization of the classical HDAC family. *Biochemical Journal*, **370**, 737–749.

7 Xu, W.S., Parmigiani, R.B. and Marks, P.A. (2007) Histone deacetylase inhibitors: molecular mechanisms of action. *Oncogene*, **26**, 5541–5552.

8 Abel, T. and Zukin, R.S. (2008) Epigenetic targets of HDAC inhibition in neurodegenerative and psychiatric disorders. *Current Opinion in Pharmacology*, **8**, 57–64.

9 Finnin, M.S., Donigian, J.R., Cohen, A., Richon, V.M., Rifkind, R.A., Marks, P.A. *et al.* (1999) Structures of a HDAC homologue bound to the TSA and SAHA inhibitors. *Nature*, **401**, 188–193.

10 (a) Vannini, A., Volpari, C., Filocamo, G., Casavola, E.C., Brunetti, M., Renzoni, D. *et al.* (2004) Crystal structure of a eukaryotic zinc-dependent histone deacetylase, human HDAC8, complexed with a hydroxamic acid inhibitor. *Proceedings of the National Academy of Sciences of the United States of America*, **101**, 15064–15069; (b) Vannini, A., Volpari, C., Gallinari, P., Jones, P., Mattu, M., Carfi, A. *et al.* (2007) Substrate binding to histone deacetylases as shown by the crystal structure of the HDAC8–substrate complex. *EMBO Reports*, **8**, 879–884.

11 Somoza, J.R., Skene, R.J., Katz, B.A., Mol, C., Ho, J.D., Jennings, A.J. *et al.* (2004) Structural snapshots of human HDAC8 provide insights into the class I histone deacetylases. *Structure (London, England: 1993)*, **12**, 1325–1334.

12 Jones, P., Bottomley, M.J., Carfí, A., Cecchetti, O., Ferrigno, F., Lo Surdo, P. *et al.* (2008) 2-Trifluoroacetylthiophenes, a novel series of potent and selective class II histone deacetylase inhibitors. *Bioorganic & Medicinal Chemistry Letters*, **18**, 3456–3461.

13 Leder, A. and Leder, P. (1975) Butyric acid, a potent inducer of erythroid differentiation in cultured erythroleukemic cells. *Cell*, **5**, 319–322.

14 Riggs, M.G., Whittaker, R.G., Neumann, J.R. and Ingram, V.M. (1977) Butyrate causes histone modification in HeLa and Friend erythroleukemia cells. *Nature*, **268**, 462–464.

15 Rephaeli, A., Zhuk, R. and Nudelman, A. (2000) Prodrugs of butyric acid from bench to bedside: synthetic design, mechanisms of action, and clinical applications. *Drug Development Research*, **50**, 379–391.

16 Phiel, C.J., Zhang, F., Huang, E.Y., Guenther, M.G., Lazar, M.A. and Klein, P.S. (2001) Histone deacetylase is a direct target of valproic acid, a potent anticonvulsant, mood stabilizer, and teratogen. *The Journal of Biological Chemistry*, **276**, 36734–36741.

17 (a) Miller, T.A., Witter, D.J. and Belvedere, S. (2003) Histone deacetylase inhibitors. *Journal of Medicinal Chemistry*, **46**, 5097–5116; (b) Paris, M., Porcelloni, M., Binaschi, M., Fattori, D. (2008) Histone deacetylase inhibitors: from bench to clinic. *Journal of Medicinal Chemistry*, **51**, 1505–1529; (c) Jones, P., Steinkühler, C. (2008) From natural products to small molecule ketone histone deacetylase inhibitors: development of new class specific agents. *Current Pharmaceutical Design*, **14**, 545–561.

18 Tsuji, N., Kobayashi, M., Nagashima, K., Wakisaka, Y. and Koizumi, K. (1976) A new

antifungal antibiotic, trichostatin. *Journal of Antibiotics (Tokyo)*, **29**, 1–6.
19 Yoshida, M., Kijima, M., Akita, M. and Beppu, T. (1990) Potent and specific inhibition of mammalian HDAC both in vivo and in vitro by TSA. *The Journal of Biological Chemistry*, **265**, 17174–17179.
20 Marks, P.A. and Breslow, R. (2007) Dimethyl sulfoxide to vorinostat: development of this histone deacetylase inhibitor as an anticancer drug. *Nature Biotechnology*, **25**, 84–90.
21 Richon, V.M., Webb, Y., Merger, R., Sheppard, T., Jursic, B., Ngo, L. *et al.* (1996) Second generation hybrid polar compounds are potent inducers of transformed cell differentiation. *Proceedings of the National Academy of Sciences of the United States of America*, **93**, 5705–5708.
22 Richon, V.M., Emiliani, S., Verdin, E., Webb, Y., Breslow, R., Rifkind, R.A. *et al.* (1998) A class of hybrid polar inducers of transformed cell differentiation inhibits histone deacetylases. *Proceedings of the National Academy of Sciences of the United States of America*, **95**, 3003–3007.
23 Richon, V.M. (2006) Cancer biology: mechanism of antitumour action of vorinostat (suberoylanilide hydroxamic acid), a novel histone deacetylase inhibitor. *British Journal of Cancer*, **95**, S2–S6.
24 Duvic, M. and Zhang, C. (2006) Clinical and laboratory experience of vorinostat (suberoylanilide hydroxamic acid) in the treatment of cutaneous T-cell lymphoma. *British Journal of Cancer*, **95**, S13–S19.
25 Olsen, E.A., Kim, Y.H., Kuzel, T.M., Pacheco, T.R., Foss, F.M., Parker, S. *et al.* (2007) Phase IIB multicenter trial of vorinostat in patients with persistent, progressive, or treatment refractory cutaneous T-cell lymphoma. *Journal of Clinical Oncology*, **25**, 3109–3115.
26 Kim, Y.B., Lee, K.-H., Sugita, K., Yoshida, M. and Horinouchi, S. (1999) Oxamflatin is a novel antitumor compound that inhibits mammalian histone deacetylase. *Oncogene*, **18**, 2461–2470.
27 Jung, M., Hoffmann, K., Brosch, G. and Loidl, P. (1997) Analogues of trichostatin A and trapoxin B as histone deacetylase inhibitors. *Bioorganic & Medicinal Chemistry Letters*, **7**, 1655–1658.
28 Jung, M., Brosch, G., Kolle, D., Scherf, H., Gerhauser, C. and Loidl, P. (1999) Amide analogues of trichostatin A as inhibitors of histone deacetylase and inducers of terminal cell differentiation. *Journal of Medicinal Chemistry*, **42**, 4669–4679.
29 (a) Remiszewski, S.W., Sambucetti, L.C., Atadja, P., Bair, K.W., Cornell, W.D., Green, M.A. *et al.* (2002) Inhibitors of human histone deacetylase: synthesis and enzyme and cellular activity of straight chain hydroxamates. *Journal of Medicinal Chemistry*, **45**, 753–757; (b) Woo, S.H., Frechette, S., Khalil, E.A., Bouchain, G., Vaisburg, A., Bernstein, N. *et al.* (2002) Structurally simple trichostatin A-like straight chain hydroxamates as potent histone deacetylase inhibitors. *Journal of Medicinal Chemistry*, **45**, 2877–2885.
30 Curtin, M.L., Garland, R.B., Heyman, H.R., Frey, R.R., Michaelides, M.R., Li, J. *et al.* (2002) Succinimide hydroxamic acids as potent inhibitors of histone deacetylase (HDAC). *Bioorganic & Medicinal Chemistry Letters*, **12**, 2919–2923.
31 Dai, Y., Guo, Y., Guo, J., Pease, L.J., Li, J., Marcotte, P.A. *et al.* (2003) Indole amide hydroxamic acids as potent inhibitors of histone deacetylases. *Bioorganic & Medicinal Chemistry Letters*, **13**, 1897–1901.
32 Dai, Y., Guo, Y., Curtin, M.L., Li, J., Pease, L.J., Guo, J. *et al.* (2003) A novel series of histone deacetylase inhibitors incorporating hetero aromatic ring systems as connection units. *Bioorganic & Medicinal Chemistry Letters*, **13**, 3817–3820.
33 Wu, T.Y.H., Hassig, C., Wu, Y., Ding, S. and Schultz, P.G. (2004) Design, synthesis, and activity of HDAC inhibitors with a *N*-formyl hydroxylamine head group. *Bioorganic & Medicinal Chemistry Letters*, **14**, 449–453.
34 Remiszewski, S.W., Sambucetti, L.C., Bair, K.W., Bontempo, J., Cesarz, D.,

Chandramouli, N. *et al.* (2003) *N*-Hydroxy-3-phenyl-2-propenamides as novel inhibitors of human HDAC with in vivo antitumor activity: discovery of NVP-LAQ824. *Journal of Medicinal Chemistry*, **46**, 4609–4624.

35 Giles, F., Fischer, T., Cortes, J., Garcia-Manero, G., Beck, J., Ravandi, F. *et al.* (2006) A phase I study of intravenous LBH589, a novel cinnamic hydroxamic acid analogue histone deacetylase inhibitor, in patients with refractory hematologic malignancies. *Clinical Cancer Research*, **12**, 4628–4635.

36 Revill, P., Mealy, N., Serradell, N., Bolós, J. and Rosa, E. (2007) Panobinostat. *Drugs of the Future*, **32**, 315–322.

37 Lavoie, R., Bouchain, G., Frechette, S., Woo, S.H., Khalil, E.A., Leit, S. *et al.* (2001) Design and synthesis of a novel class of histone deacetylase inhibitors. *Bioorganic & Medicinal Chemistry Letters*, **11**, 2847–2850.

38 Finn, P.W., Bandara, M., Butcher, C., Finn, A., Hollinshead, R., Khan, N. *et al.* (2005) Novel sulfonamide derivatives as inhibitors of histone deacetylase. *Helvetica Chimica Acta*, **88**, 1630–1657.

39 Plumb, J.A., Finn, P.W., Williams, R.J., Bandara, M.J., Romero, M.R., Watkins, C.J. *et al.* (2003) Pharmacodynamic response and inhibition of growth of human tumor xenografts by the novel histone deacetylase inhibitor PXD101. *Molecular Cancer Therapeutics*, **2**, 721–728.

40 (a) Buggy, J.J., Cao, Z.A., Bass, K.E., Verner, E., Balasubramanian, S., Liu, L. *et al.* (2006) CRA-024781: a novel synthetic inhibitor of HDAC enzymes with antitumor activity *in vitro* and *in vivo*. *Molecular Cancer Therapeutics*, **5**, 1309–1317; (b) Balasubramanian, S., Ramos, J., Luo, W., Sirisawad, M., Verner, E., Buggy, J.J. (2008) A novel histone deacetylase 8 (HDAC8)-specific inhibitor PCI-34051 induces apoptosis in T-cell lymphomas. *Leukemia*, **22**, 1026–1034.

41 Golay, J., Cuppini, L., Leoni, F., Micò, C., Barbui, V., Domenghini, M. *et al.* (2007) The histone deacetylase inhibitor ITF2357 has anti-leukemic activity *in vitro* and *in vivo* and inhibits IL-6 and VEGF production by stromal cells. *Leukemia*, **21**, 1892–1900.

42 Arts, J., Angibaud, P., Mariën, A., Floren, W., Janssens, B., King, P. *et al.* (2007) R306465 is a novel potent inhibitor of class I HDACs with broad-spectrum antitumoral activity against solid and haematological malignancies. *British Journal of Cancer*, **97**, 1344–1353.

43 (a) Price, S., Bordogna, W., Braganza, R., Bull, R.J., Dyke, H.J., Gardan, S. *et al.* (2007) Identification and optimisation of a series of substituted 5-pyridin-2-yl-thiophene-2-hydroxamic acids as potent histone deacetylase (HDAC) inhibitors. *Bioorganic & Medicinal Chemistry Letters*, **17**, 363–369; (b) Price, S., Bordogna, W., Bull, R.J., Clark, D.E., Crackett, P.H., Dyke, H.J. *et al.* (2007) Identification and optimisation of a series of substituted 5-(1*H*-pyrazol-3-yl)-thiophene-2-hydroxamic acids as potent histone deacetylase (HDAC) inhibitors. *Bioorganic & Medicinal Chemistry Letters*, **17**, 370–375.

44 Witter, D.J., Belvedere, S., Chen, L., Secrist, J.P., Mosley, R.T. and Miller, T.A. (2007) Benzo[*b*]thio phene-based histone deacetylase inhibitors. *Bioorganic & Medicinal Chemistry Letters*, **17**, 4562–4567.

45 Mai, A., Massa, S., Pezzi, R., Simeoni, S., Rotili, D., Nebbioso, A. *et al.* (2005) Class II (IIa)-selective histone deacetylase inhibitors. 1. Synthesis and biological evaluation of novel (aryloxopropenyl) pyrrolyl hydroxyamides. *Journal of Medicinal Chemistry*, **48**, 3344–3353.

46 Berger, M.R., Bischoff, H., Fritschi, E., Henne, T., Hermann, M., Pool, B.L. *et al.* (1985) Synthesis, toxicity, and therapeutic efficacy of 4-amino-*N*-(2′-aminophenyl)-benzamide: a new compound preferentially active in slowly growing tumors. *Cancer Treatment Reports*, **69**, 1415–1424.

47 Kraker, A.J., Mizzen, C.A., Hartl, B.G., Miin, J., Allis, C.D. and Merriman, R.L.

(2003) Modulation of Histone Acetylation by [4-(Acetylamino)-*N*-(2-Amino-phenyl) Benzamide] in HCT-8 Colon Carcinoma. *Molecular Cancer Therapeutics*, **2**, 401–408.

48 Hauschild, A. (2006) A phase II multicenter study on the HDACi MS-275, comparing two dosage schedules in metastatic melanoma. Abs. 8044, Annual Meeting of the American Society of Clinical Oncology, Atlanta, Ga.

49 Suzuki, T., Ando, T., Tsuchiya, K., Fukazawa, N., Saito, A., Mariko, Y. *et al.* (1999) Synthesis and histone deacetylase inhibitory activity of new benzamide derivatives. *Journal of Medicinal Chemistry*, **42**, 3001–3003.

50 Saito, A., Yamashita, T., Mariko, Y., Nosaka, Y., Tsuchiya, K., Ando, T. *et al.* (1999) A synthetic inhibitor of HDAC, MS-27-275, with marked in vivo antitumor activity against human tumors. *Proceedings of the National Academy of Sciences of the United States of America*, **96**, 4592–4597.

51 Hess-Stump, H., Bracker, T.U., Henderson, D. and Politz, O. (2007) MS-275, a potent orally available inhibitor of histone deacetylases—The development of an anticancer agent. *The International Journal of Biochemistry & Cell Biology*, **39**, 1388–1405.

52 Kell, J. and Serradell, N. (2008) MGCD-0103. *Drugs of the Future*, **33**, 323–327.

53 Fournel, M., Bonfils, C., Hou, Y., Yan, P.T., Trachy-Bourget, M.-C., Kalita, A. *et al.* (2008) MGCD0103, a novel isotype-selective histone deacetylase inhibitor, has broad spectrum antitumor activity in vitro and in vivo. *Molecular Cancer Therapeutics*, **7**, 759–768.

54 Fournel, M., Trachy-Bourget, M.-C., Yan, P.T., Kalita, A., Bonfils, C., Beaulieu, C. *et al.* (2002) Sulfonamide anilides, a novel class of histone deacetylase inhibitors, are antiproliferative against human tumors. *Cancer Research*, **62**, 4325–4330.

55 Bouchain, G., Leit, S., Frechette, S., Khalil, E.A., Lavoie, R., Moradei, O. *et al.* (2003) Development of potential antitumor agents. Synthesis and biological evaluation of a new set of sulfonamide derivatives as histone deacetylase inhibitors. *Journal of Medicinal Chemistry*, **46**, 820–830.

56 Moradei, O., Leit, S., Zhou, N., Frechétte, S., Paquin, I., Raeppel, S. *et al.* (2006) Substituted *N*-(2-aminophenyl)-benzamides, (*E*)-*N*-(2-aminophenyl)-acrylamides and their analogues: Novel classes of histone deacetylase inhibitors. *Bioorganic & Medicinal Chemistry Letters*, **16**, 4048–4052.

57 Vaisburg, A., Paquin, I., Bernstein, N., Frechette, S., Gaudette, F., Leit, S. *et al.* (2007) *N*-(2-Amino-phenyl)-4-(heteroarylmethyl)-benzamides as new histone deacetylase inhibitors. *Bioorganic & Medicinal Chemistry Letters*, **17**, 6729–6733.

58 Fréchette, S., Leit, S., Woo, S.H., Lapointe, G., Jeannotte, G., Moradei, O. *et al.* (2008) 4-(Heteroarylaminomethyl)-*N*-(2-aminophenyl)-benzamides and their analogs as a novel class of histone deacetylase inhibitors. *Bioorganic & Medicinal Chemistry Letters*, **18**, 1502–1506.

59 Hamblett, C.L., Methot, J.L., Mampreian, D.M., Sloman, D.L., Stanton, M.G., Kral, A.M. *et al.* (2007) The discovery of 6-amino nicotinamides as potent and selective histone deacetylase inhibitors. *Bioorganic & Medicinal Chemistry Letters*, **17**, 5300–5309.

60 Andrews, D.M., Gibson, K.M., Graham, M.A., Matusiak, Z.S., Roberts, C.A., Stokes, E.S.E. *et al.* (2008) Design and campaign synthesis of pyridine-based histone deacetylase inhibitors. *Bioorganic & Medicinal Chemistry Letters*, **18**, 2525–2529.

61 Andrews, D.M., Stokes, E.S.E., Carr, G.R., Matusiak, Z.S., Roberts, C.A., Waring, M.J. *et al.* (2008) Design and campaign synthesis of piperidine- and thiazole-based histone deacetylase inhibitors. *Bioorganic & Medicinal Chemistry Letters*, **18**, 2580–2584.

62 (a) Moradei, O.M., Mallais, T.C., Frechette, S., Paquin, I., Tessier, P.E., Leit, S.M. *et al.* (2007) Novel aminophenyl benzamide-type histone deacetylase inhibitors with enhanced potency and selectivity. *Journal of Medicinal Chemistry*, **50**, 5543–5546; (b) Witter, D.J., Harrington, P., Wilson, K.J., Chenard, M., Fleming, J.C., Haines, B. *et al.* (2008) Optimization of biaryl Selective HDAC1&2 Inhibitors (SHI-1:2). *Bioorganic & Medicinal Chemistry Letters*, **18**, 726–731; (c) Methot, J.L., Chakravarty, P.K., Chenard, M., Close, J., Cruz, J.C., Dahlberg, W.K. *et al.* (2008) Exploration of the internal cavity of histone deacetylase (HDAC) with selective HDAC1/HDAC2 inhibitors (SHI-1:2). *Bioorganic & Medicinal Chemistry Letters*, **18**, 973–978.

63 Haggarty, S.J., Koeller, K.M., Wong, J.C., Grozinger, C.M. and Schreiber, S.L. (2003) Domain-selective small-molecule inhibitor of HDAC6-mediated tubulin deacetylation. *Proceedings of the National Academy of Sciences of the United States of America*, **100**, 4389–4394.

64 Frey, R.R., Wada, C.K., Garland, R.B., Curtin, M.L., Michaelides, M.R., Li, J. *et al.* (2002) Trifluoromethyl ketones as inhibitors of HDAC. *Bioorganic & Medicinal Chemistry Letters*, **12**, 3443–3447.

65 Vasudevan, A., Ji, Z., Frey, R.R., Wada, C.K., Steinman, D., Heyman, H.R. *et al.* (2003) Heterocyclic ketones as inhibitors of HDAC. *Bioorganic & Medicinal Chemistry Letters*, **13**, 3909–3913.

66 Wada, C.K., Frey, R.R., Ji, Z., Curtin, M.L., Garland, R.B., Holms, J.H. *et al.* (2003) α-Keto amides as inhibitors of HDAC. *Bioorganic & Medicinal Chemistry Letters*, **13**, 3331–3335.

67 (a) Lahm, A., Paolini, C., Pallaoro, M., Nardi, M.C., Jones, P., Neddermann, P. *et al.* (2007) Unraveling the hidden catalytic activity of vertebrate class IIA histone deacetylases. *Proceedings of the National Academy of Sciences of the United States of America*, **104**, 17335–17340; (b) Jones, P., Altamura, S., De Francesco, R., Gallinari, P., Lahm, A., Neddermann, P. *et al.* (2008) Probing the elusive catalytic activity of vertebrate class IIa histone deacetylases. *Bioorganic & Medicinal Chemistry Letters*, **18**, 1814–1819.

68 Ueda, M., Manda, T., Matsumoto, S., Mukumoto, S., Nishigaki, F., Kawamura, I. *et al.* (1994) FR901228, a novel antitumor bicyclic depsipeptide produced by *Chromobacterium violaceum* No. 968. III. Antitumor activities on experimental tumors in mice. *Journal of Antibiotics (Tokyo)*, **47**, 315–323.

69 Nakajima, H., Kim, Y.B., Terano, H., Yoshida, M. and Horinouchi, S. (1998) FR901228, a potent antitumor antibiotic, is a novel histone deacetylase inhibitor. *Experimental Cell Research*, **241**, 126–133.

70 Furumai, R., Matsuyama, A., Kobashi, N., Lee, K.-H., Nishiyama, M., Nakajima, H. *et al.* (2002) FK228 (depsipeptide) as a natural prodrug that inhibits class I HDACs. *Cancer Research*, **62**, 4916–4921.

71 Whittaker, S., Scarisbrick, J., Kim, Y.H., Reddy, S., Kim, E.J., Rook, A.H. *et al.* (2008) Romidepsin activity and clinical benefit in refractory CTCL: results from an international multicenter study. Abstract 444, 5th Joint Meeting of the JSID, SID and ESDR, Kyoto.

72 Walton, J.D. (2006) HC-toxin. *Phytochemistry*, **67**, 1406–1413.

73 Brosch, G., Ransom, R., Lechner, T., Walton, J.D. and Loidl, P. (1995) Inhibition of maize histone deacetylases by HC toxin, the host-selective toxin of *Cochliobolus carbonum*. *Plant Cell*, **7**, 1941.

74 Closse, A. and Huguenin, R. (1974) Isolierung und strukturaufklärung von chlamydocin. *Helvetica Chimica Acta*, **57**, 533–545.

75 De Schepper, S., Bruwiere, H., Verhulst, T., Steller, U., Andries, L., Wouters, W. *et al.* (2003) Inhibition of histone deacetylases by chlamydocin induces apoptosis and proteasome-mediated degradation of survivin. *The Journal of Pharmacology and Experimental Therapeutics*, **304**, 881–888.

76 Itazaki, H., Nagashima, K., Sugita, K., Yoshida, H., Kawamura, Y., Yasuda, Y. *et al.* (1990) Isolation and structural elucidation of new cyclotetrapeptides, trapoxins

A and B, having detransformation activities as antitumor agents. *Journal of Antibiotics (Tokyo)*, **43**, 1524–1532.

77 Kijima, M., Yoshida, M., Sugita, K., Horinouchi, S. and Beppu, T. (1993) Trapoxin, an antitumor cyclic tetrapeptide, is an irreversible inhibitor of mammalian histone deacetylase. *The Journal of Biological Chemistry*, **268**, 22429–22435.

78 Taunton, J., Collins, J.L. and Schreiber, S.L. (1996) Synthesis of natural and modified trapoxins, useful reagents for exploring histone deacetylase function. *Journal of the American Chemical Society*, **118**, 10412–10422.

79 Mori, H., Urano, Y., Abe, F., Furukawa, S., Furukawa, S., Tsurumi, Y. *et al.* (2003) FR235222, a fungal metabolite, is a novel immunosuppressant that inhibits mammalian histone deacetylase (HDAC). I. Taxonomy, fermentation, isolation and biological activities. *Journal of Antibiotics (Tokyo)*, **56**, 72–79.

80 Mori, H., Yoshimura, S., Takase, S. and Hino, M. (2000) Inhibitor of histone deacetylase, WO2000/08048.

81 Darkin-Rattray, S.J., Gurnett, A.M., Myers, R.W., Dulski, P.M., Crumley, T.M., Allocco, J.J. *et al.* (1996) Apicidin: A novel antiprotozoal agent that inhibits parasite HDAC. *Proceedings of the National Academy of Sciences of the United States of America*, **93**, 13143–13147.

82 Han, J.-W., Ahn, S.H., Park, S.H., Wang, S.Y., Bae, G.-U., Seo, D.-W. *et al.* (2000) Apicidin, a histone deacetylase inhibitor, inhibits proliferation of tumor cells via induction of $p21^{WAF1/Cip1}$ and gelsolin. *Cancer Research*, **60**, 6068–6074.

83 Nakao, Y., Yoshida, S., Matsunaga, S., Shindoh, N., Terada, Y., Nagai, K. *et al.* (2006) Azumamides A-E: histone deacetylase inhibitory cyclic tetrapeptides from the marine sponge. *Mycale izuensis Angewandte Chemie (International Edition in English)*, **45**, 7553–7557.

84 Pina, I.C., Gautschi, J.T., Wang, G.-Y.-S., Sanders, M.L., Schmitz, F.J., France, D. *et al.* (2003) Psammaplins from the sponge *Pseudoceratina purpurea:* inhibition of both histone deacetylase and DNA methyltransferase. *The Journal of Organic Chemistry*, **68**, 3866–3873.

85 Furumai, R., Komatsu, Y., Nishino, N., Khochbin, S., Yoshida, M. and Horinouchi, S. (2001) Potent histone deacetylase inhibitors built from trichostatin A and cyclic tetrapeptide antibiotics including trapoxin. *Proceedings of the National Academy of Sciences of the United States of America*, **98**, 87–92.

86 Komatsu, Y., Tomizaki, K., Tsukamoto, M., Kato, T., Nishino, N., Sato, S. *et al.* (2001) Cyclic hydroxamic-acid-containing peptide 31, a potent synthetic histone deacetylase inhibitor with antitumor activity. *Cancer Research*, **61**, 4459–4466.

87 Nishino, N., Jose, B., Okamura, S., Ebisusaki, S., Kato, T., Sumida, Y. *et al.* (2003) Cyclic tetrapeptides bearing a sulfhydryl group potently inhibit histone deacetylases. *Organic Letters*, **5**, 5079–5082.

88 Jones, P., Altamura, S., Chakravarty, P.K., Cecchetti, O., De Francesco, R., Gallinari, P. *et al.* (2006) A series of novel, potent, and selective histone deacetylase inhibitors. *Bioorganic & Medicinal Chemistry Letters*, **16**, 5948–5952.

89 Jones, P., Altamura, S., De Francesco, R., Gonzalez Paz, O., Kinzel, O., Mesiti, G. *et al.* (2008) A novel series of potent and selective ketone histone deacetylase inhibitors with antitumor activity in vivo. *Journal of Medicinal Chemistry*, **51**, 2350–2353.

90 Suzuki, T., Nagano, Y., Kouketsu, A., Matsuura, A., Maruyama, S., Kurotaki, M. *et al.* (2005) Novel Inhibitors of human histone deacetylases: design, synthesis, enzyme inhibition, and cancer cell growth inhibition of SAHA-based non-hydroxamates. *Journal of Medicinal Chemistry*, **48**, 1019–1032.

91 (a) Suzuki, T., Kouketsu, A., Itoh, Y., Hisakawa, S., Maeda, S., Yoshida, M. *et al.* (2006) Highly potent and selective histone deacetylase 6 inhibitors designed based on a small-molecular substrate. *Journal of*

Medicinal Chemistry, **49**, 4809–4812; (b) Itoh, Y., Suzuki, T., Kouketsu, A., Suzuki, N., Maeda, S., Yoshida, M. *et al.* (2007) Design, synthesis, structure-selectivity relationship, and effect on human cancer cells of a novel series of histone deacetylase 6-selective inhibitors. *Journal of Medicinal Chemistry*, **50**, 5425–5438.

92 Chen, B., Petukhov, P.A., Jung, M., Velena, A., Eliseeva, E., Dritschilo, A. and Kozikowski, A.P. (2005) Chemistry and biology of mercaptoacetamides as novel histone deacetylase inhibitors. *Bioorganic & Medicinal Chemistry Letters*, **15**, 1389–1392.

93 Kozikowski, A.P., Chen, Y., Gaysin, A., Chen, B., D'Annibale, M.A., Suto, C.M. *et al.* (2007) Functional differences in epigenetic modulators-superiority of mercaptoacetamide-based histone deacetylase inhibitors relative to hydroxamates in cortical neuron neuroprotection studies. *Journal of Medicinal Chemistry*, **50**, 3054–3061.

94 Hassig, C.A., Symons, K.T., Guo, X., Nguyen, P.-M., Annable, T., Wash, P.L. *et al.* (2008) KD5170, a novel mercaptoketone-based histone deacetylase inhibitor that exhibits broad spectrum antitumor activity *in vitro* and *in vivo Mol. Cancer Therapeutics*, **7**, 1054–1065.

10
NAD-Dependent Deacetylases as Therapeutic Targets

Hongzhe Li, Julian Simon, and Antonio Bedalov

10.1
Historical Perspective and Functions of Sir2 in Yeast

The founding member of the sirtuin family, SIR2, was characterized in the mid-1980s as a gene required for the transcriptional [1] repression of the silent mating-type loci and mating competence [2–4]. While the subsequent work led to recognition of SIR2 as a key epigenetic regulator in yeast [5], a major breakthrough occurred in 2000 with the discovery that Sir2 possesses NAD-dependent histone deacetylase activity [6–8]. At the mating type loci and at telomeres, the two regions that exhibit characteristics of heterochromatin in yeast, Sir2 forms a complex with Sir3 and Sir4 (silent information regulator, SIR), which is recruited to chromatin through protein–protein interactions with DNA-binding proteins [1]. After recruitment, Sir2 deacetylates histone tails, which is thought to promote spreading of the SIR complex along the chromatin and to confer transcriptional repression over the region. In addition, Sir2 associates with different proteins at the rDNA locus [9], where its main role is suppression of recombination of tandem copies of rRNA genes [10]. The function of Sir2 at the rDNA locus was found to be critical for promoting replicative lifespan of mother cells [11, 12]. Yeast cells divide asymmetrically with a larger mother cell giving rise to a smaller daughter. Mother cells have limited replicative potential and die after producing 20–40 daughter cells. Therefore, while a culture of yeast cells is immortal, the lifespan of each mother cell is limited. One of the events that limits a mothers' lifespan is the accumulation of rDNA circles that are excised during recombination at the rDNA locus and are preferentially retained in mother cells during cell division [11]. By controlling the rate of recombination at the rDNA locus, loss of SIR2 shortens and increased SIR2 dosage extends the lifespan of mother cells [11]. The observation that increased activity of Sir2 in budding yeast suppresses senescence led to studies in multicellular eukaryotes such as nematodes [13] and fruit flies [14], which showed that increased gene dosage of the Sir2 orthologs extends lifespan. Because nematodes and flies do not show accumulation of rDNA circles during aging, and yet Sir2 orthologs promote longevity in these

Epigenetic Targets in Drug Discovery. Edited by Wolfgang Sippl and Manfred Jung

ISBN: 978-3-527-32355-5

organisms, it was proposed that the longevity control role of sirtuins was retained during evolution despite differences in the specific degenerative processes that occur during aging in different species. One intervention shown to be universal in its ability to extend longevity across species is calorie restriction. This led to the hypothesis that the beneficial effects of calorie restriction in different species during aging are mediated through a conserved molecular pathway that involves calorie restriction induced increase in sirtuin activity [15]. Despite ongoing controversy whether calorie restriction-mediated lifespan extension requires Sir2 [16], this hypothesis generated a high level of enthusiasm for studies from many laboratories that evaluated the role of Sir2 orthologs on various aspects of aging (e.g. neurodegeneration, type II diabetes) in metazoan organisms including mice. Genetic and pharmacologic manipulations of sirtuin activity showed beneficial effects in a surprisingly broad spectrum of aging-associated conditions and diseases, suggesting that the Sir2-family of enzymes presents an attractive pharmacological target.

10.2
Sirtuin Enzymatic Activity and its Modulation by Endogenous Molecules

The sirtuin family is defined by a homology with *Saccharomyces cerevisiae* Sir2 and is broadly conserved from bacteria to humans. Different species carry widely different number of enzymes with two members in *Escherichia coli*, five members in *S. cerevisiae*, three in *Schizosaccharomyces pombe*, five in *Drosophila melanogaster* and seven in mammals (SIRT1–7) [17]. The conserved catalytic domain contains approximately 250 residues and functions as an NAD-dependent protein deacetylase or mono-ADP-ribosyltransferase, or both (reviewed in [18]). The catalytic reaction carried out by sirtuin family of enzymes, or class III histone deacetylases (HDAC), is distinct from that carried out by class I, II and IV HDACs that use a Zn ion at the active site to activate a water molecule for amide bond hydrolysis. During Sir2-mediated deacetylation cleavage of the glycosidic bond between nicotinamide and ribose is coupled to transfer of the acetyl group from lysine onto the ribose moiety of ADP-ribose to generate lysine, O-acetyl-ADP-ribose and nicotinamide [19]. Alternatively the enzyme can transfer the ADP-ribose to a protein to generate a mono-ADP-ribosylated protein. Among human enzymes, deacetylase activity has been demonstrated for SIRT1, SIRT2, SIRT3, SIRT5 and SIRT6. These enzymes differ in respect to their cellular localization, substrate specificity and biological functions [20, 21]. SIRT1, which has been most extensively studied, is a nuclear protein implicated in regulation of stress response [22, 23], differentiation [24], glucose homeostasis [25], cholesterol mobilization [26], HIV transcription [27], mitochondrial respiration [28] and ribosome biogenesis [29] through deacetylation of specific set of substrates that, beside histones, include transcription factors and repressors (e.g. p53, FOXOs, MyoD, NF-kappa B, LXR, BCL6, E2F1) [30], transcriptional coactivators (e.g. PGC1α), chromatin modifying enzymes (e.g. histone methyltransferase SUV39H1) [31] and other proteins (e.g. Ku70) [32]. SIRT6 is also a nuclear protein and is implicated in DNA damage repair [33], SIRT7 is localized in the nucleolus [34], SIRT2 is predominantly cytoplasmic [35] and SIRT3–5 are located in the mitochondria [36–39]. With the exception of SIRT6, these enzymes do not exhibit high *in vitro* specificity, as shown by their ability deacetylate a wide range of acetylated substrates [40]. Because individual sirtuins have distinct N-acetyl lysine substrates, specificity appears to be achieved at the level of protein–protein association and cellular localization rather than inherent active site specificity. In contrast to other deacetylases, SIRT6 has been shown to specifically deacetylate histone H3 lysine 9 residue both *in vitro* and *in vivo* with no detectable activity against other histone residues [41] or other tested substrates [42]. In addition, SIRT4 and SIRT6 both have robust ADP-ribosyl transferase activity [37, 39, 42]. While no *in vitro* enzymatic activity has been demonstrated for the nucleolar sirtuin, SIRT7, using the available substrates, the observation that the mutations known to abolish enzymatic activity of other sirtuins led to the loss of SIRT7 biological functions suggests that SIRT7 also functions as an enzyme [41].

Nicotinamide produced during sirtuin-mediated deacetylation inhibits sirtuin activity and the physiological concentration of nicotinamide has been shown to be sufficient to modulate cellular sirtuin activity in the cell [43–45]. Accordingly, the enzymes that participate in the removal of nicotinamide have been shown to influence sirtuin activity *in vivo*. Furthermore, cellular NAD levels also affect sirtuin activity. NAD can be synthesized *de novo* in several enzymatic steps from tryptophan via the kynurenine pathway, or it can be generated through reutilization of its breakdown product by the salvage pathway. In yeast, the Sir2 homolog Hst1 acts as cellular NAD sensor that controls transcription of the genes in the kynurenine pathway and thus *de novo* NAD biosynthesis and cellular NAD levels [46]. In addition to regenerating NAD, the salvage pathway also reutilizes and thus removes nicotinamide. Both of these two outcomes can promote SIR2 activity [47–49].

The redox state in cells and concomitant alterations of the NAD/NADH ratio are implicated in the regulation of cellular sirtuin activity and control of several processes including calorie restriction-induced lifespan extension in yeast [50], muscle differentiation [51] and neurogenesis [52]. An alteration in the NAD/NADH ratio was proposed to influence sirtuin activity by modulating the level of NAD, and conversely by altering cellular NADH, which inhibits Sir2 activity. However, detailed characterization of coenzyme specificity of Sir2-proteins failed to generate biochemical support for the role of cellular NAD/NADH alterations as cellular regulators of sirtuin activity [53]. First, given that only a fraction of the total cellular NAD/NADH pool is in the reduced state (NADH) (i.e. NAD/NADH ratio is estimated to be high), even if the total pool were converted to NAD, the result would be only a minor increase in the available NAD. Second, NADH has been shown to be an extremely inefficient sirtuin inhibitor (IC_{50} 15 mM) [53]. Because cellular NADH levels are at least two orders of magnitude lower than the measured IC_{50} of NADH, it is unlikely that cellular NADH level has a significant direct influence on sirtuin enzymatic activity. There is however evidence that cellular redox state regulates SIRT1 protein level at the transcriptional and posttranscriptional level. Cellular NADH levels and thus the NAD/NADH ratio are proposed to control SIRT1 transcription though a regulatory circuit that involves redox sensor CtBP and HIC1, an inhibitor of SIRT1 transcription [54]. Furthermore, a separate study suggests that glucose deprivation and cellular pyruvate control SIRT1 protein, even though the level of SIRT1 mRNA does not change [25]. These studies suggest that overall cellular SIRT1 activity may be influenced by NAD/NADH ratio through alterations in SIRT1 protein level rather than through direct control of SIRT1 enzymatic activity.

10.3
Small Molecule Inhibitors of Sirtuins

The first small molecule inhibitors of NAD-dependent histone deacetylases, beta-naphthol containing compounds, sirtinol (**1**) and splitomicin (**2**) [55, 56], were identified through cell-based screens in the yeast *S. cerevisiae* for compounds that abrogate telomeric silencing (Figure 10.1). Splitomicin was shown to create a conditional phenocopy of a *sir2* deletion with loss of silencing at telomeres, silent mating loci and ribosomal DNA. Several point mutants in the Sir2 small helical domain adjacent to peptide binding site conferred resistance to splitomicin *in vivo* and attenuated inhibition of Sir2 NAD-dependent deacetylase activity with splitomicin *in vitro*, thus identifying a potential binding site [55]. Subsequent work with cambinol (**3**), which inhibits human SIRT1 and SIRT2, showed that this class of molecules is competitive with the peptide binding and is consistent with the location of the identified point mutants [57]. One of the limitations of splitomicins was the instability of the lactone ring, which led to a short half-life, particularly at physiological pH [58]. However, several splitomicin derivatives were described that have not only increased potency (e.g. HR73; **4** [27]) but also retained inhibitory activity despite the replacement of the lactone with the lactam ring [59]. Provided that the lactams retain the *in vivo* activity, their stability makes them highly suited for further development as sirtuins inhibitors. Despite the limitations, splitomicin and its derivatives proved to be useful tools for dissection the cellular roles of sirtuins in chromatin biology [46, 55, 60] not only in yeast but also in mammalian cells [27, 61, 62].

Several other classes of SIRT1 and SIRT2 inhibitors have been identified including indole derivatives (e.g. EX-527) (**5**) [63], suramin and its derivatives [64, 65], adenosine mimetics (i.e. kinase inhibitors) [66] and phloroglucinol derivatives (e.g. guttiferone G, aristoforin, hyperforin) [67]. In addition, several inhibitors were derived from compounds identified using virtual screening [68–70]. Among these compounds, EX-527 is the most potent against SIRT1, with an IC_{50} value in the 100 nM range and 20-fold lower activity against SIRT2. This compound was shown to be cell permeable and capable of inhibiting cellular SIRT1. The identification of suramin and several related adenosine antagonists as SIRT1 inhibitors [64, 65] led to the investigation of other drugs that bind to ATP binding pockets including kinase inhibitors as lead structures that might inhibit sirtuin activity by interfering with the binding of the adenosine moiety of NAD to the enzyme. Several known kinase inhibitors including CDK inhibitors (paullones) and bisindolylmaleimides (BIMs) were found to be relatively potent sirtuin inhibitors [66]. One of the BIM derivatives had a fivefold selectivity against SIRT2 over SIRT1 and was shown to inhibit cellular SIRT2. These

SIRT Inhibitors

SIRT Activators

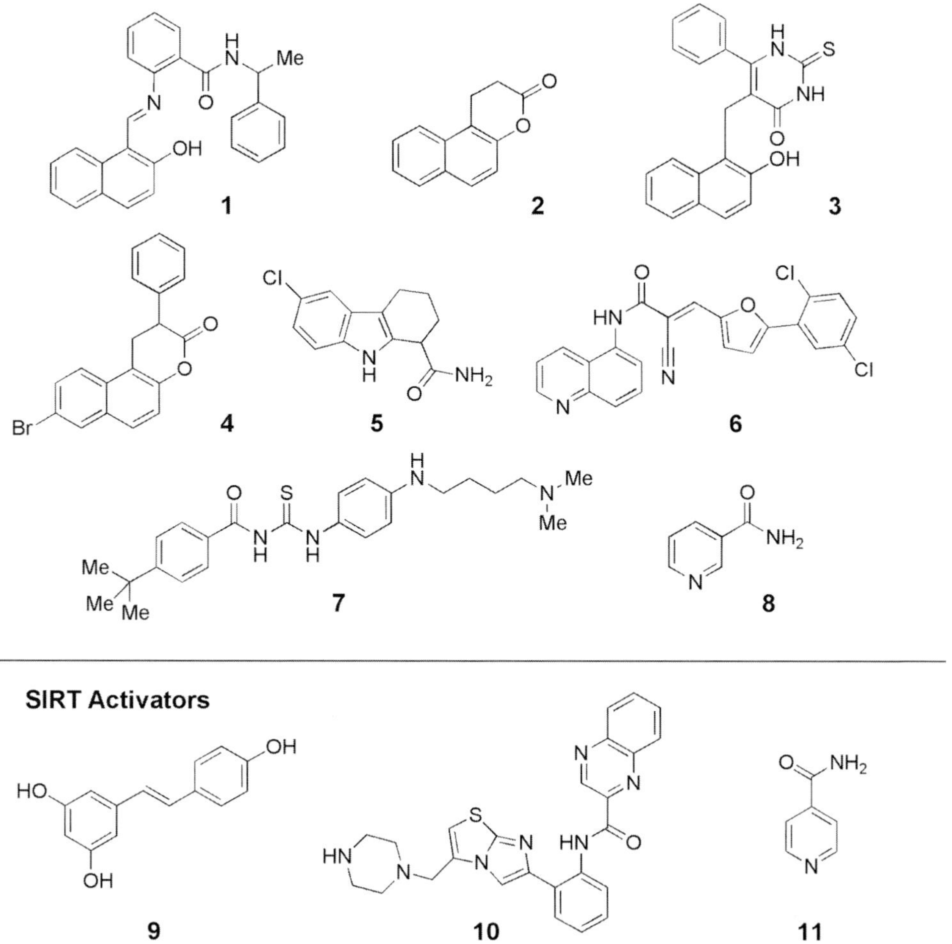

Figure 10.1 Inhibitors and activators of sirtuins. Inhibitors: **1**, sirtinol; **2**, splitomicin; **3**, cambinol; **4**, HR-73; **5**, EX-527; **6**, AGK-2; **7**, tenovin-6; **8**, nicotinamide. Activators: **9**, resveratrol; **10**, SRT-1720; **11**, isonicotinamide.

findings also suggest that small molecules that bind adenosine binding pockets such as kinase inhibitors may cross-react with this enzyme class.

Several compounds that were identified in unbiased mammalian cell-based screens for phenotypes that are not directly linked to chromatin biology were later identified as SIRT1 and/or SIRT2 inhibitors. The SIRT2 inhibitor AGK2 (**6**) and related compounds were identified in cell-based screens screen that alter aggregation patterns and diminish toxicity of polyglutamine repeat containing huntingtin and alpha-synuclein protein fragments in a search for possible treatments of Huntington and Parkinson disease [71]. Tenovins (**7**) are nonselective SIRT1 and SIRT2 inhibitors with anticancer activity that were identified in a screen for compounds that activate p53-dependent transcriptional reporter [72]. The sirtuin inhibitors identified through these unbiased chemical genetic approaches not only expand the armamentarium of cell-permeable small molecules that inhibit cellular sirtuins, but more importantly, they identify unexpected links of human diseases processes to sirtuin function and directly validate sirtuin inhibition as a potential therapeutic strategy for these conditions.

While different sirtuins and the members of class I and II deacetylases (HDACs) have distinct substrates that define their cellular roles, the division of labor among these enzymes is not absolute. Several acetylated proteins have been found to be deacetylated by more than one member within a family or by enzymes belonging to different families. For example, lysine 16 of the histone H4 has been shown to be deacetylated both with SIRT1 and SIRT2 [73, 74], whereas tubulin is deacetylated by both SIRT2 and HDAC6 [35, 75]. The functional and substrate overlap among different deacetylases has important implications in designing and using small molecule inhibitors of these enzymes for therapeutic purposes and for dissecting biology, as the inhibitors that are highly specific may not fully ablate specific cellular roles of a given deacetylase. Therefore, less selective inhibitors may be advantageous for altering cellular function and bringing therapeutic benefit. By the same token, cancer therapies may involve the combination of inhibitors of different deacetylase classes (e.g. sirtuin and HDACs). In contrast, highly selective inhibitors may be advantageous over nonselective ones as their side-effects are expected to be lessened by the relatively unperturbed function of the backup systems. Therefore, it will be important to develop both highly selective as well broadly active inhibitors for evaluating sirtuins as therapeutic targets.

10.4 Small Molecule Activators of Sirtuins

First activators of sirtuins identified were plant polyphenols among which resveratrol (**9**) was the most highly active [64]. At concentrations of 10 μM resveratrol led to an approximately twofold increase in SIRT1 deacetylase activity. A number of beneficial effects of resveratrol have been demonstrated in a variety of pre-clinical models (see below). The elucidation of the specific molecular mechanism by which resveratrol exerts these effects is complicated by the multitude of its biological activities (reviewed in [76]) and the unique interaction between this compound and the substrate used in the deacetylase assay. The screen that led to identification of these compounds employed as a substrate an acetyl-lysine-containing peptide with a fluorophore [64]. SIRT1 deacetylation of the peptide enabled trypsin to cleave the peptide, releasing the fluorophore, which was then capable of light emission. Resveratrol promoted deacetylation of the substrate by increasing the affinity of the substrate peptide for the enzyme acting as an allosteric activator. *In vivo*, resveratrol was shown to extend the lifespan in yeast, flies and in mice fed high-fat diet [64, 77, 78]. Subsequent work showed that the peptide containing the fluorophore has significantly lower affinity for SIRT1 compared to the same peptide without a fluorophore [79, 80]. Resveratrol specifically increases the affinity and deacetylation of the fluorophore-containing peptide, while having no influence on the same peptide without the fluorophore. Recently, structurally unrelated synthetic compounds were also found to activate SIRT1 (e.g. SRT1720; **10**). These compounds carry out activation of SIRT1 at submicromolar concentrations and increase SIRT1 activity several hundred-fold [81]. Furthermore, these compounds were found to be orally bioavailable and led to improvement of several metabolic parameters in mice fed a high-fat diet and other diabetes models in mice. Similarly to resveratrol, these compounds acted as allosteric enzyme activators by increasing binding of the peptide substrates and mapping studies using truncated forms of the enzyme revealed that the small helical domain of SIRT1 was required for their activity. Because these compounds were identified and characterized using fluorophore containing substrates, it will be important to determine whether they discriminate between unmodified and fluorophore-containing substrates.

In addition to resveratrol and other compounds that activate SIRT1 by promoting peptide binding, a different mechanism has been described for isonicotinamide (**11**), which was shown to activate yeast Sir2 through relief of nicotinamide inhibition [45]. As discussed previously, nicotinamide is an endogenous sirtuin inhibitor that promotes the chemical reversal of the covalent reaction intermediates and generation of NAD and acetyl lysine, resulting in nicotinamide exchange. Isonicotinmide is competitive with nicotinamide in the exchange reaction thus promoting deacetylation both *in vitro* and *in vivo*.

10.5
SIRT1 as a Therapeutic Target in Metabolic Syndrome and Type 2 Diabetes

The metabolic syndrome comprises a set of disorders including central (abdominal) obesity, insulin resistance, hypertension, proinflammatory and prothrombotic state which markedly increases the risk of cardiovascular disease. It is estimated that up to 25% of the population in western societies is affected with this condition. Calorie excess and physical inactivity have been proposed to be the main causes for this epidemic. The health detriment brought on by calorie excess and the health benefits created by calorie restriction have been proposed to be mediated through shared genetic circuitry that includes SIRT1 [82]. SIRT1 has been implicated in the control of several critical metabolic processes in various tissues including insulin secretion in beta cells in the pancreas (SIRT1 promotes insulin secretion) [83, 84], gluconeogenesis in the liver (SIRT1 promotes gluconeogenesis) [25], fatty acid oxidation and mitochondrial respiration in skeletal muscle (SIRT1 promotes both processes) [28] and fatty acid mobilization and differentiation in the adipose tissue [24]. These activities of SIRT1 raised the possibility that pharmacologic manipulations of its activity could be used for obesity-associated metabolic syndrome and type 2 diabetes (DM). The interest in SIRT1 activation as a therapeutic strategy in DM has been stimulated by the initial observation that activation of SIRT1 by resveratrol prevents physiological decline and extends survival in mice fed high-fat diet [78, 85], a finding that was later replicated using synthetic small molecule SIRT1 activators [81] and in SIRT1 overexpression mouse models [86, 87]. The activation of SIRT1 with resveratrol was thought to mimic calorie restriction-induced activation of SIRT1 and its beneficial effects in several tissues, including muscle where SIRT1 promotes fatty acid oxidation and mitochondrial respiration and in fat tissue, where SIRT1 promotes fat mobilization. However, studies addressing the specific roles of SIRT1 in different metabolic tissues indicate that the function of SIRT1 in metabolism is more complex than previously thought. One of the well established deacetylation targets of SIRT1 that mediates tissue specific metabolic processes in response to nutritional changes is the transcriptional coactivator PGC-1alpha (peroxisome proliferator-activated receptor gamma-coactivated receptor transcriptional coactivator-1alpha) [25]. PGC-1alpha is a key regulator of glucose production in the liver and is activated through SIRT1-mediated deacetylation. SIRT1 protein levels have been shown to increase in response to fasting, in turn promoting PGC-1alpha deacetylation and stimulating gluconeogenesis [25]. SIRT1 knockdown in the liver achieved by adenoviral delivery of SIRT1-specific shRNA leads improved glucose tolerance and reduced fasting glucose level in the mouse model of diabetes [88]. Because increased glucose production in the liver during fasting is one of the hallmarks of diabetes, it appears that pharmacologic inhibition of SIRT1 function in the liver would be beneficial for reversing hyperglycemia in diabetes. Consistent with the beneficial effects of reducing SIRT1 activity in the liver in obesity, a separate study showed that liver specific SIRT1 knockout protects animals from high-fat diet-induced weight gain and hepatic steatosis [89]. Another important recent observation is that calorie restriction increases SIRT1 in some tissues (e.g. muscle, white fat) and decreases SIRT1 activity in other tissues such as liver [89], which argues against a simple model whereby calorie restriction equates with increased SIRT1 activity. Together, these observations suggest that, while it may be desirable to activate SIRT1 in some tissues, its inhibition would be beneficial in others.

The multitude of the protein targets and physiological roles that SIRT1 has in different tissues as well as complex regulation of SIRT1 protein level by nutritional cues makes it difficult to predict the net benefit of promoting or inhibiting SIRT1 activity on metabolism in diabetes. It should be noted however that, while extremely valuable, rodent models have only limited value in prediction the utility of drug targets in metabolic diseases in humans. The role of SIRT1 inhibitors and activators in the treatment of diabetes and obesity-associated metabolic syndrome will ultimately be decided though clinical trials. Given the rapid progress in the field and interest of the pharmaceutical industry, as illustrated by the fact that clinical trials with resveratrol have already been initiated, it is likely that the optimal therapeutic strategy for targeting SIRT1 in the treatment of DM will be defined in the very near future.

10.5.1 Sirtuins and Cancer

The wide spectrum of biological activities exhibited by the sirtuins linking transcriptional repression and activation, metabolic state and stress response strongly suggests that this class of enzymes could play an important role in tumorigenesis and cancer therapy. SIRT1 has been found to control the function of several tumor suppressor proteins (e.g. p53, Rb) and oncoproteins (e.g. BCL6) [90–92]. Furthermore, SIRT1 has been implicated in aberrant silencing of tumor suppressor genes (TSGs). Inhibition of SIRT1 activity with splitomicin resulted in reactivation of silenced TSG [62], suggesting that sirtuin inhibitors may constitute a new class of epigenetic therapies that may complement DNA demethylating drugs and HDAC inhibitors that are already in clinical use.

Among the first activities of human sirtuins to be described is the deacetylation and downregulation of the DNA damage response and cell cycle control protein p53 by SIRT1 [91, 93]. In response to DNA damage, p53 activates a transcriptional program of cell cycle arrest and DNA repair and, in some cases, apoptosis. The NAD-dependent deacetylation of p53 promotes survival under conditions of DNA damage and, conversely, inhibition of SIRT1 activity sensitizes cells to the cytotoxic effects of DNA damaging agents. In a number of model systems, inhibition of SIRT1 leads to hyperacetylation of p53 and increased sensitivity to DNA damage. Interestingly, the sensitization of cells treated with SIRT1 inhibitors is only partially dependent on p53 as a number of p53-null cell lines are sensitized as well [57], suggesting the involvement of other regulatory pathways. Retinoblastoma tumor suppressor pRb is regulated by phosphorylation and acetylation [92]. SIRT1 activity downregulates pRb activity and inhibition of SIRT1 by nicotinamide leads to increased pRb acetylation and cell cycle inhibitory activity. Furthermore, the forkhead transcription factors are involved in mobilizing a cellular response to stress and as with p53, SIRT1 deacetylation of FOXO3a dampens this protein's ability to activate apoptosis programs, but leaves intact its ability to induce cell cycle arrest [22, 23]. These findings suggest that inhibition of SIRT1 may sensitize cancer cells to genotoxic stress through several pathways besides p53.

The transcriptional repressor BCL6 plays a critical role in maintaining B-cell progenitors in an undifferentiated state and suppressing DNA damage checkpoints, as these cells undergo rapid expansion and immunoglobulin gene rearrangement and somatic hypermutation in the germinal centers after encountering an antigen [94]. Aberrant BCL6 activity allows many B-cell-derived lymphomas to avoid terminal differentiation and attain limitless replication. Like p53, BCL6 is a substrate for SIRT1, but unlike p53, the repressive activity of BCL6 is enhanced by deacetylation [90]. Thus treatment of cells with inhibitors of NAD-dependent deacetylases leads to hyperacetylation and inactivation of BCL6. Indeed, treatment of a panel of BCL6-expressing germinal center-derived lymphomas with cambinol, an equipotent inhibitor of SIRT1 and SIRT2 led to BCL6 hyperacetylation and induction of apoptosis. Cambinol showed *in vivo* antitumor activity in lymphoma xenograft model [57]. Dual SIRT1 and SIRT inhibitors, tenovins, were also recently shown to be active in a xenograft model of melanoma [72].

An endogenous SIRT1 modulator and several targets have been described that hint at potential therapeutic benefits from pharmacological SIRT1 inhibition in a number of cancer models. The gene product of deleted in breast cancer 1 (DBC1) interacts with and inhibits SIRT1 [95, 96]. Downregulation of DBC1 expression in normal mammary epithelium cells leads to SIRT1-mediated downregulation of p53 and increased resistance to genotoxic stress. This finding strongly suggests that pharmacological inhibition to SIRT1 in DBC1 null breast cancer cells should lead to increased sensitivity to standard chemotherapeutic agents.

Conversely, transcriptional repression by antagonists of the androgen receptor (AR) requires SIRT1 activity. The androgen receptor, when occupied by a pharmacological antagonist recruits SIRT1 to AR-responsive gene promoters and promotes histone H3 deacetylation [97]. Prostate cancer cells treated with SIRT1 inhibitors are simultaneously more sensitive to androgen stimulation and insensitive to AR antagonists. This finding suggests that stimulation of SIRT1 activity may have a therapeutically beneficial effect in prostate cancer.

In addition to data describing the cellular functions of sirtuins and their targets, more circumstantial data link sirtuin expression and tumorigenesis. For example, mouse and human prostate adenocarcinoma have been shown to overexpress SIRT1 [98]. In addition, a significant fraction of node-positive breast cancers overexpress SIRT3 (mitochondrial) and SIRT7 (nucleolar) [99]. The role of overexpressed sirtuins in these tumor types remains to be elucidated but these results suggest that multiple sirtuin isoforms may be valid therapeutic targets for human cancer.

Together these findings predict a major role for sirtuin modulators, both activators and inhibitors, in the treatment of cancer.

10.6
Neurological Diseases

The roles of SIRT1 in nervous system include alleviating neural degeneration, guiding neurogenesis and mediating neuronal oxidative resistance. Similar to the paradoxical SIRT1 functions in other organs and in the regulation of metabolism, both upregulation and downregulation of SIRT1 may result into neural protection.

The proposed role of sirtuins as "longevity genes" coupled with the recognition of neurodegenerative disorders such as Alzheimer's disease (AD) and Parkinson's disease as hallmarks of aging, led several laboratories to explore of the possible link between sirtuins and neurodegeneration. A first hint for possible role of SIRT1 in nervous system came from a study that demonstrated that SIRT1 function is involved in slowing down axonal degeneration in Wallerian degeneration slow (Wlds) mice that overexpress a fusion protein containing NAD salvage enzyme nicotinamide mononucleotide adenylyltransferase (Nmnat1) [100]. SIRT1 was later shown to reduce amyloid-beta toxicity by inhibiting NF-kB signaling in microglia [101] and to attenuate neurodegeneration in mouse AD models. Impaired function of PGC-1 alpha in the central nervous tissue and the resulting mitochondrial dysfunction and the lack of adequate oxidative stress defense are proposed to play an important role in pathogenesis of Huntington disease (HD) and other neurodegenerative diseases. The known role of SIRT1 as a deacetylase that promotes PGC-1alpha function suggests that SIRT1 activation may alleviate neurodegeneration in HD through this mechanism. Intriguingly, inhibition of SIRT2 was shown to be another therapeutic strategy in HD. AGK2, an inhibitor of SIRT2 has been identified as a compound that alters the aggregation pattern of huntingtin and alpha-synuclein and alleviate the resulting proteasome dysfunction and toxicity. These opposing effects by the two related sirtuins, SIRT1 and SIRT2, in HD underscore the importance of developing small molecules that are highly specific for each enzyme.

There are several neurological disorders where inhibition of SIRT1 may be used as a therapeutic strategy. Fragile X-mental retardation syndrome is caused by trinucleotide repeat tracts in the 5′ UTR region of the FRM1 gene on the X-chromosome, which leads to alterations in DNA methylation, histone hypoacetylation, transcriptional silencing of the locus and thus loss of FRM1 function [102]. Inhibition of SIRT1 with splitomicin resulted in transcriptional activation of the fragile X allele [61]. Importantly, SIRT1 inhibition-mediated abrogation of silencing of the FRM1 occurred in absence of DNA replication or DNA demethylation, suggesting that activation of FRM1 through SIRT1 inhibition may be possible in nondividing cells, including neurons.

The SIRT1 protein is highly expressed in the brain during embryonic neurogenesis. Its expression level peaks between embryonic day 10.5 to day 13.5 in mice, coinciding with rapid cortical expansion. During neural progenitor differentiation SIRT1 promotes glial over neuronal differentiation [52] and inhibition of SIRT1 promotes neuronal differentiation. This finding raises the expectation that SIRT1 inhibition could promote neurogenesis and prevent excessive glial scarring as it occurs during traumatic or vascular injury in the brain and spinal cord.

Consistent with a protective role conferred by SIRT1 inhibition in the brain, a separate study demonstrated that downregulation of SIRT1 protects neuronal cells against oxidative damage [103]. This protective effect was linked to the role of cytoplasmic SIRT1 in promoting IGF-1 and RAS/ERK1/2 signaling through deacetylation of insulin receptor substrate 2 (IRS2), an adaptor molecule that links IGF-1 and insulin receptors and its downstream effectors. Conversely, inhibiting SirT1 increases IRS-2 acetylation and decreases its phosphorylation, which in turn suppresses the downstream targets, MEK/ERK1/2, resulting in neuronal protection against oxidative stress. In addition to the effect on IGF-1 that are mediated through cytoplasmic SIRT1, nuclear SIRT1 may regulate IGF-1 signaling by downregulating major IGF-1 binding proteins, such as IGFBP1 [104]. With SirT1 inhibition, IGF-1 signaling is likely inhibited by the abundance of secretive IGFBP1 and/or nonfunctioning supra-acetylated IRS-2. The blockade of IGF-1 signaling is likely responsible for the reduced oxidative damage in SirT1 knockout mice brain, similar to its role in blocking the epithelial ductal morphogenesis in SirT1 knockout virgin mammary tissue. IGF-1 signaling, including its upstream effector, estrogen, also plays crucial role in adult neurogenesis.

10.7 Conclusion

The diverse and at times contradictory roles of NAD-dependent deacetylases in human diseases make it difficult to predict with certainty whether inhibition or activation of a particular sirtuin or group of sirtuins will ultimately lead to a beneficial therapeutic outcome. Only rigorous testing of both isoform-specific and pan-sirtuin inhibitors and activators in appropriate animal models and ultimately human clinical trials will determine the clinical utility of sirtuin modulators.

References

1 Rusche, L.N., Kirchmaier, A.L. and Rine, J. (2003) The establishment, inheritance, and function of silenced chromatin in Saccharomyces cerevisiae. *Annual Review of Biochemistry*, **72**, 481–516.

2 Ivy, J.M., Klar, A.J. and Hicks, J.B. (1986) Cloning and characterization of four SIR genes of Saccharomyces cerevisiae. *Molecular and Cellular Biology*, **6**, 688–702.

3 Rine, J. and Herskowitz, I. (1987) Four genes responsible for a position effect on expression from HML and HMR in Saccharomyces cerevisiae. *Genetics*, **116**, 9–22.

4 Shore, D., Squire, M. and Nasmyth, K.A. (1984) Characterization of two genes required for the position-effect control of yeast mating-type genes. *The EMBO Journal*, **3**, 2817–2823.

5 Braunstein, M., Rose, A.B., Holmes, S.G., Allis, C.D. and Broach, J.R. (1993) Transcriptional silencing in yeast is associated with reduced nucleosome acetylation. *Genes & Development*, **7**, 592–604.

6 Imai, S., Armstrong, C.M., Kaeberlein, M. and Guarente, L. (2000) Transcriptional silencing and longevity protein Sir2 is an NAD-dependent histone deacetylase. *Nature*, **403**, 795–800.

7 Lin, S.J., Defossez, P.A. and Guarente, L. (2000) Requirement of NAD and SIR2 for life-span extension by calorie restriction in Saccharomyces cerevisiae. *Science*, **289**, 2126–2128.

8 Smith, J.S., Brachmann, C.B., Celic, I., Kenna, M.A., Muhammad, S., Starai, V.J., Avalos, J.L., Escalante-Semerena, J.C., Grubmeyer, C., Wolberger, C. and Boeke, J.D. (2000) A phylogenetically conserved NAD^+-dependent protein deacetylase activity in the Sir2 protein family. *Proceedings of the National Academy of Sciences of the United States of America*, **97**, 6658–6663.

9 Straight, A.F., Shou, W., Dowd, G.J., Turck, C.W., Deshaies, R.J., Johnson, A.D. and Moazed, D. (1999) Net1, a Sir2-associated nucleolar protein required for rDNA silencing and nucleolar integrity. *Cell*, **97**, 245–256.

10 Gottlieb, S. and Esposito, R.E. (1989) A new role for a yeast transcriptional silencer gene, SIR2, in regulation of recombination in ribosomal DNA. *Cell*, **56**, 771–776.

11 Sinclair, D.A. and Guarente, L. (1997) Extrachromosomal rDNA circles a cause–of aging in yeast. *Cell*, **91**, 1033–1042.

12 Kaeberlein, M., McVey, M. and Guarente, L. (1999) The SIR2/3/4 complex and SIR2 alone promote longevity in Saccharomyces cerevisiae by two different mechanisms. *Genes & Development*, **13**, 2570–2580.

13 Tissenbaum, H.A. and Guarente, L. (2001) Increased dosage of a sir-2 gene extends lifespan in Caenorhabditis elegans. *Nature*, **410**, 227–230.

14 Rogina, B. and Helfand, S.L. (2004) Sir2 mediates longevity in the fly through a pathway related to calorie restriction. *Proceedings of the National Academy of Sciences of the United States of America*, **101**, 15998–16003.

15 Bordone, L. and Guarente, L. (2005) Calorie restriction, SIRT1 and metabolism: understanding longevity.

Nature Reviews. Molecular Cell Biology, **6**, 298–305.

16 Kaeberlein, M., Kirkland, K.T., Fields, S. and Kennedy, B.K. (2004) Sir2-independent life span extension by calorie restriction in yeast. *PLoS Biology*, **2**, E296.

17 Frye, R.A. (2000) Phylogenetic classification of prokaryotic and eukaryotic Sir2-like proteins. *Biochemical & Biophysical Research Communications*, **273**, 793–798.

18 Sauve, A.A., Wolberger, C., Schramm, V.L. and Boeke, J.D. (2006) The Biochemistry of Sirtuins. *Annual Review of Biochemistry*.

19 Tanner, K.G., Landry, J., Sternglanz, R. and Denu, J.M. (2000) Silent information regulator 2 family of NAD- dependent histone/protein deacetylases generates a unique product, 1-O-acetyl-ADP-ribose. *Proceedings of the National Academy of Sciences of the United States of America*, **97**, 14178–14182.

20 Blander, G. and Guarente, L. (2004) The Sir2 family of protein deacetylases. *Annual Review of Biochemistry*, **73**, 417–435.

21 Michishita, E., Park, J.Y., Burneskis, J.M., Barrett, J.C. and Horikawa, I. (2005) Evolutionarily conserved and nonconserved cellular localizations and functions of human SIRT proteins. *Molecular Biology of the Cell*, **16**, 4623–4635.

22 Brunet, A., Sweeney, L.B., Sturgill, J.F., Chua, K.F., Greer, P.L., Lin, Y., Tran, H., Ross, S.E., Mostoslavsky, R., Cohen, H.Y., Hu, L.S., Cheng, H.L., Jedrychowski, M.P., Gygi, S.P., Sinclair, D.A., Alt, F.W. and Greenberg, M.E. (2004) Stress-dependent regulation of FOXO transcription factors by the SIRT1 deacetylase. *Science*, **303**, 2011–2015.

23 Motta, M.C., Divecha, N., Lemieux, M., Kamel, C., Chen, D., Gu, W., Bultsma, Y., McBurney, M. and Guarente, L. (2004) Mammalian SIRT1 represses forkhead transcription factors. *Cell*, **116**, 551–563.

24 Picard, F., Kurtev, M., Chung, N., Topark-Ngarm, A., Senawong, T., Machado De Oliveira, R., Leid, M., McBurney, M.W. and Guarente, L. (2004) Sirt1 promotes fat mobilization in white adipocytes by repressing PPAR-gamma. *Nature*, **429**, 771–776.

25 Rodgers, J.T., Lerin, C., Haas, W., Gygi, S.P., Spiegelman, B.M. and Puigserver, P. (2005) Nutrient control of glucose homeostasis through a complex of PGC-1alpha and SIRT1. *Nature*, **434**, 113–118.

26 Li, X., Zhang, S., Blander, G., Tse, J.G., Krieger, M. and Guarente, L. (2007) SIRT1 deacetylates and positively regulates the nuclear receptor LXR. *Molecular Cell*, **28**, 91–106.

27 Pagans, S., Pedal, A., North, B.J., Kaehlcke, K., Marshall, B.L., Dorr, A., Hetzer-Egger, C., Henklein, P., Frye, R., McBurney, M.W., Hruby, H., Jung, M., Verdin, E. and Ott, M. (2005) SIRT1 regulates HIV transcription via Tat deacetylation. *PLoS Biology*, **3**, e41.

28 Gerhart-Hines, Z., Rodgers, J.T., Bare, O., Lerin, C., Kim, S.H., Mostoslavsky, R., Alt, F.W., Wu, Z. and Puigserver, P. (2007) Metabolic control of muscle mitochondrial function and fatty acid oxidation through SIRT1/PGC-1alpha. *The EMBO Journal*, **26**, 1913–1923.

29 Murayama, A., Ohmori, K., Fujimura, A., Minami, H., Yasuzawa-Tanaka, K., Kuroda, T., Oie, S., Daitoku, H., Okuwaki, M., Nagata, K., Fukamizu, A., Kimura, K., Shimizu, T. and Yanagisawa, J. (2008) Epigenetic control of rDNA loci in response to intracellular energy status. *Cell*, **133**, 627–639.

30 Yeung, F., Hoberg, J.E., Ramsey, C.S., Keller, M.D., Jones, D.R., Frye, R.A. and Mayo, M.W. (2004) Modulation of NF-kappaB-dependent transcription and cell survival by the SIRT1 deacetylase. *The EMBO Journal*, **23**, 2369–2380.

31 Vaquero, A., Scher, M., Erdjument-Bromage, H., Tempst, P., Serrano, L. and Reinberg, D. (2007) SIRT1 regulates the histone methyl-transferase SUV39H1 during heterochromatin formation. *Nature*, **450**, 440–444.

32 Cohen, H.Y., Miller, C., Bitterman, K.J., Wall, N.R., Hekking, B., Kessler, B., Howitz, K.T., Gorospe, M., de Cabo, R. and Sinclair, D.A. (2004) Calorie restriction promotes mammalian cell survival by inducing the SIRT1 deacetylase. *Science*, **305**, 390–392.

33 Mostoslavsky, R., Chua, K.F., Lombard, D.B., Pang, W.W., Fischer, M.R., Gellon, L., Liu, P., Mostoslavsky, G., Franco, S., Murphy, M.M., Mills, K.D., Patel, P., Hsu, J.T., Hong, A.L., Ford, E., Cheng, H.L., Kennedy, C., Nunez, N., Bronson, R., Frendewey, D., Auerbach, W., Valenzuela, D., Karow, M., Hottiger, M.O., Hursting, S., Barrett, J.C., Guarente, L., Mulligan, R., Demple, B., Yancopoulos, G.D. and Alt, F.W. (2006) Genomic instability and aging-like phenotype in the absence of mammalian SIRT6. *Cell*, **124**, 315–329.

34 Ford, E., Voit, R., Liszt, G., Magin, C., Grummt, I. and Guarente, L. (2006) Mammalian Sir2 homolog SIRT7 is an activator of RNA polymerase I transcription. *Genes and Development*, **20**, 1075–1080.

35 North, B.J., Marshall, B.L., Borra, M.T., Denu, J.M. and Verdin, E. (2003) The human Sir2 ortholog, SIRT2, is an NAD dependnet tubulin deacetylase. *Molecular Cell*, **11**, 437–444.

36 Schwer, B., North, B.J., Frye, R.A., Ott, M. and Verdin, E. (2002) The human silent information regulator (Sir)2 homologue hSIRT3 is a mitochondrial nicotinamide adenine dinucleotide-dependent deacetylase. *The Journal of Cell Biology*, **158**, 647–657.

37 Haigis, M.C., Mostoslavsky, R., Haigis, K.M., Fahie, K., Christodoulou, D.C., Murphy, A.J., Valenzuela, D.M., Yancopoulos, G.D., Karow, M., Blander, G., Wolberger, C., Prolla, T.A., Weindruch, R., Alt, F.W. and Guarente, L. (2006) SIRT4 inhibits glutamate dehydrogenase and opposes the effects of calorie restriction in pancreatic beta cells. *Cell*, **126**, 941–954.

38 Schwer, B., Bunkenborg, J., Verdin, R.O., Andersen, J.S. and Verdin, E. (2006) Reversible lysine acetylation controls the activity of the mitochondrial enzyme acetyl-CoA synthetase 2. *Proceedings of the National Academy of Sciences of the United States of America*, **103**, 10224–10229.

39 Ahuja, N., Schwer, B., Carobbio, S., Waltregny, D., North, B.J., Castronovo, V., Maechler, P. and Verdin, E. (2007) Regulation of insulin secretion by SIRT4, a mitochondrial ADP-ribosyltransferase. *The Journal of Biological Chemistry*, **282**, 33583–33592.

40 Blander, G., Olejnik, J., Krzymanska-Olejnik, E., McDonagh, T., Haigis, M., Yaffe, M.B. and Guarente, L. (2005) SIRT1 shows no substrate specificity in vitro. *The Journal of Biological Chemistry*, **280**, 9780–9785.

41 Michishita, E., McCord, R.A., Berber, E., Kioi, M., Padilla-Nash, H., Damian, M., Cheung, P., Kusumoto, R., Kawahara, T.L., Barrett, J.C., Chang, H.Y., Bohr, V.A., Ried, T., Gozani, O. and Chua, K.F. (2008) SIRT6 is a histone H3 lysine 9 deacetylase that modulates telomeric chromatin. *Nature*, **452**, 492–496.

42 Liszt, G., Ford, E., Kurtev, M. and Guarente, L. (2005) Mouse Sir2 homolog SIRT6 is a nuclear ADP-ribosyltransferase. *The Journal of Biological Chemistry*, **280**, 21313–21320.

43 Bitterman, K.J., Anderson, R.M., Cohen, H.Y., Latorre-Esteves, M. and Sinclair, D.A. (2002) Inhibition of silencing and accelerated aging by nicotinamide, a putative negative regulator of yeast sir2 and human SIRT1. *Journal of Biological Chemistry*, **277**, 45099–45107.

44 Denu, J.M. (2005) Vitamin B3 and sirtuin function. *Trends in Biochemical Sciences*, **30**, 479–483.

45 Sauve, A.A., Moir, R.D., Schramm, V.L. and Willis, I.M. (2005) Chemical activation of Sir2-dependent silencing by

relief of nicotinamide inhibition. *Molecular Cell*, **17**, 595–601.

46 Bedalov, A., Hirao, M., Posakony, J., Nelson, M. and Simon, J. (2003) NAD-dependent deacetylase Hst1p controls biosynthesis and cellular NAD levels in Saccharomyces cerevisiae. *Molecular and Cellular Biology*, **23**.

47 Anderson, R.M., Bitterman, K.J., Wood, J.G., Medvedik, O., Cohen, H., Lin, S.S., Manchester, J.K., Gordon, J.I. and Sinclair, D.A. (2002) Manipulation of a nuclear NAD^+ salvage pathway delays aging without altering steady-state NAD^+ levels. *Journal of Biological Chemistry*, **277**, 18881–18890.

48 Anderson, R.M., Bitterman, K.J., Wood, J.G., Medvedik, O. and Sinclair, D.A. (2003) Nicotinamide and PNC1 govern lifespan extension by calorie restriction in Saccharomyces cerevisiae. *Nature*, **423** (6936), 181–185.

49 Revollo, J.R., Grimm, A.A. and Imai, S. (2004) The NAD biosynthesis pathway mediated by nicotinamide phosphoribosyltransferase regulates Sir2 activity in mammalian cells. *The Journal of Biological Chemistry*, **279**, 50754–50763.

50 Lin, S.J., Ford, E., Haigis, M., Liszt, G. and Guarente, L. (2004) Calorie restriction extends yeast life span by lowering the level of NADH. *Genes and Development*, **18**, 12–16.

51 Fulco, M., Schiltz, R.L., Iezzi, S., King, T.M., Zhao, P., Kashiwaya, Y., Hoffman, E., Veech, R.L. and Sartorelli, V. (2003) Sir2 regulates skeletal muscle differentiation as a potential sensor of the redox state. *Molecular Cell*.

52 Prozorovski, T., Schulze-Topphoff, U., Glumm, R., Baumgart, J., Schroter, F., Ninnemann, O., Siegert, E., Bendix, I., Brustle, O., Nitsch, R., Zipp, F. and Aktas, O. (2008) Sirt1 contributes critically to the redox-dependent fate of neural progenitors. *Nature Cell Biology*, **10**, 385–394.

53 Schmidt, M.T., Smith, B.C., Jackson, M.D. and Denu, J.M. (2004) Coenzyme specificity of Sir2 protein deacetylases: implications for physiological regulation. *The Journal of Biological Chemistry*, **279**, 40122–40129.

54 Zhang, Q., Wang, S.Y., Fleuriel, C., Leprince, D., Rocheleau, J.V., Piston, D.W. and Goodman, R.H. (2007) Metabolic regulation of SIRT1 transcription via a HIC1:CtBP corepressor complex. *Proceedings of the National Academy of Sciences of the United States of America*, **104**, 829–833.

55 Bedalov, A., Gatbonton, T., Irvine, W.P., Gottschling, D.E. and Simon, J.A. (2001) Identification of a small molecule inhibitor of Sir2p. *Proceedings of the National Academy of Sciences of the United States of America*, **98**, 15113–15118.

56 Grozinger, C.M., Chao, E.D., Blackwell, H.E., Moazed, D. and Schreiber, S.L. (2001) Identification of a class of small molecule inhibitors of the sirtuin family of NAD-dependent deacetylases by phenotypic screening. *The Journal of Biological Chemistry*, **276**, 38837–38843.

57 Heltweg, B., Gatbonton, T., Schuler, A.D., Posakony, J., Li, H., Goehle, S., Kollipara, R., DePinho, R.A., Gu, Y., Simon, J.A. and Bedalov, A. (2006) Antitumor activity of a small molecule inhibitor of human Sir2 enzymes. *Cancer Research*, **66**, 4368–4377.

58 Posakony, J., Hirao, M., Stevens, S., Simon, J.A. and Bedalov, A. (2004) Inhibitors of Sir2: evaluation of splitomicin analogues. *Journal of Medicinal Chemistry*, **47**, 2635–2644.

59 Neugebauer, R.C., Uchiechowska, U., Meier, R., Hruby, H., Valkov, V., Verdin, E., Sippl, W. and Jung, M. (2008) Structure-activity studies on splitomicin derivatives as sirtuin inhibitors and computational prediction of binding mode. *Journal of Medicinal Chemistry*, **51**, 1203–1213.

60 Chang, C.R., Wu, C.S., Hom, Y. and Gartenberg, M.R. (2005) Targeting of cohesin by transcriptionally silent chromatin. *Genes and Development*, **19**, 3031–3042.

61 Biacsi, R., Kumari, D. and Usdin, K. (2008) SIRT1 inhibition alleviates gene silencing in Fragile X mental retardation syndrome. *PLoS Genetics*, **4**, e1000017.

62 Pruitt, K., Zinn, R.L., Ohm, J.E., McGarvey, K.M., Kang, S.H., Watkins, D.N., Herman, J.G. and Baylin, S.B. (2006) Inhibition of SIRT1 reactivates silenced cancer genes without loss of promoter DNA hypermethylation. *PLoS Genetics*, **2**, e40.

63 Napper, A.D., Hixon, J., McDonagh, T., Keavey, K., Pons, J.F., Barker, J., Yau, W.T., Amouzegh, P., Flegg, A., Hamelin, E., Thomas, R.J., Kates, M., Jones, S., Navia, M.A., Saunders, J.O., DiStefano, P.S. and Curtis, R. (2005) Discovery of indoles as potent and selective inhibitors of the deacetylase SIRT1. *Journal of Medicinal Chemistry*, **48**, 8045–8054.

64 Howitz, K.T., Bitterman, K.J., Cohen, H.Y., Lamming, D.W., Lavu, S., Wood, J.G., Zipkin, R.E., Chung, P., Kisielewski, A., Zhang, L.L., Scherer, B. and Sinclair, D.A. (2003) Small molecule activators of sirtuins extend Saccharomyces cerevisiae lifespan. *Nature*, **425**, 191–196.

65 Trapp, J., Meier, R., Hongwiset, D., Kassack, M.U., Sippl, W. and Jung, M. (2007) Structure-activity studies on suramin analogues as inhibitors of NAD^+-dependent histone deacetylases (sirtuins). *ChemMedChem*, **2**, 1419–1431.

66 Trapp, J., Jochum, A., Meier, R., Saunders, L., Marshall, B., Kunick, C., Verdin, E., Goekjian, P., Sippl, W. and Jung, M. (2006) Adenosine mimetics as inhibitors of NAD^+-dependent histone deacetylases, from kinase to sirtuin inhibition. *Journal of Medicinal Chemistry*, **49**, 7307–7316.

67 Gey, C., Kyrylenko, S., Hennig, L., Nguyen, L.H., Buttner, A., Pham, H.D. and Giannis, A. (2007) Phloroglucinol derivatives guttiferone G, aristoforin, and hyperforin: inhibitors of human sirtuins SIRT1 and SIRT2. *Angewandte Chemie (International Edition in English)*, **46**, 5219–5222.

68 Huhtiniemi, T., Suuronen, T., Rinne, V.M., Wittekindt, C., Lahtela-Kakkonen, M., Jarho, E., Wallen, E.A., Salminen, A., Poso, A. and Leppanen, J. (2008) Oxadiazole-carbonylaminothioureas as SIRT1 and SIRT2 inhibitors. *Journal of Medicinal Chemistry*, **51**, 4377–4380.

69 Kiviranta, P.H., Leppanen, J., Rinne, V.M., Suuronen, T., Kyrylenko, O., Kyrylenko, S., Kuusisto, E., Tervo, A.J., Jarvinen, T., Salminen, A., Poso, A. and Wallen, E.A. (2007) N-(3-(4-Hydroxyphenyl)-propenoyl)-amino acid tryptamides as SIRT2 inhibitors. *Bioorganic & Medicinal Chemistry Letters*, **17**, 2448–2451.

70 Tervo, A.J., Kyrylenko, S., Niskanen, P., Salminen, A., Leppanen, J., Nyronen, T.H., Jarvinen, T. and Poso, A. (2004) An in silico approach to discovering novel inhibitors of human sirtuin type 2. *Journal of Medicinal Chemistry*, **47**, 6292–6298.

71 Outeiro, T.F., Kontopoulos, E., Altmann, S.M., Kufareva, I., Strathearn, K.E., Amore, A.M., Volk, C.B., Maxwell, M.M., Rochet, J.C., McLean, P.J., Young, A.B., Abagyan, R., Feany, M.B., Hyman, B.T. and Kazantsev, A.G. (2007) Sirtuin 2 inhibitors rescue alpha-synuclein-mediated toxicity in models of Parkinson's disease. *Science*, **317**, 516–519.

72 Lain, S., Hollick, J.J., Campbell, J., Staples, O.D., Higgins, M., Aoubala, M., McCarthy, A., Appleyard, V., Murray, K.E., Baker, L., Thompson, A., Mathers, J., Holland, S.J., Stark, M.J., Pass, G., Woods, J., Lane, D.P. and Westwood, N.J. (2008) Discovery, in vivo activity, and mechanism of action of a small-molecule p53 activator. *Cancer Cell*, **13**, 454–463.

73 Vaquero, A., Scher, M., Lee, D., Erdjument-Bromage, H., Tempst, P. and Reinberg, D. (2004) Human SirT1 interacts with histone H1 and promotes formation of facultative heterochromatin. *Molecular Cell*, **16**, 93–105.

74 Vaquero, A., Scher, M.B., Lee, D.H., Sutton, A., Cheng, H.L., Alt, F.W.,

Serrano, L., Sternglanz, R. and Reinberg, D. (2006) SirT2 is a histone deacetylase with preference for histone H4 Lys 16 during mitosis. *Genes and Development*, **20**, 1256–1261.

75 Hubbert, C., Guardiola, A., Shao, R., Kawaguchi, Y., Ito, A., Nixon, A., Yoshida, M., Wang, X.F. and Yao, T.P. (2002) HDAC6 is a microtubule-associated deacetylase. *Nature*, **417**, 455–458.

76 Harikumar, K.B. and Aggarwal, B.B. (2008) Resveratrol: a multitargeted agent for age-associated chronic diseases. *Cell Cycle (Georgetown, Tex)*, **7**, 1020–1035.

77 Wood, J.G., Rogina, B., Lavu, S., Howitz, K., Helfand, S.L., Tatar, M. and Sinclair, D. (2004) Sirtuin activators mimic caloric restriction and delay ageing in metazoans. *Nature*, **430**, 686–689.

78 Lagouge, M., Argmann, C., Gerhart-Hines, Z., Meziane, H., Lerin, C., Daussin, F., Messadeq, N., Milne, J., Lambert, P., Elliott, P., Geny, B., Laakso, M., Puigserver, P. and Auwerx, J. (2006) Resveratrol improves mitochondrial function and protects against metabolic disease by activating SIRT1 and PGC-1alpha. *Cell*, **127**, 1109–1122.

79 Kaeberlein, M., McDonagh, T., Heltweg, B., Hixon, J., Westman, E.A., Caldwell, S.D., Napper, A., Curtis, R., DiStefano, P.S., Fields, S., Bedalov, A. and Kennedy, B.K. (2005) Substrate-specific activation of sirtuins by resveratrol. *The Journal of Biological Chemistry*, **280**, 17038–17045.

80 Borra, M.T., Smith, B.C. and Denu, J.M. (2005) Mechanism of human SIRT1 activation by resveratrol. *The Journal of Biological Chemistry*, **280**, 17187–17195.

81 Milne, J.C., Lambert, P.D., Schenk, S., Carney, D.P., Smith, J.J., Gagne, D.J., Jin, L., Boss, O., Perni, R.B., Vu, C.B., Bemis, J.E., Xie, R., Disch, J.S., Ng, P.Y., Nunes, J.J., Lynch, A.V., Yang, H., Galonek, H., Israelian, K., Choy, W., Iffland, A., Lavu, S., Medvedik, O., Sinclair, D.A., Olefsky, J.M., Jirousek, M.R., Elliott, P.J. and Westphal, C.H. (2007) Small molecule activators of SIRT1 as therapeutics for the treatment of type 2 diabetes. *Nature*, **450**, 712–716.

82 Guarente, L. (2006) Sirtuins as potential targets for metabolic syndrome. *Nature*, **444**, 868–874.

83 Bordone, L., Motta, M.C., Picard, F., Robinson, A., Jhala, U.S., Apfeld, J., McDonagh, T., Lemieux, M., McBurney, M., Szilvasi, A., Easlon, E.J., Lin, S.J. and Guarente, L. (2006) Sirt1 regulates insulin secretion by repressing UCP2 in pancreatic beta cells. *PLoS Biology*, **4**, e31.

84 Moynihan, K.A., Grimm, A.A., Plueger, M.M., Bernal-Mizrachi, E., Ford, E., Cras-Meneur, C., Permutt, M.A. and Imai, S. (2005) Increased dosage of mammalian Sir2 in pancreatic beta cells enhances glucose-stimulated insulin secretion in mice. *Cell Metabolism*, **2**, 105–117.

85 Baur, J.A., Pearson, K.J., Price, N.L., Jamieson, H.A., Lerin, C., Kalra, A., Prabhu, V.V., Allard, J.S., Lopez-Lluch, G., Lewis, K., Pistell, P.J., Poosala, S., Becker, K.G., Boss, O., Gwinn, D., Wang, M., Ramaswamy, S., Fishbein, K.W., Spencer, R.G., Lakatta, E.G., Le Couteur, D., Shaw, R.J., Navas, P., Puigserver, P., Ingram, D.K., de Cabo, R. and Sinclair, D.A. (2006) Resveratrol improves health and survival of mice on a high-calorie diet. *Nature*, **444**, 337–342.

86 Bordone, L., Cohen, D., Robinson, A., Motta, M.C., van Veen, E., Czopik, A., Steele, A.D., Crowe, H., Marmor, S., Luo, J., Gu, W. and Guarente, L. (2007) SIRT1 transgenic mice show phenotypes resembling calorie restriction. *Aging Cell*, **6**, 759–767.

87 Pfluger, P.T., Herranz, D., Velasco-Miguel, S., Serrano, M. and Tschop, M.H. (2008) Sirt1 protects against high-fat diet-induced metabolic damage. *Proceedings of the National Academy of Sciences of the United States of America*, **105**, 9793–9798.

88 Rodgers, J.T. and Puigserver, P. (2007) Fasting-dependent glucose and lipid metabolic response through hepatic sirtuin 1. *Proceedings of the National Academy of Sciences of the United States of America*, **104**, 12861–12866.

89 Chen, D., Bruno, J., Easlon, E., Lin, S.J., Cheng, H.L., Alt, F.W. and Guarente, L. (2008) Tissue-specific regulation of SIRT1 by calorie restriction. *Genes and Development*, **22**, 1753–1757.

90 Bereshchenko, O.R., Gu, W. and Dalla-Favera, R. (2002) Acetylation inactivates the transcriptional repressor BCL6. *Nature Genetics*, **32**, 606–613.

91 Vaziri, H., Dessain, S.K., Ng Eaton, E., Imai, S.I., Frye, R.A., Pandita, T.K., Guarente, L. and Weinberg, R.A. (2001) hSIR2(SIRT1) functions as an NAD-dependent p53 deacetylase. *Cell*, **107**, 149–159.

92 Wong, S. and Weber, J.D. (2007) Deacetylation of the retinoblastoma tumour suppressor protein by SIRT1. *The Biochemical Journal*, **407**, 451–460.

93 Luo, J., Nikolaev, A.Y., Imai, S., Chen, D., Su, F., Shiloh, A., Guarente, L. and Gu, W. (2001) Negative control of p53 by Sir2alpha promotes cell survival under stress. *Cell*, **107**, 137–148.

94 Phan, R.T. and Dalla-Favera, R. (2004) The BCL6 proto-oncogene suppresses p53 expression in germinal-centre B cells. *Nature*, **432**, 635–639.

95 Zhao, W., Kruse, J.P., Tang, Y., Jung, S.Y., Qin, J. and Gu, W. (2008) Negative regulation of the deacetylase SIRT1 by DBC1. *Nature*, **451**, 587–590.

96 Kim, J.E., Chen, J. and Lou, Z. (2008) DBC1 is a negative regulator of SIRT1. *Nature*, **451**, 583–586.

97 Dai, Y., Ngo, D., Forman, L.W., Qin, D.C., Jacob, J. and Faller, D.V. (2007) Sirtuin 1 is required for antagonist-induced transcriptional repression of androgen-responsive genes by the androgen receptor. *Molecular Endocrinology*, **21**, 1807–1821.

98 Huffman, D.M., Grizzle, W.E., Bamman, M.M., Kim, J.S., Eltoum, I.A., Elgavish, A. and Nagy, T.R. (2007) SIRT1 is significantly elevated in mouse and human prostate cancer. *Cancer Research*, **67**, 6612–6618.

99 Ashraf, N., Zino, S., Macintyre, A., Kingsmore, D., Payne, A.P., George, W.D. and Shiels, P.G. (2006) Altered sirtuin expression is associated with node-positive breast cancer. *British Journal of Cancer*, **95**, 1056–1061.

100 Araki, T., Sasaki, Y. and Milbrandt, J. (2004) Increased nuclear NAD biosynthesis and SIRT1 activation prevent axonal degeneration. *Science*, **305**, 1010–1013.

101 Chen, J., Zhou, Y., Mueller-Steiner, S., Chen, L.F., Kwon, H., Yi, S., Mucke, L. and Gan, L. (2005) SIRT1 protects against microglia-dependent amyloid-beta toxicity through inhibiting NF-kappaB signaling. *The Journal of Biological Chemistry*, **280**, 40364–40374.

102 Orr, H.T. and Zoghbi, H.Y. (2007) Trinucleotide repeat disorders. *Annual Review of Neuroscience*, **30**, 575–621.

103 Li, Y., Xu, W., McBurney, M.W. and Longo, V.D. (2008) SirT1 inhibition reduces IGF-I/IRS-2/Ras/ERK1/2 signaling and protects neurons. *Cell Metabolism*, **8**, 38–48.

104 Li, H., Rajendran, G.K., Liu, N., Ware, C., Rubin, B.P. and Gu, Y. (2007) SirT1 modulates the estrogen-insulin-like growth factor-1 signaling for postnatal development of mammary gland in mice. *Breast Cancer Research*, **9**, R1.

11
Inhibitors of Histone Acetyltransferases: Discovery and Biomedical Perspectives

Margarete von Wantoch Rekowski and Athanassios Giannis

11.1
Introduction

In 1963 J.H. Rubinstein and H. Taybi reported a rare human disease that induced mental retardation, an increased risk of neoplasia and physical abnormalities, including broad thumbs, big and broad toes, short stature and craniofacial anomalies. The molecular basis of the Rubinstein–Taybi syndrome (RTS) was later discovered to be a disruption of one copy of the human CREB binding protein (CBP or CREB-BP) gene that encodes the histone acetyltransferase CBP [3]. In addition to CBP, all mammals have a closely related acetyltransferase, p300. Retrospectively, RTS was the first disease found to be due to a defective acetylation process [1–3].

CBP and p300 represent a family among nuclear transcription factors possessing an intrinsic histone acetyltransferase (HAT) activity. These proteins feature a distinct but closely related structure and an extensive homology that is characterized not only by overlapping but also by unique functions. Further proteins with such a functionality are known and grouped into different classes by sequence homologies and similarities in their biological functions (Table 11.1).

HATs catalyze the post-translational acetylation of amino-terminal lysine tails of core histones, which results in disruption of the repressive chromatin folding and an increased DNA accessibility to regulatory proteins. The level of histone acetylation is highly controlled and balanced by the activity of histone deacetylases (HDACs), the opponents of HATs. Generally, acetylation is correlated with activation and deacetylation with repression of gene expression. Therefore, the dynamic equilibrium of these proteins represents a key mechanism of gene regulation.

It should be noted that HATs and HDACs are not only limited to histones, but rather various nonhistone proteins can be acetylated/deacetylated as well [2, 4]. Many regulators of DNA repair, recombination and replication, viral proteins, classic metabolic enzymes (e.g. bacterial and mammalian acetyl-CoA synthases) and

Epigenetic Targets in Drug Discovery. Edited by Wolfgang Sippl and Manfred Jung

ISBN: 978-3-527-32355-5

Table 11.1 HAT families and functions of selected members.

Family	HAT	Organism	Targets	Function
GNAT	Gcn5	Yeast, human	H2B, H4, cMYC	Coactivator
	PCAF	Human	H3, H4, cMYC, p53, MYOD, E2F	Coactivator
	Elp3	Yeast	H2A, H2B, H3, H4	Elongation
	ATF-2	Yeast, human		Activator
MYST	MOZ	Human	H3, H4	Coactivator
	Ybf2/Sas3	Yeast	H3, H4	Elongation
	Sas2	Yeast	H3, H4	Silencing
	Tip60	Human	H2A, H3, H4, cMYC, androgen receptor (AR)	DNA repair, apoptosis
	Esa1	Yeast	H2A, H3, H4	Cell cycle progression
	MOF	Fruit fly	H3, H4	Dosage compensation
CBP/p300	CBP	Human	H2A, H2B, H3, H4, pRb, E2F, p53, AR, c-MYB, MYOD, FOXO	Global coactivator
	p300	Human	H2A, H2B, H3, H4, pRb, E2F, p53, AR, c-MYB, MYOD, FOXO	Global coactivator

recently kinases, phosphatases and other signaling regulators are substrates for these enzymes. Hence, multiple cellular processes such as transcription, cell division, differentiation, transformation, apoptosis and embryonic development are due to the activity of HATs and HDACs (Figure 11.1) [5, 6].

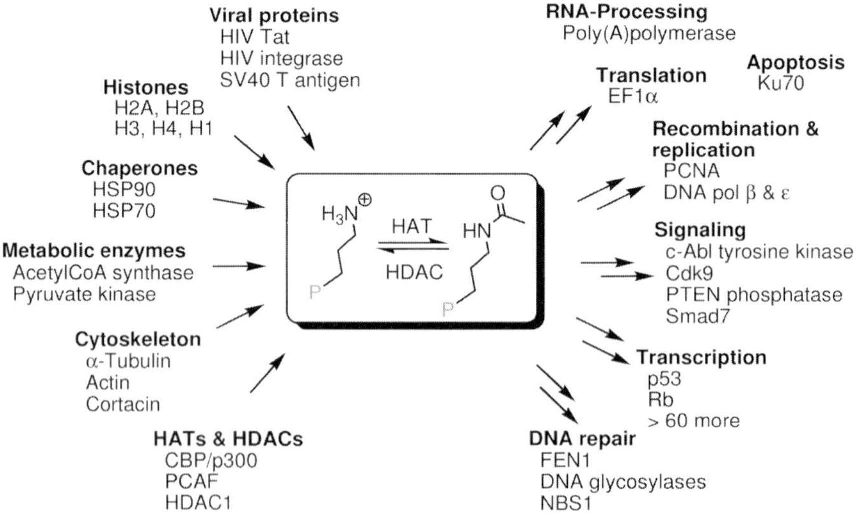

Figure 11.1 Substrates of HATs/HDACs and processes that are initiated by their acetylation level, modified from Yang [7] (P denotes protein).

Acetylation of several nonhistone proteins is tightly related to their functions. For example, acetylated α-tubulin can be found in stabilized microtubule structures, suggesting that this modificated form plays an important role in the regulation of microtubule dynamics. Furthermore, CBP/p300 participates in various tumor-suppressor pathways (i.e. wnt, p53) and contributes to the actions of many cellular and viral oncogenes (i.e. *c-jun*, *c-fos*, *c-myb*, *v-myb*) [8]. Missense and deletion mutations in the *p300* gene have been found in breast, colorectal, gastric and epithelial cancers, whereas loss of heterozygosity of *p300* gene has been related to glioblastoma and other malignancies. Several viruses encode proteins such as the adenoviral E1a, the HTLV-1 Tax and the simian virus 40 large T protein which specifically bind CBP/p300, preventing cell growth and enhancing DNA synthesis. CBP displays important functions during central nervous system development and increasing evidence suggests that CBP loss of function is involved not only in RTS but also in further neurodegenerative diseases, such as polyglutamine-related pathologies (Huntington's disease), Alzheimer's disease and amyotrophic lateral sclerosis [9].

In recent years great effort has been taken to get a deeper insight into the biochemistry and biology of HATs. Although a lot of knowledge has accumulated leading to the causative connection between these enzymes and various diseases, the processes behind are only poorly understood. In order to bridge this gap, cell-permeable, small molecules that act as specific inhibitors of HATs are urgently required. Such compounds would help to elucidate molecular mechanisms of HAT functions in cells. Furthermore, they can be regarded as valuable tools in the area of epigenetics, as well as anticancer and antiviral drug candidates.

11.2 HAT Inhibitors

The first reported selective inhibitors of the HATs p300 and PCAF were peptides representing structurally simple bi-substrate analogs of H3 and acetyl-CoA [10, 11]. Hence, p300 was inhibited by Lys-CoA **1** and the more specific PCAF by the 20-amino-acid peptide H3-CoA-20 **2** (Figure 11.2). Unfortunately, these inhibitors showed low cell permeability and high metabolic instability, which decreases their suitability for investigations *in vivo* [12].

In 2003 screening of plant extracts with antitumor activity gave rise to anacardic acid **3** (Figure 11.2) which shows *in vitro* inhibitory effects on both HATs p300 and PCAF ($IC_{50} = 8.5$ and $5.0\,\mu M$, respectively). This natural product was the first small molecule acting as a noncompetitive HAT inhibitor [13]. Beyond, recent investigations demonstrated that anacardic acid inhibited Tip60 (a human HAT of the MYST family, see Table 11.1) *in vitro* and thus blocked Tip60-dependent activation of ATM and DNA-PK protein kinases by DNA damage *in vivo*. Treatment of human cancer cells with anacardic acid increased their sensitivity to ionizing radiation, providing a novel therapeutic approach to the radiosensitization of tumor cells [14].

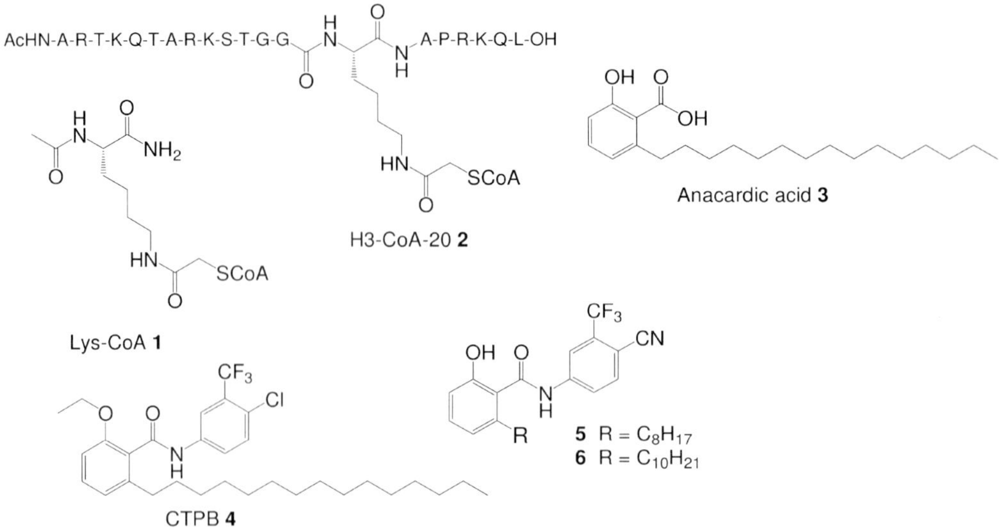

Figure 11.2 Di-substrate analogs Lys-CoA **1**, H3-CoA-20 **2**, the natural product anacardic acid **3**, its analogs cyano-benzamides **5** and **6** and the p300 activator CTPB **4**.

However, anarcadic acid was also found to be poorly cell permeable, thus limiting its practical application.

Contradictory results were obtained from studies with benzamide analogs of anacardic acid. While CTPB **4** (Figure 11.2) was reported to be an activator of p300 [13], the related cyano-benzamides **5** and **6** (Figure 11.2) acted as cell-permeable inhibitors of p300, exhibiting a similar profile to anacardic acid [15].

A further series of HAT inhibitors using anacardic acid as lead structure was synthesized by Jung *et al.* Biological studies of these compounds showed that analog **7** (Figure 11.3), having the longest alkyl side-chain of all tested compounds, was the most potent, cell-penetrating inhibitor ($IC_{50} = 14\,\mu M$). It showed significantly less toxicity than other structurally related compounds to the normal human cell lines Hs-68 and NHP-5 at the concentrations sufficient to kill cancer cells. Beyond, it was also the least efficient in suppressing p300 HAT activity in luciferase assay. Nevertheless these compounds suffer from low solubility in aqueous medium and very high lipophilicity. However, the effects of these new HATi on protein acetylation and HAT activity *in vivo* represent a promising approach for the design of more potent and specific inhibitors [16].

Recently, a cell-permeable inhibitor of the human Gcn5 named MB-3 **8** was discovered (Figure 11.3). This compound is structurally related to the α-methylene-γ-butyrolactone class of compounds, a common structural element in a plethora of natural products. MB-3 was developed by appropriate derivatization of the basic γ-butyrolactone motif without the arbitrary screening of large compound libraries. Interestingly, the length of the aliphatic side-chain is crucial for biological activity [17, 18].

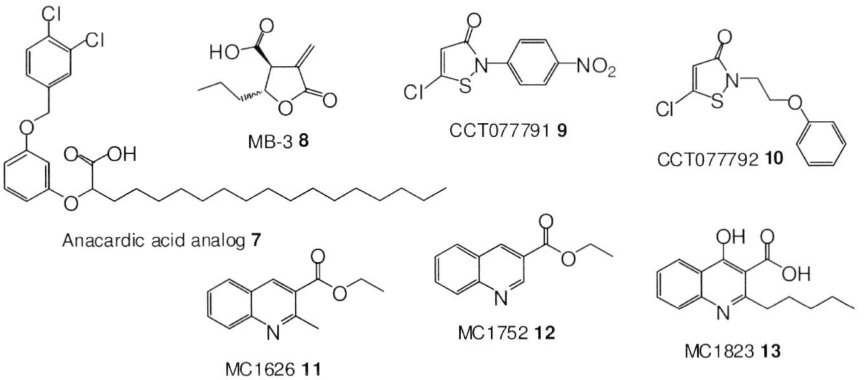

Figure 11.3 Anacardic acid analog **7**, γ-butyrolactone MB-3 **8**, isothiazolones CCT077791 **9** and CCT077792 **10** and the quinolines **11**, **12** and **13**.

The isothiazolone class of HAT inhibitors was disclosed by high-throughput screening. These compounds inhibited enzymatic activity of both PCAF and p300 and also blocked cellular proliferation of a panel of human colon and ovarian tumor cell lines. In particular, derivatives CCT077791 **9** and CCT077792 **10** (Figure 11.3) decreased protein acetylation in a time and concentration-dependent manner in HCT116 and in HT29 human colon tumor cell lines. CCT077791 reduced total acetylation of histones H3 and H4 and acetylation of α-tubulin. Still, the compounds also seem to have considerable off-target effects, which may be attributable to their high chemical reactivity of these Michael-acceptors with thiol groups [19].

Mai *et al.* recently reported the discovery of quinolines MC1752 **11** and MC1626 **12** (Figure 11.3). These derivatives were able to inhibit yeast cell growth, Gcn5-dependent gene transcription and acetylation of histone H3 *in vivo*. Further studies showed that both quinolines led to hypoacetylated histones H3 and α-tubulin in human cells (leukaemia U937) at the millimolar level. Due to these effects Mai *et al.* prepared a series of second generation inhibitors combining the structural features of MC1626 and MC1752 with those of anacardic acid and MB-3. As a result MC1823 **13** (Figure 11.3) was shown to be 10-fold more potent than the first generation inhibitors and anacardic acid, but less potent than MB-3 [20].

Further HAT inhibitors are the naturally occurring compounds curcumin **14** and garcinol **15** (Figure 11.4). They show equal activity *in vitro* and *in vivo*.

Curcumin represents a covalent inhibitor of CBP. Beyond, it showed anti-angiogenic effects and is currently in phase II/III of clinical trials for cancer therapy, as well as in phase II for Alzheimer's disease and psoriasis [21, 22]. Garcinol, a potent inhibitor of PCAF and p300 ($IC_{50} = 5$ and 7 μM, respectively) was found to induce apoptosis and alter global gene expression in HeLa cells. It was identified to repress chromatin transcription. None of these inhibitors had effects on HDAC activity or on histone-free DNA transcription [23].

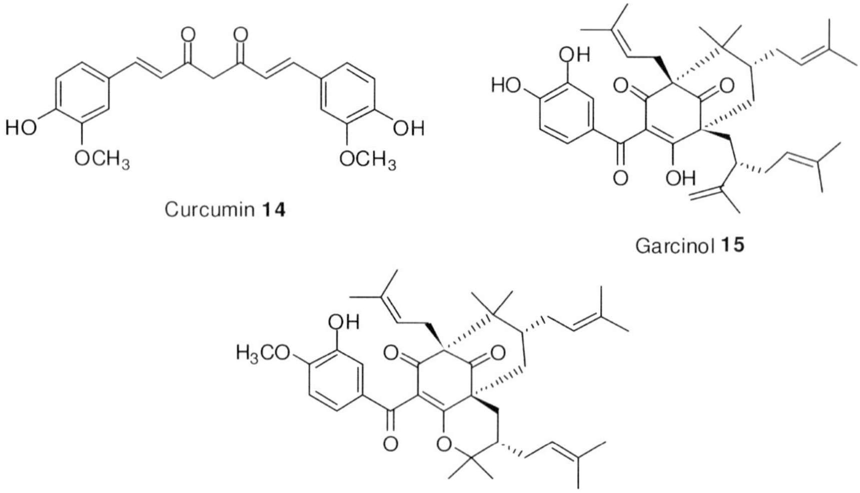

Figure 11.4 Inhibitors of HATs curcumin **14**, garcinol **15** and LTK-14 **16**.

Starting from garcinol **15**, Mantelingu *et al.* developed analog LTK-14 **16** (Figure 11.4), a specific inhibitor of p300-HAT. Contrary to the parent compound garcinol, LTK-14 was found to be nontoxic to T cells. Interestingly, it inhibits histone acetylation of HIV infected cells, repressing the replication of HIV in these cells. SAR studies performed by these authors showed that the low toxicity of LTK-14 is due to the introduction of a methyl group at the aromatic moiety of garcinol. The alkylation of one of the two phenolic groups in garcinol prevents an oxidation to ortho-quinones which causes lower toxicity. Furthermore, cyclization at the south-east part of garcinol induces the specificity of LTK-14 towards p300 and inactivity against PCAF, a member of the GNAT family. Microarray analysis showed that inhibition of p300-mediated acetylation by LTK-14 down-regulates 118 genes and up-regulates six genes. Further, derivative LTK-14 is able to inhibit HIV replication in SupT1 cells by histone acetylation at the viral long-term repeat (LTR) promoter which requires the virally encoded transactivator of transcription (Tat) to be activated, Tat induces the association of p300 and the CBP with the LTR promoter [24, 25]. In the light of the very recent discovery that the similar phloroglucinols like hyperforin and aristoforin are potent inhibitors of the HDACs SIRT1 and SIRT2 [26], it is necessary to investigate whether LTK-14 has similar properties [27].

11.3 Summary

In summary, during the past five years several inhibitors of HATs have been developed and biologically investigated. They represent interesting tools in the emerging area of epigenetics and may also find applications in experimental antiviral therapy, as well as in the study of processes like cancer, ageing, neurodegenerative diseases, obesity and diabetes.

References

1 Rubinstein, J.H. and Taybi, H. (1963) Broad thumbs and toes and facial abnormalities. A possible mental retardation syndrome. *American Journal of Diseases of Children*, **105**, 588–608.

2 Petrij, F., Giles, R.H., Dauwerse, H.G., Saris, J.J., Hennekam, R.C.M., Masuno, M. *et al.* (1995) Rubinstein-Taybi-syndrome caused by mutations in the transcriptional co-activator CBP. *Nature*, **376**, 348–351.

3 Chan, H.M. and La Thangue, N.B. (2001) p300/CBP proteins: HATs for transcriptional bridges and scaffolds. *Journal of Cell Science*, **114**, 2363–2673.

4 Biel, M., Wascholowski, V. and Giannis, A. (2005) Epigenetics-an epicenter of gene regulation: histones and histone-modifying enymes. *Angewandte Chemie-International Edition*, **44**, 3186–3216.

5 Roth, S.Y., Denu, J.M. and Allis, C.D. (2001) Histone acetyltransferases. *Annual Review of Biochemistry*, **70**, 81–120.

6 Zhang, Y., Li, N., Caron, C., Matthias, G., Hess, D., Khochbin, S. and Matthias, P. (2003) HDAC-6 interacts with and deacetylates tubulin and microtubules in vivo. *The EMBO Journal*, **22**, 1168–1179.

7 Yang, J.-X. and Seto, E. (2007) HATs and HDACs: from structure, function and regulation to novel strategies for therapy and prevention. *Oncogene*, **26**, 5310–5318.

8 Goodman, R.H. and Smolik, S. (2000) CBP/p300 in cell growth, transformation, and development. *Genes & Development*, **14**, 1553–1577.

9 Lau, O.D., Kundu, T.K., Soccio, R.E., Alt-Si-Ali, S., Khalil, E.M., Vassilev, A. *et al.* (2000) HATs off: selective synthetic inhibitors of the histone acetyltransferases p300 and PCAF. *Molecular Cell*, **5**, 589–595.

10 Thompson, P.R., Kurooka, H., Nakatani, Y. and Cole, P.A. (2001) Transcriptional coactivator protein p300. Kinetic characterization of its histone acetyltransferase activity. *The Journal of Biological Chemistry*, **276**, 33721–33729.

11 Poux, A.N., Cebrat, M., Kim, C.M., Cole, P.A. and Marmorstein, R. (2002) Structure of the GCN5 histone acetyltransferase bound to a bisubstrate inhibitor. *Proceedings of the National Academy of Sciences of the United States of America*, **99**, 14065–14070.

12 Costanzo, A., Merlo, P., Pediconi, N., Fulco, M., Sartorelli, V., Cole, P.A. *et al.* (2002) DNA damage-dependent acetylation of p73 dictates the selective activation of apoptotic target genes. *Molecular Cell*, **9**, 175–186.

13 Balsubramanyam, K., Swaminathan, V., Ranganathan, A. and Kundu, T.K. (2003) Small molecule modulators of histone acetyltransferase p300. *The Journal of Biological Chemistry*, **278**, 19134–19140.

14 Sun, Y.L., Jiang, X.F., Chen, S.J. and Price, B.D. (2006) Inhibition of histone acetyltransferase activity by anacardic acid sensitizes tumor cells to ionizing radiation. *FEBS Letters*, **580**, 4353–4356.

15 Souto, J.A., Conte, M., Alvarez, R., Nebbioso, A., Carafa, V., Altucci, L. *et al.* (2008) Synthesis of benzamides related to anacardic acid and their histone acetyltransferase (HAT) inhibitory activities. *ChemMedChem*, **3**, 1435–1442.

16 Eliseeva, E.D., Valkov, V., Jung, M. and Jung, M.O. (2007) Characterization of novel inhibitors of histone acetyltransferases. *Molecular Cancer Therapeutics*, **6**, 2391–2398.

17 Biel, M., Kretsovali, N., Karatzali, E., Papamatheakis, J. and Giannis, A. (2004)

Design, synthesis, and biological evaluation of a small-molecule inhibitor of the histone acetyltransferase Gcn5. *Angewandte Chemie*, **116**, 4065–4067; (2004) *Angewandte Chemie International Edition in English*, **43**, 3974–3976.

18 Hoffmann, H.M.R. and Rabe, J. (1985) Synthese und biologische Aktivität von α-methylen-γ-butyrolactonen. *Angewandte Chemie*, **97**, 96–112; (1985) *Angewandte Chemie International Edition in English*, **24**, 94–110.

19 Stimson, L., Rowlands, M.G., Newbatt, Y.M., Smith, N.F., Raynaud, F.I., Rogers, P. *et al.* (2005) Isothiazolones as inhibitors of PCAF and p300 histone acetyltransferase activity. *Molecular Cancer Therapeutics*, **4**, 1521–1532.

20 Mai, A. (2007) The therapeutic uses of chromatin-modifying agents. *Expert Opinion on Therapeutic Targets*, **11**, 835–851.

21 Marcu, M.G., Jung, Y.J., Lee, S., Chung, E.J., Lee, M.J., Trepel, J. *et al.* (2006) Curcumin is an inhibitor of p300 histone acetyltransferase. *Medicinal Chemistry*, **2**, 169–174.

22 Balasubramanyam, K., Varier, R.A. and Altaf, M. (2004) Curcumin, a novel p300/CREB-binding protein-specific inhibitor of acetyltransferase, represses the acetylation of histone/nonhistone proteins and histone acetyltransferase-dependent chromatin transcription. *The Journal of Biological Chemistry*, **279**, 51163–51171.

23 Balasubramanyam, K., Altaf, M. and Varier, R.A. (2004) Polyisoprenylated benzophenone, garcinol, a natural histone acetyltransferase inhibitor, represses chromatin transcription and alters global gene expression. *The Journal of Biological Chemistry*, **279**, 33716–33726.

24 Mantelingu, K., Reddy, B.A.A., Swaminathan, V., Kishore, A.H., Siddappa, N.B., Kumar, G.V. *et al.* (2007) Specific inhibition of p300-HAT alters global gene expression and represses HIV replication. *Chemistry & Biology*, **14**, 645–657.

25 Marzio, G. and Giacca, M. (1999) Chromatin control of HIV-1 gene expression. *Genetica*, **106**, 125–130.

26 Gey, C., Kyrylenko, S., Hennig, L., Nguyen, L.H., Büttner, A., Pham, H.D. *et al.* (2007) Phloroglucinol derivatives guttiferone G, aristoforin, and hyperforin: inhibitors of human sirtuins SIRT1 and SIRT2. *Angewandte Chemie*, **119**, 5311–5314.

27 Ciochina, R. and Grossman, R.B. (2006) Polycyclic polyprenylated acylphloroglucinols. *Chemical Reviews*, **106**, 3963–3986.

12
Histone Methyltransferases as Novel Drug Targets

Manfred Jung

12.1
Introduction

The N-terminal tails of histone proteins are rich in arginine and lysine residues and undergo various types of posttranslational modifications. There are small modifications such as acetylation, methylation, phosphorylation but also the attachment of larger peptide groups such as ubiquitinylation and sumoylation [1]. This has an impact on chromatin structure and subsequently on gene transcription and the epigenetic maintenance of altered transcription after cell division [2].

Most data has accumulated on reversible histone acetylation. Acetylation levels are regulated by histone acetyltransferases (HATs) and histone deacetylases (HDACs) [3, 4]. Small molecule inhibitors of HDACs affect gene regulation but also signal transduction via the hyperacetylation of nonhistone substrate proteins. The HDAC inhibitor vorinostat is used as a drug for the treatment of cancer and several other HDAC inhibitors are in clinical trials [5, 6]. Histone methyltransferases have emerged in just the past few years as potential therapeutic targets in the epigenetic field and only a few inhibitors are available so far [7].

12.2
Protein Methylation

Histone methylation participates in the regulation of gene expression patterns. Unlike histone acetylation, histone methylation does not alter the charge of the amino acid and hence the histone tail. There are changes in the basicity and the hydrophobicity which are relatively small when viewed at the scale of the histone but still influence the affinity of the histone tails to certain proteins, for example transcription factors, which in turn result in certain signaling events. The histone methyltransferases are usually subdivided into three classes: SET domain lysine methyltransfeases, nonSET domain lysine methyltransferases and arginine methyltransferases (PRMTs). All of them utilize S-adenosylmethionine (SAM) as cosubstrate for the methylation reaction.

Epigenetic Targets in Drug Discovery. Edited by Wolfgang Sippl and Manfred Jung

ISBN: 978-3-527-32355-5

In contrast to, for example HDACs, histone methyltransferases are regarded to be highly site-specific [8–12]. First reports on a greater variety of nonhistone substrates for the lysine methyltransferase G9a [13] indicate that the specificity might be somewhat less restrictive than previously thought but still in histones mainly only one residue is modified [14]. Histone tails can be mono-, di- or trimethylated on the ε-amino group of lysine residues and can be mono- or dimethylated on arginine residues with two possible patterns of dimethylation (see below).

12.2.1
Arginine Methylation

PRMTs lead to the methylation of certain arginine residues in histones as depicted in Table 12.1. They are not restricted to histone substrates but also catalyze the methylation of other proteins that play a role in signal transduction and cell proliferation [15]. Usually glycine–alanine–arginine patches (called GAR motifs)

Table 12.1 Selected arginine methyltransferases and links to disease.

Enzyme	Links to disease (examples)	Major target site(s)[a]
Type I enzmyes (asymmetric dimethylation)		
PRMT1	Coactivator of hormone receptor function [53] Essential component of the MLL oncogenic transcriptional complex [58]	H4R3, NAB2p, NPL3p, many others
PRMT2	Coactivator for the androgen receptor [57]	Catalytically inactive
PRMT4 (CARM1)	Involved in estrogen-driven cell cycle progression in breast cancer [83] Knockdown impedes androgen receptor signaling [56] Aberrant expression in prostate tumor cells [84] Methylation of CBP contributes to its coactivation [19]	H3R2, H3R17, H3R26 (and others); CBP/p300R2142 [85]
Type II enzymes (symmetric dimethylation)		
PRMT5	Expression of tumor suppressor genes in fibroblasts is hampered [60]	H3R8, H4R3; MBD2 [86]
PRMT7	Downregulation sensitizes cancer cells to camptothecin treatment [87]	Not yet known

[a] If no reference is cited, source is Ref. [46].

are methylated except by CARM1 [16]. This subtype and PRMT5 show an affinity towards proline–glycine–methionine–arginine sequences (called PGM motifs) [17] but also other motifs, for example RGG [18], are possible. In the latter case, incubation of the Ewing sarcoma (EWS) protein *in vitro* with PRMT resulted in a methylation of 27 arginine residues. Generally, it needs to be established which of the *in vitro* results in terms of substrate sites actually plays a role *in vivo*. Nonhistone protein methylation also has an impact on other epigenetic modulators because arginine methylation of the histone acetyltransferase CBP by the enzyme CARM1 contributes to the coactivating effects of CBP [19]. An important group of substrates for arginine methylation are the different proteins involved in RNA maturation [17, 20]; and DNA repair is also affected [21]. The latter casts doubt on the safety of PRMT inhibitors as potential drugs. It has been shown that the function of the protein MRE 11 that is involved in DNA damage control is dependent on arginine methylation [22]. A more detailed overview of PRMT substrates can be found in other review articles, for example Ref. [23]. The arginine methylation status of proteins is sensed by proteins with a so-called Tudor domain. These are bound by methylated peptide sequences depending on the state and the pattern (asymmetric vs symmetric) of methylation [17, 24]. The regulation of PRMT activity may occur via PRMT-binding proteins or posttranslational modifications [16]. For example the protein BTG1 [25] and the BTG1-binding protein hCAF1 [26] regulate PRMT1 activity and phosphorylation of CARM1 decreases its activity [27].

12.2.2 Lysine Methylation

Lysine methyltransferases are usually also highly specific in terms of histone methylation. The biological consequences of the histone methylation depend on the target site where they occur. In the case of histones, methylation of K4, K36 and K79 on H3 are implicated in activation of transcription whereas methylation on H3K9, H3K27 and H4K20 are considered repressive marks [14]. But such posttranslational modifications may vary in their biological effect, depending on the cellular context or neighboring modifications [28]. The construction of designed histone modification patterns by means of protein ligation [29, 30] or chemical modification [31] are therefore important tools for further dissection of the "histone code" [32], which may actually be a "nucleosome code" [28]. Opposing effects of lysine methylation are also observed in nonhistone proteins, as the monomethylation of p53 at K372 by the lysine methyltransferase Set9 leads to transcriptional activation [33] and methylation on K370 by Smyd2 [34] or K382 by SET8 [35] inhibits transcriptional activity of p53. Generally, much less is known about nonhistone protein lysine methylation as compared to arginine methylation and as mentioned the tumor suppressor protein p53 is the most prominent example [36]. Lately, additional lysine methylation targets have been discovered by probing the specificity of the methyltransferase G9a by peptide arrays and subsequent sequence searches [13]. The methylation of the viral tat protein indicates that diseases other than cancer may also provide lysine methyltransferases as future drug targets [37].

12.3
Histone Demethylation

The existence of a reversal of histone methylation was doubted for quite some time but has lately been described. Mono- and dimethylated lysines are demethylated by an amine oxidase type protein called LSD1 [38, 39]. Trimethylated lysine residues can only be demethylated by oxygenating enzymes such as a group of proteins with a so-called Jumanji (JmJ) domain. These do not depend on presence of a electron pair on the ε-amino group of the lysine [40–43] like LSD1 does. The JmJ proteins can also demethylate dimethylated lysines and it was discovered that JMJD6 is also able to reverse arginine methylation [44]. PADI4, an arginine deiminase, catalyzes the conversion of unmethylated and to some extent monomethylated arginines to citrullines [45]. A detailed overview over histone demethylation is the subject of another chapter in this book.

12.4
Histone Methyltransferases

So far nine arginine methyltransferases [46] and more than 20 lysine methyltransferases [11] have been identified in humans. Many of them show links to cancer. We discuss several of these subtypes below and an overview can be found in Tables 12.1 and 12.2. For lysine methyltransferases traditionally individual names have been used for the various subtypes. Lately, a common nomenclature for chromatin modifying enzymes has been proposed. For the human lysine methyltransferases the name KMTs should be used in analogy to (P)RMTs and eight groups (KMT1–8) with different subtypes suggested for some members [47]. But this nomenclature is not used consistently even throughout the recent literature so we provide both names if available in Table 12.2.

12.4.1
Arginine Methyltransferases

Protein arginine methylation is catalyzed by two classes of enzymes: type I methyltransferases and type II methyltransferases (PRMTs). Type I enzymes lead to the formation of asymmetric ω-N_G,N_G-dimethylarginines and Type II enzymes maintain the formation of symmetric ω-N_G,N_G-dimethylarginine tails (Figure 12.1). PRMTs 1–4, 6, 8 belong to the PRMTs of type I and PRMTs 5, 7, 9 are considered to be type II enzymes. Additionally, two putative PRMTs 10 and 11 have been found in the genome but a clear demonstration of their ability to act as methyltransferases needs yet to be established [46]. For PRMT7 opposing reports on its catalytic activity exist. The exclusive formation of monomethylarginine has been described in one report but it was also shown to be a type II enzyme when a different substrate was used [48, 49]. For PRMTs 2 and 9 so far no enzymatic activity has been monitored yet.

Table 12.2 Selected lysine methyltransferases and links to cancer.

Enzyme	Links to cancer (examples)	Major target site(s)[a]
SUV39H1/2 (KMT1A/B)	Protein overexpression in dietary induced tumors [88] Increased mRNA levels in colon cancer samples [65]	H3K9
G9a (KMT1C)	Contributes to H3K9 dimethylation and is involved in suppressor gene silencing [89]	H3K9; various non-histone proteins (e.g. CDYL1, WIZ, CSB, HDAC1) automethylation [13]
	Knockdown inhibited cancer cell growth [66]	
Eu-HMTase1 (KMT1D)	Overexpression in gland tumors cells [90]	H3K9
SETDB1/ESET (KMT1E)	Cooperation with DNA methyl-transferase silencing of promotor regions in tumor cells [91]	H3K9
MLL1 (KMT2A)	Mutations/rearrangements observed in leukemogenesis [63]	H3K4
MLL4 (KMT2D)	Involvement in viral (hepatitis B) liver carcinogenesis [92]	H3K4
SMYD2 (KMT3C)	Suppressor of p53 transcriptional activity [34]	H3K56, p53K370
SMYD3	Overexpression and enhanced breast cancer cell growth [93]	
	Overexpression also in colorectal and hepatocellular carcinoma [94]	
DOT1L (KMT4)	Role in leukemogenesis [68]	H3K79
SET8/PR-SET7 (KMT5A)	Suppressor of p53-dependent transcription [35]	H4K20, p53K372, p53K382 [95]
MMSET	Transcriptional corepressor, its knockdown impedes myeloma viability [67]	H4K20 (H3K4) [67]

[a]If no reference is cited, source is Ref. [47].

PRMT1 provides the major source of arginine methylation in cells [50]. Like PRMT4 (CARM1) it is a coactivator of androgen and estrogen receptors [51, 52] and both subtpyes therefore represent a potential target for an indirect antihormone therapy. Consequently, PRMT1 inhibitors have been shown to block sexual hormone receptor activation in reporter gene models [53, 54]. PRMT1 also methylates the estrogen receptor which contributes to these effects [55]. CARM1 is overexpressed in hormone dependent breast and prostate tumors and its knockdown impedes androgen receptor signaling [56]. Despite its apparent lack of catalytic activity also PRMT2 has been

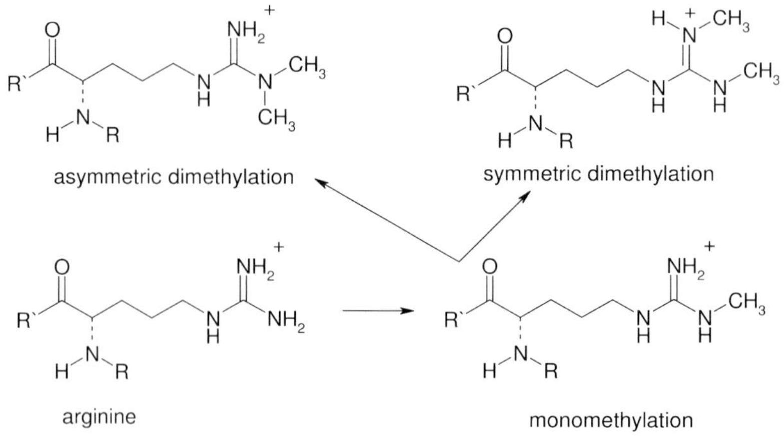

Figure 12.1 Protein arginine methylation pathways.

shown to be a coactivator for the androgen receptor [57], so protein–protein interactions should also be involved in coactivator functions of PRMTs. PRMT1 is a necessary component for the oncogenic transformation caused by a mixed lineage leukemia (MLL) complex and its knockdown-suppressed MLL-mediated transformation [58]. PRMT1 is not necessary for viability but was shown to be important for proper differentiation during embryogenesis. Therefore, knockout mutant mice die in an early embryonic stage [59]. PRMT5 methylates the same arginine as PRMT1 (H4R3) but towards a symmetric and not an unsymmetric product. Therefore, the significance of Western blot analyses targeted against H4R3 highly depends on the selectivity of the antibody between those two closely related products. PRMT5 negatively regulates the transcription of tumor suppressor genes in fibroblasts and maintains a tumorigenic state [60], but PRMT5 overexpression leads to growth inhibition in cancer cell lines [46]. PRMT1 and PRMT3 are overexpressed in myocardial tissue of patients with coronary heart disease [61] and therefore may also be interesting targets for cardiovascular indications. But PRMT5 is required for proper myogenesis [62] which might be a cause of side-effects for unselective PRMT inhibitors.

12.4.2
Lysine Methyltransferases

Lysine methyltransferases have been linked in various cases to the pathogenesis of cancer. Examples can be found for KMTs that induce repressive marks as well as for those that lead to an activating methylation pattern. Possible reasons for a disturbed regulation of methylation may result in mutations of enzymes or overexpression in cancer cells. An indication for a therapeutic benefit of potential inhibitors is often derived from siRNA knockdown of the requisite isotype. Mutations of MLL1 for example are thought to be responsible for various forms of acute leukemia [63]. Overexpression of EZH2 was linked to breast or prostate cancer [64] and increased levels in human cancers have also been observed for G9a. Increased mRNA levels for the isotype SUV39H1 have been described in patients with primary colorectal cancer [65]. siRNA-mediated knockdown of G9a inhibited cell growth [66] and MMSET knockdown was also effective in suppressing viability in myeloma cells [67]. The human homolog of the yeast methyltransferase Dot1, hDOT1L, has been linked to cancer in recent studies. It interacts with the protein AF10, which acts as a MLL fusion partner in leukemia cells. Hypermethylation of H3K79 was observed in AF10-MLL cells. Again, antisense knockdown of hDOT1L expression blocked cell proliferation [68].

12.5 Histone Methyltransferase Inhibitors

Various epigenetic targets have been investigated in drug discovery approaches. So far only HDAC and DNA methyltransferase (DNMT) inhibitors are approved for the treatment of human cancer or are currently investigated in clinical studies [69]. The search for histone methyltransferase inhibitors is far less developed.

Generally, for enzymes that involve a peptidic substrate and a cosubstrate (SAM), competitive inhibitors can be found either among compounds mimicking either one of these substrate or among ligands that bind to parts of both the peptide and the cosubstrate pocket. For example, for kinases it is very common to use inhibitors that compete for the binding of the cosubstate (ATP) and by addressing additional binding regions selectivity may still be obtained [70]. For histone methyltransferases so far only rather unselective analogs of SAM are available. Examples are methylthioadenosine, S-adenosyl-homocysteine (SAH) and sinefungin [71]. The latter is a SAM analog from bacteria and is very unselective. Therefore, therapeutic applications of such compounds are not very likely. Thus, as far as is known or can be deduced from docking studies, the available specific histone methyltransferase inhibitors either compete mostly with the protein substrate or are bisubstrate inhibitors.

In terms of strategy, all available druglike histone methyltransferase inhibitors were discovered by screening approaches, or were derived from such screening hits subsequently by chemical synthesis. Either the screening campaigns were performed as random screening projects or an enrichment by means of virtual screening was performed initially.

12.5.1 Arginine Methyltransferase Inhibitors

The first inhibitors of arginine methyltransferases were found in 2004 [53]. Random screening of 9000 compounds was performed with the yeast enzyme Hmt1p and the nonhistone protein substrate Npl3. Nine compounds with activity in the low micromolar region were identified and subsequently tested against human PRMT1. The inhibitors, called arginine methyltransferase inhibitors (AMIs), were not selective versus PRMT3, 4, 6; but two compounds, called AMI-1 and -6, were selective *in vitro* against several lysine methyltransferases (Suv39H1, Suv39H2, SET7/9, DOT1; Figure 12.2). AMI-1, but not -6, showed an *in vivo* effect on the methylation of Npl3 and also an inhibitory effect on the activation of estrogen and androgen receptors [53]. Eosin (AMI-5; Figure 12.2), for example, is an unselective histone methyltransferase inhibitor. The *in vitro* results for some of the AMIs have not been verified in cell culture and caution is warranted for some of them, for example AMI-2 and -9, contain partial structures of well known promiscous enzyme inhibitors that act *in vitro* by aggregation or precipitation [72].

Later, AMI-5 was used as a lead compound in the design of new inhibitors. Initial structure activity studies were presented with compound **6e** showing the best activity [73] (Figure 12.3). The lead structure was further modified and simplified to curcumin-like scaffolds with bromo- or dibromophenol substructures. For example, compound **4b** showed an IC_{50} value of 14 μM against the *Aspergillus* homolog of PMRT1 that is called RmtA [74]. **4b** also inhibited CARM1 and SET7. Compound **8e** from this paper was selective at 100 μM for CARM1 over PRMT1. As curcumin is known to be a HAT inhibitor [75] and the dibromophenol GW5074 shows sirtuin inhibitory properties [76], the new PRMT inhibitors were also tested against these targets. Indeed, inhibition of HAT and sirtuin activity was also observed for several compounds *in vitro*. But whereas cellular histone hypomethylation was demonstrated for some of the inhibitors, it is unclear yet whether an effect on cellular protein acetylation occurs in the same range of concentration. Compound **7b** (Figure 12.3) was optimized from the high-throughput screening hit **1** (Figure 12.2) into a potent selective inhibitor of CARM1 [77].

Our group presented the first target-based approach to inhibitors of histone arginine methyltransferase in 2007. A hPRMT1 homology model was created as a basis for a virtual screening of compound libraries. The screening procedure was set up in a way so that we were selecting potential ligands for the arginine and not for the cosubstrate binding site. Manual inspection of the screening hits for binding to an active site glutamate led to a subset of the NCI diversity set of about 40 compounds which were chosen for *in vitro* testing. The procedure resulted in seven compounds with IC_{50} values below 55 μM. Two inhibitors, stilbamidine and a compound we called allantodapsone, also induced hypomethylation at the PRMT1 target H4R3 in HepG2 cells. Additionally, kinetic studies were performed and both compounds were found to be competitive with regard to the histone substrate. Selectivity studies with SET7/9 revealed that allantodapsone also processed an inhibitory effect *in vitro* towards this enzyme. Both inhibitors showed a dose-dependent block of the activation of the estrogen receptor by estradiol in a reporter gene model in MCF7a cells [54].

As an alternative strategy we performed a fragment-based virtual screening looking for molecules with inhibitory properties and a molecular weight below 200 g/mol. We discovered an α-methylthioglycolic amide that inhibited PRMT1 but lacked chemical stability and did not have a druglike structure. As a consequence, by means of a similarity search, compounds which posessed this α-methylthioglycolic amide substructure were identified and tested against RmtA and PRMT1. This resulted in the finding of a compound (RM65; see Figure 12.2) that inhibited both the *Aspergillus* and the human enzyme with equal strength. In contrast, the original lead compound showed a pronounced selectivity for the fungal enzyme. RM65 was selective for arginine methyltransferases as compared to its action on SET7/9. Again, a cellular hypomethylation could be observed in HepG2 cells. Although we had started with a

Random screening hits

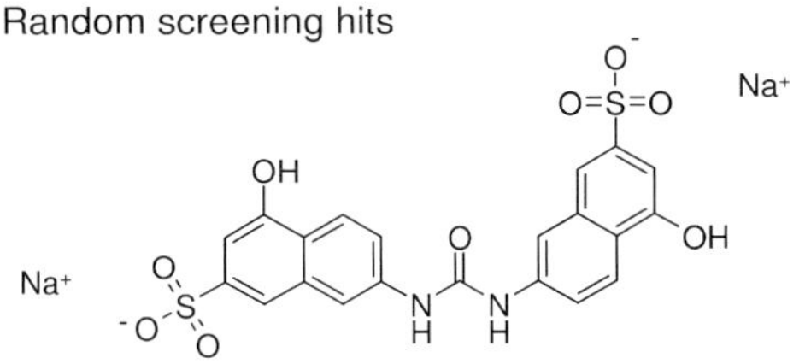

AMI-1 (9 µM)

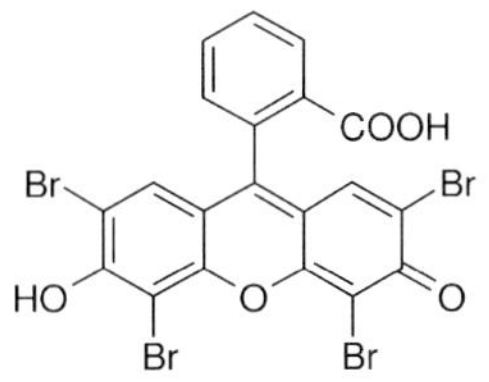

AMI-5 (eosin, 1 µM)

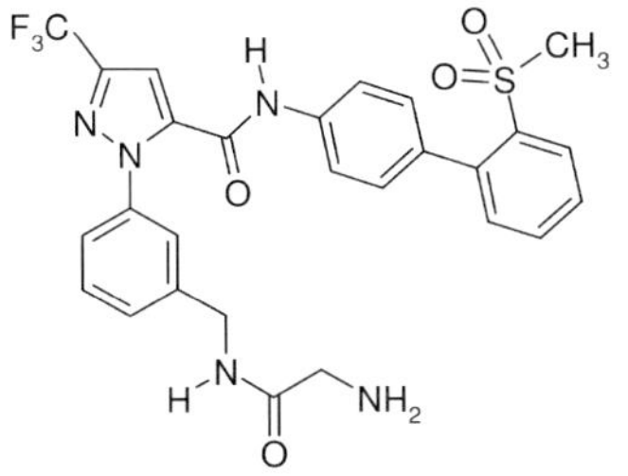

Inhibitor **1** (1.8 µM, CARM1)

Virtual screening hits

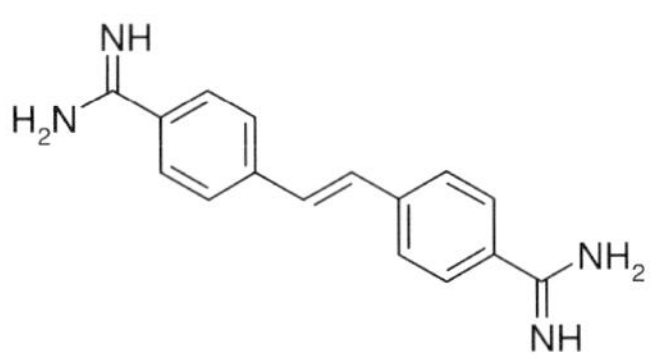

Stilbamidine (57 µM)

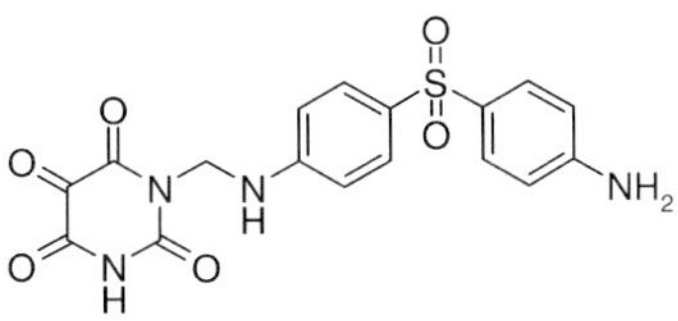

Allantodapsone (2 µM)

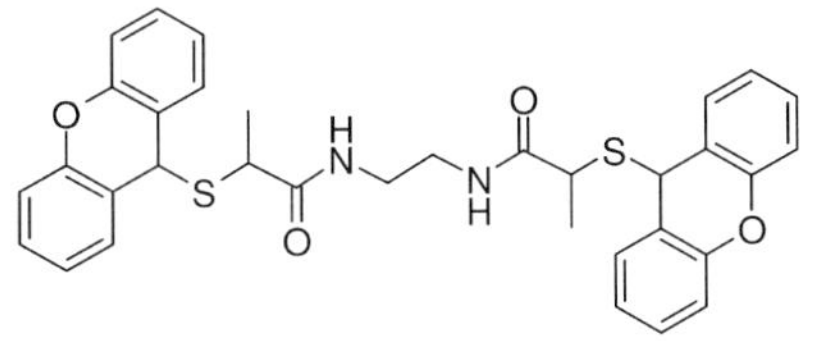

RM-65 (55 µM)

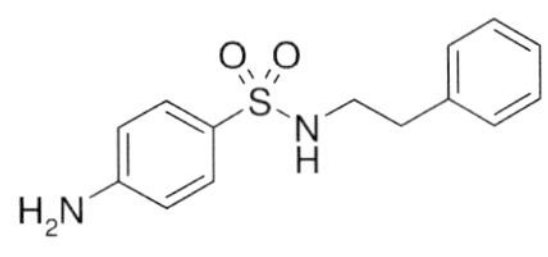

Inhibitor **6** (13 µM)

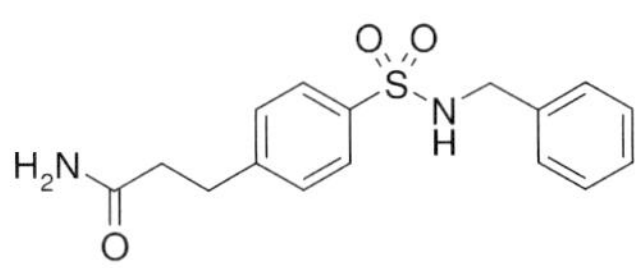

Inhibitor **7** (15 µM)

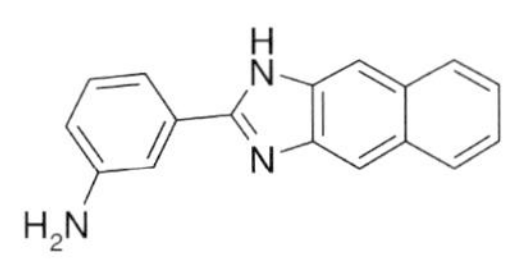

Inhibitor **9** (14 µM)

Figure 12.2 Arginine methyltransferase inhibitors from random and virtual screening campaigns (IC_{50} values in brackets; if no enzyme is mentioned, against hPRMT1).

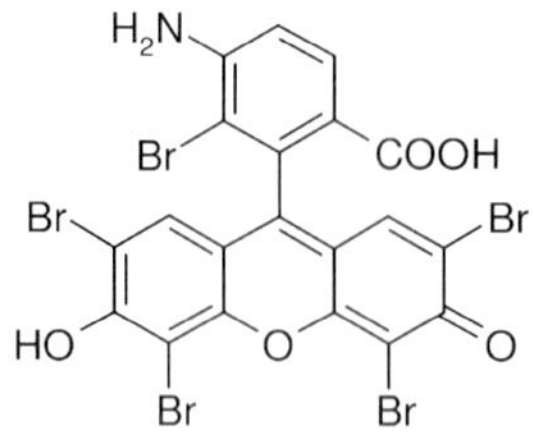

Inhibitor **6e** (5 μM)

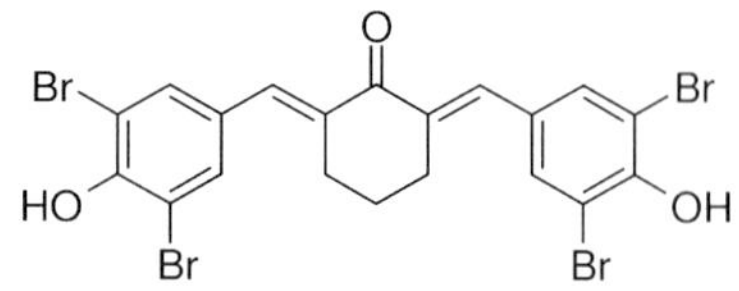

Inhibitor **4b** (14 μM, RmtA)

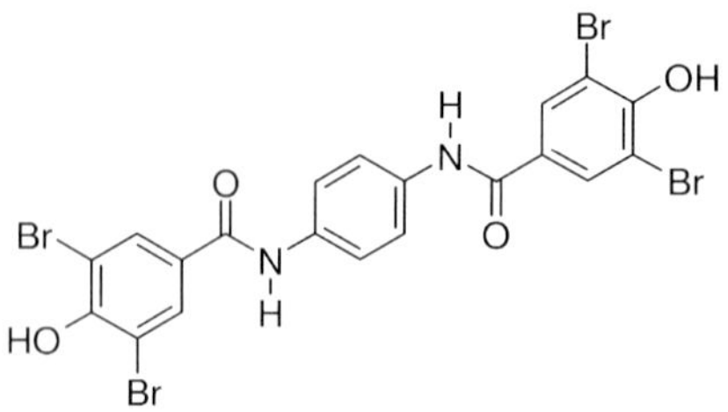

Inhibitor **8e**

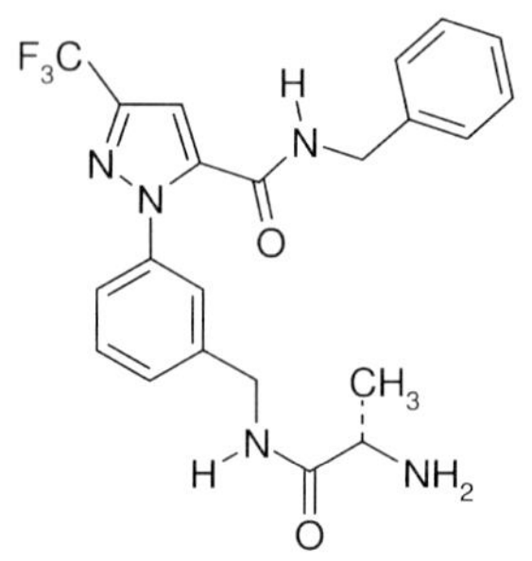

Inhibitor **7b** (80 nM, CARM1)

Figure 12.3 Arginine methyltransferase inhibitors obtained by synthetic variation of screening hits (IC_{50} values in brackets; if no enzyme is mentioned, against hPRMT1).

fragment that binds to the arginine binding site, docking showed that the inhibitor RM65 most likely acts as a bisubstrate mimic that targets both the histone and the cosubstrate binding site [78]. In both studies, docking of all members of the virtual libraries was performed. This was only possible due to the limited size of the libraries in question (2000–6000). For virtual screening of a larger database (Chembridge, ~330 000 compounds) we prefiltered the library with a simple pharmacophore and the resulting sublibrary with about 6000 members was then used for the docking procedures (see Chapter 3 in this book for further details). These efforts led to additional new lead structures with PRMT1 inhibition down to 13 μM (Figure 12.2) [79].

As an alternative approach an adenosine-derived mustard was developed as a PRMT inhibitor by a strategy that was based on the mechanism of the enzyme. This compound is an alkylating agent which is covalently attached to a peptide substrate only upon incubation with PRMT1 [80]. It is not very druglike and is more of a chemical tool.

12.5.2
Lysine Methyltransferase Inhibitors

For lysine methyltransferases few specific inhibitors have been reported so far and all were discovered by random screening procedures. The first inhibitor that was

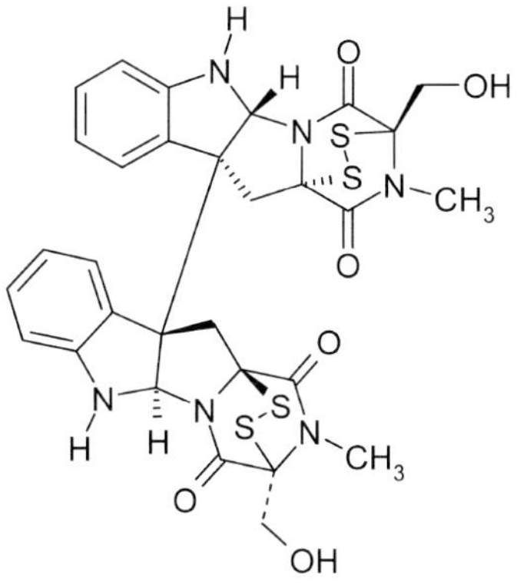

Chaetocin (0.8 μM, Su(var)3-9)

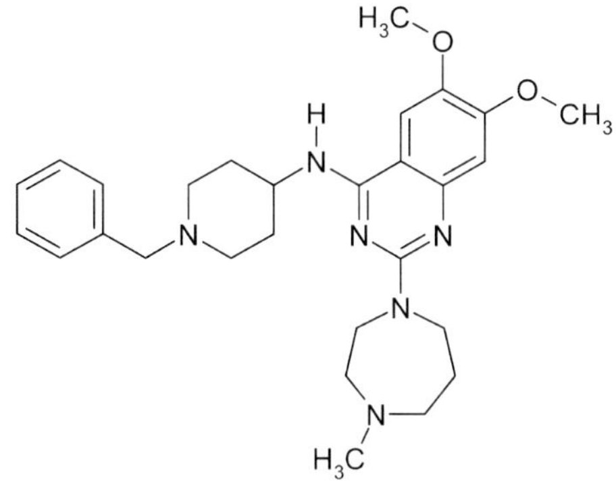

Bix-01294 (3 μM, G9a)

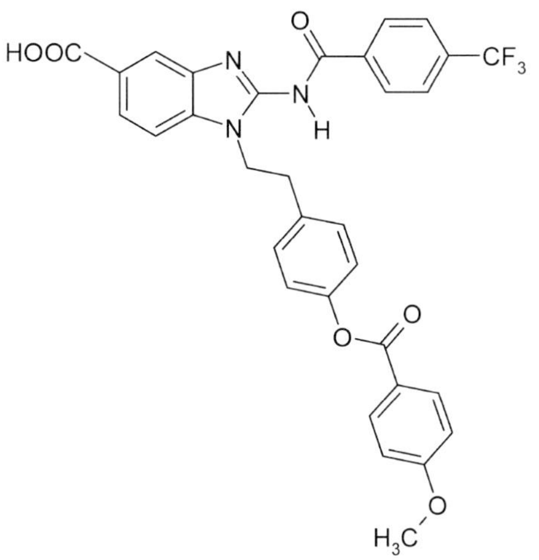

Bix-01338 (5 μM, G9a; 6 μM, PRMT1)

Figure 12.4 Lysine methyltransferase inhibitors (all from random screening, IC_{50} values and enzymes in brackets).

discovered is the fungal mycotoxin chaetocin (Figure 12.4). It inhibits the histone methyltransferase Su(var)3–9 from *Drosophila melanogaster* with an IC_{50} of 0.8 μM. Inhibition of G9a is also observed (IC_{50} 2.5 μM), whereas the lysine methyltransferases EZH2 and SET7/9 were not inhibited below 90 μM. Chaetocin also inhibited hSu(var)3–9 in cells and cytotoxic effects were observed [81].

The compound BIX-01294 was identified as an inhibitor of G9a in the low micromolar region and a selectivity against SUV39H1 and PRMT1 was shown. BIX-01294 also showed a reduction of the methylation levels of H3K9 dimethylation. Known sites of other lysine methyltransferases like H3K27 or H4K20 were not affected. In the same study dual inhibitors of arginine and lysine methyltransferases like BIX-01338 were reported [82].

12.6 Concluding Remarks

Although the field of histone methyltransferase inhibitors is still in its infancy in terms of drug discovery, a lot of knowledge in terms of their biological roles has been acquired. Test systems for *in vitro* and *in vivo* evaluation are available and model approaches have been presented already that led to inhibitors of these enzymes with promising cellular activity. Therefore, a dynamic development of the field can be expected which hopefully will lead to clinical candidates in the upcoming years.

References

1 Schäfer, S. and Jung, M. (2005) Chromatin modifications as targets for new anticancer drugs. *Archives of Pharmarcy Chemistry and Life Sciences*, **338**, 347–357.

2 Biel, M., Wascholowski, V. and Giannis, A. (2005) Epigenetics - An epicenter of gene regulation: Histones and histone-modifying enzymes. *Angewandte Chemie (International Edition in English)*, **44**, 3186–3216.

3 Yang, X.J. and Seto, E. (2007) HATs and HDACs: from structure, function and regulation to novel strategies for therapy and prevention. *Oncogene*, **26**, 5310–5318.

4 Minucci, S. and Pelicci, P.G. (2006) Histone deacetylase inhibitors and the promise of epigenetic (and more) treatments for cancer. *Nature Reviews. Cancer*, **6**, 38–51.

5 Herranz, M. and Esteller, M. (2006) New therapeutic targets in cancer: the epigenetic connection. *Clinical Transplants and Oncology*, **8**, 242–249.

6 Paris, M., Porcelloni, M., Binaschi, M. and Fattori, D. (2008) Histone deacetylase inhibitors: from bench to clinic. *Journal of Medicinal Chemistry*, **51**, 1505–1529.

7 Spannhoff, A., Sippl, W. and Jung, M. (2008) Cancer treatment of the future: inhibitors of histone methyltransferases. *The International Journal of Biochemistry & Cell Biology*, 10.1016/j.biocel.2008.1007.1024.

8 Rice, J.C. and Allis, C.D. (2001) Histone methylation versus histone acetylation: new insights into epigenetic regulation. *Current Opinion in Cell Biology*, **13**, 263–273.

9 Kouzarides, T. (2002) Histone methylation in transcriptional control. *Current Opinion in Genetics & Development*, **12**, 198–209.

10 Trievel, R.C. (2004) Structure and function of histone methyltransferases. *Critical Reviews in Eukaryotic Gene Expression*, **14**, 147–169.

11 Qian, C. and Zhou, M.M. (2006) SET domain protein lysine methyltransferases: Structure, specificity and catalysis. *Cellular and Molecular Life Sciences*, **63**, 2755–2763.

12 Morgunkova, A. and Barlev, N.A. (2006) Lysine methylation goes global. *Cell Cycle (Georgetown, Tex)*, **5**, 1308–1312.

13 Rathert, P., Dhayalan, A., Murakami, M., Zhang, X., Tamas, R., Jurkowska, R., Komatsu, Y., Shinkai, Y., Cheng, X. and Jeltsch, A. (2008) Protein lysine methyltransferase G9a acts on non-histone targets. *Nature Chemical Biology*, **4**, 344–346.

14 Kouzarides, T. (2007) Chromatin modifications and their function. *Cell*, **128**, 693–705.

15 Bedford, M.T. and Richard, S. (2005) Arginine methylation an emerging regulator of protein function. *Molecular Cell*, **18**, 263–272.

16 Bedford, M.T. (2007) Arginine methylation at a glance. *Journal of Cell Science*, **120**, 4243–4246.

17 Cheng, D., Cote, J., Shaaban, S. and Bedford, M.T. (2007) The arginine methyltransferase CARM1 regulates the coupling of transcription and mRNA processing. *Molecular Cell*, **25**, 71–83.

18 Pahlich, S., Bschir, K., Chiavi, C., Belyanskaya, L. and Gehring, H. (2005) Different methylation characteristics of protein arginine methyltransferase 1 and 3 toward the Ewing Sarcoma protein and a peptide. *Proteins*, **61**, 164–175.

19 Chevillard-Briet, M., Trouche, D. and Vandel, L. (2002) Control of CBP co-activating activity by arginine methylation. *The EMBO Journal*, **21**, 5457–5466.

20 Brahms, H., Meheus, L., de Brabandere, V., Fischer, U. and Luhrmann, R. (2001) Symmetrical dimethylation of arginine residues in spliceosomal Sm protein B/B′ and the Sm-like protein LSm4, and their interaction with the SMN protein. *RNA (New York, NY)*, **7**, 1531–1542.

21 Dery, U., Coulombe, Y., Rodrigue, A., Stasiak, A., Richard, S. and Masson, J.Y. (2008) A glycine-arginine domain in control of the human MRE11 DNA repair protein. *Molecular and Cellular Biology*, **28**, 3058–3069.

22 Boisvert, F.M., Dery, U., Masson, J.Y. and Richard, S. (2005) Arginine methylation of MRE11 by PRMT1 is required for DNA damage checkpoint control. *Genes and Development*, **19**, 671–676.

23 Pahlich, S., Zakaryan, R.P. and Gehring, H. (2006) Protein arginine methylation: Cellular functions and methods of analysis. *Biochimica et Biophysica Acta*, **1764**, 1890–1903.

24 Cote, J. and Richard, S. (2005) Tudor domains bind symmetrical dimethylated arginines. *The Journal of Biological Chemistry*, **280**, 28476–28483.

25 Lin, W.J., Gary, J.D., Yang, M.C., Clarke, S. and Herschman, H.R. (1996) The mammalian immediate-early TIS21 protein and the leukemia-associated BTG1 protein interact with a protein-arginine N-methyltransferase. *The Journal of Biological Chemistry*, **271**, 15034–15044.

26 Robin-Lespinasse, Y., Sentis, S., Kolytcheff, C., Rostan, M.C., Corbo, L. and Le Romancer, M. (2007) hCAF1, a new regulator of PRMT1-dependent arginine methylation. *Journal of Cell Science*, **120**, 638–647.

27 Higashimoto, K., Kuhn, P., Desai, D., Cheng, X. and Xu, W. (2007) Phosphorylation-mediated inactivation of coactivator-associated arginine methyltransferase 1. *Proceedings of the National Academy of Sciences of the United States of America*, **104**, 12318–12323.

28 Ruthenburg, A.J., Li, H., Patel, D.J. and Allis, C.D. (2007) Multivalent engagement of chromatin modifications by linked binding modules. *Nature Reviews. Molecular Cell Biology*, **8**, 983–994.

29 Shogren-Knaak, M.A. and Peterson, C.L. (2004) Creating designer histones by native chemical ligation. *Methods in Enzymology*, **375**, 62–76.

30 Shogren-Knaak, M.A., Fry, C.J. and Peterson, C.L. (2003) A native peptide ligation strategy for deciphering nucleosomal histone modifications. *The Journal of Biological Chemistry*, **278**, 15744–15748.

31 Simon, M.D., Chu, F., Racki, L.R., de la Cruz, C.C., Burlingame, A.L., Panning, B., Narlikar, G.J. and Shokat, K.M. (2007) The site-specific installation of methyl-lysine analogs into recombinant histones. *Cell*, **128**, 1003–1012.

32 Jenuwein, T. and Allis, C.D. (2001) Translating the histone code. *Science*, **293**, 1074–1080.

33 Chuikov, S., Kurash, J.K., Wilson, J.R., Xiao, B., Justin, N., Ivanov, G.S., McKinney, K., Tempst, P., Prives, C., Gamblin, S.J., Barlev, N.A. and Reinberg, D. (2004) Regulation of p53 activity through lysine methylation. *Nature*, **432**, 353–360.

34 Huang, J., Sengupta, R., Espejo, A.B., Lee, M.G., Dorsey, J.A., Richter, M., Opravil, S., Shiekhattar, R., Bedford, M.T., Jenuwein, T. and Berger, S.L. (2007) p53 is regulated by the lysine demethylase LSD1. *Nature*, **449**, 105–108.

35 Shi, X., Kachirskaia, I., Yamaguchi, H., West, L.E., Wen, H., Wang, E.W., Dutta, S., Appella, E. and Gozani, O. (2007) Modulation of p53 function by SET8-mediated methylation at lysine 382. *Molecular Cell*, **27**, 636–646.

36 Huang, J. and Berger, S.L. (2008) The emerging field of dynamic lysine methylation of non-histone proteins. *Current Opinion in Genetics & Development*, **18**, 152–158.

37 Van Duyne, R., Easley, R., Wu, W., Berro, R., Pedati, C., Klase, Z., Kehn-Hall, K., Flynn, E.K., Symer, D.E. and Kashanchi, F. (2008) Lysine methylation of HIV-1 Tat regulates transcriptional activity of the viral LTR. *Retrovirology*, **5**, 40.

38 Shi, Y., Lan, F., Matson, C., Mulligan, P., Whetstine, J.R., Cole, P.A. and Casero, R.A. (2004) Histone Demethylation Mediated by the Nuclear Amine Oxidase Homolog LSD1. *Cell*, **119**, 941–953.

39 Metzger, E., Wissmann, M., Yin, N., Muller, J.M., Schneider, R., Peters, A.H., Gunther, T., Buettner, R. and Schule, R. (2005) LSD1 demethylates repressive histone marks to promote androgen-receptor-dependent transcription. *Nature*, **437**, 436–439.

40 Agger, K., Christensen, J., Cloos, P.A. and Helin, K. (2008) The emerging functions of histone demethylases. *Current Opinion in Genetics & Development*, **18**, 1–10.

41 Tsukada, Y., Fang, J., Erdjument-Bromage, H., Warren, M.E., Borchers, C.H., Tempst, P. and Zhang, Y. (2006) Histone demethylation by a family of JmjC domain-containing proteins. *Nature*, **439**, 811–816.

42 Cloos, P.A., Christensen, J., Agger, K., Maiolica, A., Rappsilber, J., Antal, T., Hansen, K.H. and Helin, K. (2006) The putative oncogene GASC1 demethylates tri- and dimethylated lysine 9 on histone H3. *Nature*, **442**, 307–311.

43 Wissmann, M., Yin, N., Muller, J.M., Greschik, H., Fodor, B.D., Jenuwein, T., Vogler, C., Schneider, R., Gunther, T., Buettner, R., Metzger, E. and Schule, R. (2007) Cooperative demethylation by JMJD2C and LSD1 promotes androgen receptor-dependent gene expression. *Nature Cell Biology*, **9**, 347–353.

44 Chang, B., Chen, Y., Zhao, Y. and Bruick, R.K. (2007) JMJD6 is a histone arginine demethylase. *Science*, **318**, 444–447.

45 Cuthbert, G.L., Daujat, S., Snowden, A.W., Erdjument-Bromage, H., Hagiwara, T., Yamada, M., Schneider, R., Gregory, P.D., Tempst, P., Bannister, A.J. and Kouzarides, T. (2004) Histone deimination antagonizes arginine methylation. *Cell*, **118**, 545–553.

46 Krause, C.D., Yang, Z.H., Kim, Y.S., Lee, J.H., Cook, J.R. and Pestka, S. (2007) Protein arginine methyltransferases: evolution and assessment of their pharmacological and therapeutic potential. *Pharmacology & Therapeutics*, **113**, 50–87.

47 Allis, C.D., Berger, S.L., Cote, J., Dent, S., Jenuwein, T., Kouzarides, T., Pillus, L., Reinberg, D., Shi, Y., Shiekhattar, R., Shilatifard, A., Workman, J. and Zhang, Y. (2007) New nomenclature for chromatin-modifying enzymes. *Cell*, **131**, 633–636.

48 Miranda, T.B., Miranda, M., Frankel, A. and Clarke, S. (2004) PRMT7 is a member of the protein arginine methyltransferase family with a distinct substrate specificity. *The Journal of Biological Chemistry*, **279**, 22902–22907.

49 Lee, J.H., Cook, J.R., Yang, Z.H., Mirochnitchenko, O., Gunderson, S.I., Felix, A.M., Herth, N., Hoffmann, R. and Pestka, S. (2005) PRMT7, a new protein arginine methyltransferase that synthesizes symmetric dimethylarginine. *The Journal of Biological Chemistry*, **280**, 3656–3664.

50 Tang, J., Frankel, A., Cook, R.J., Kim, S., Paik, W.K., Williams, K.R., Clarke, S. and Herschman, H.R. (2000) PRMT1 is the predominant type I protein arginine methyltransferase in mammalian cells. *The Journal of Biological Chemistry*, **275**, 7723–7730.

51 Koh, S.S., Chen, D., Lee, Y.H. and Stallcup, M.R. (2001) Synergistic enhancement of nuclear receptor function by p160 coactivators and two coactivators with protein methyltransferase activities. *The Journal of Biological Chemistry*, **276**, 1089–1098.

52 Koh, S.S., Li, H., Lee, Y.H., Widelitz, R.B., Chuong, C.M. and Stallcup, M.R. (2002) Synergistic coactivator function by coactivator-associated arginine methyltransferase (CARM) 1 and beta-catenin with two different classes of DNA-binding transcriptional activators. *The Journal of Biological Chemistry*, **277**, 26031–26035.

53 Cheng, D., Yadav, N., King, R.W., Swanson, M.S., Weinstein, E.J. and Bedford, M.T. (2004) Small molecule regulators of protein arginine methyltransferases. *The Journal of Biological Chemistry*, **279**, 23892–23899.

54 Spannhoff, A., Heinke, R., Bauer, I., Trojer, P., Metzger, E., Gust, R., Schüle, R., Brosch, G., Sippl, W. and Jung, M. (2007) Target-based approach to inhibitors of histone arginine methyltransferases. *Journal of Medicinal Chemistry*, **50**, 2319–2325.

55 Le Romancer, M., Treilleux, I., Leconte, N., Robin-Lespinasse, Y., Sentis, S., Bouchekioua-Bouzaghou, K., Goddard, S., Gobert-Gosse, S. and Corbo, L. (2008) Regulation of estrogen rapid signaling through arginine methylation by PRMT1. *Molecular Cell*, **31**, 212–221.

56 Majumder, S., Liu, Y., Ford, O.H. 3rd, Mohler, J.L. and Whang, Y.E. (2006) Involvement of arginine methyltransferase CARM1 in androgen receptor function and prostate cancer cell viability. *Prostate*, **66**, 1292–1301.

57 Meyer, R., Wolf, S.S. and Obendorf, M. (2007) PRMT2, a member of the protein arginine methyltransferase family, is a coactivator of the androgen receptor. *The Journal of Steroid Biochemistry and Molecular Biology*, **107**, 1–14.

58 Cheung, N., Chan, L.C., Thompson, A., Cleary, M.L. and Eric So, C.W. (2007) Protein arginine-methyltransferase-dependent oncogenesis. *Nature Cell Biology*, **9**, 1208–1215.

59 Pawlak, M.R., Scherer, C.A., Chen, J., Roshon, M.J. and Ruley, H.E. (2000) Arginine N-methyltransferase 1 is required for early postimplantation mouse development, but cells deficient in the enzyme are viable. *Molecular and Cellular Biology*, **20**, 4859–4869.

60 Pal, S., Vishwanath, S.N., Erdjument-Bromage, H., Tempst, P. and Sif, S. (2004) Human SWI/SNF-associated PRMT5 methylates histone H3 arginine 8 and negatively regulates expression of ST7 and NM23 tumor suppressor genes. *Molecular and Cellular Biology*, **24**, 9630–9645.

61 Chen, X., Niroomand, F., Liu, Z., Zankl, A., Katus, H.A., Jahn, L. and Tiefenbacher, C.P. (2006) Expression of nitric oxide related enzymes in coronary heart disease. *Basic Research in Cardiology*, **101**, 346–353.

62 Dacwag, C.S., Ohkawa, Y., Pal, S., Sif, S. and Imbalzano, A.N. (2007) The protein arginine methyltransferase Prmt5 is required for myogenesis because it facilitates ATP-dependent chromatin remodeling. *Molecular and Cellular Biology*, **27**, 384–394.

63 Hess, J.L. (2004) Mechanisms of transformation by MLL. *Critical Reviews in Eukaryotic Gene Expression*, **14**, 235–254.

64 Cooper, C.S., Campbell, C. and Jhavar, S. (2007) Mechanisms of Disease: biomarkers and molecular targets from microarray gene expression studies in prostate cancer. *Nature Clinical Practices in Urology*, **4**, 677–687.

65 Kang, M.Y., Lee, B.B., Kim, Y.H., Chang, D.K., Kyu Park, S., Chun, H.K., Song, S.Y., Park, J. and Kim, D.H. (2007) Association of the SUV39H1 histone methyltransferase with the DNA methyltransferase 1 at mRNA expression level in primary colorectal cancer. *International Journal of Cancer*, **121**, 2192–2197.

66 Kondo, Y., Shen, L., Ahmed, S., Boumber, Y., Sekido, Y., Haddad, B.R. and Issa, J.P. (2008) Downregulation of histone H3 lysine 9 methyltransferase G9a induces centrosome disruption and chromosome instability in cancer cells. *PLoS ONE*, **3**, e2037.

67 Marango, J., Shimoyama, M., Nishio, H., Meyer, J.A., Min, D.J., Sirulnik, A., Martinez-Martinez, Y., Chesi, M., Bergsagel, P.L., Zhou, M.M., Waxman, S., Leibovitch, B.A., Walsh, M.J. and Licht, J.D. (2008) The MMSET protein is a histone methyltransferase with characteristics of a transcriptional corepressor. *Blood*, **111**, 3145–3154.

68 Okada, Y., Feng, Q., Lin, Y., Jiang, Q., Li, Y., Coffield, V.M., Su, L., Xu, G. and Zhang, Y. (2005) hDOT1L links histone methylation to leukemogenesis. *Cell*, **121**, 167–178.

69 Kuendgen, A. and Lubbert, M. (2008) Current status of epigenetic treatment in myelodysplastic syndromes. *Annals of Hematology* (in press).

70 Liao, J.J. (2007) Molecular recognition of protein kinase binding pockets for design of potent and selective kinase inhibitors. *Journal of Medicinal Chemistry*, **50**, 409–424.

71 Vedel, M., Lawrence, F., Robert-Gero, M. and Lederer, E. (1978) The antifungal antibiotic sinefungin as a very active inhibitor of methyltransferases and of the transformation of chick embryo fibroblasts by Rous sarcoma virus. *Biochemical and Biophysical Research Communications*, **85**, 371–376.

72 McGovern, S.L., Caselli, E., Grigorieff, N. and Shoichet, B.K. (2002) A common mechanism underlying promiscuous inhibitors from virtual and high-throughput screening. *Journal of Medicinal Chemistry*, **45**, 1712–1722.

73 Ragno, R., Simeoni, S., Castellano, S., Vicidomini, C., Mai, A., Caroli, A., Tramontano, A., Bonaccini, C., Trojer, P., Bauer, I., Brosch, G. and Sbardella, G. (2007) Small molecule inhibitors of histone arginine methyltransferases: homology modeling, molecular docking, binding mode analysis, and biological evaluations. *Journal of Medicinal Chemistry*, **50**, 1241–1253.

74 Mai, A., Cheng, D., Bedford, M.T., Valente, S., Nebbioso, A., Perrone, A., Brosch, G., Sbardella, G., De Bellis, F., Miceli, M. and Altucci, L. (2008) Epigenetic multiple ligands: Mixed histone/protein methyltransferase, acetyltransferase, and class III deacetylase (sirtuin) inhibitors. *Journal of Medicinal Chemistry*, **51**, 2279–2290.

75 Balasubramanyam, K., Varier, R.A., Altaf, M., Swaminathan, V., Siddappa, N.B., Ranga, U. and Kundu, T.K. (2004) Curcumin, a novel p300/CREB-binding protein-specific inhibitor of acetyltransferase, represses the acetylation of histone/nonhistone proteins and histone acetyltransferase-dependent chromatin transcription. *The Journal of Biological Chemistry*, **279**, 51163–51171.

76 Trapp, J., Jochum, A., Meier, R., Saunders, L., Marshall, B., Kunick, C., Verdin, E., Goekjian, P.G., Sippl, W. and Jung, M. (2006) Adenosine mimetics as inhibitors of NAD + -dependent histone deacetylases, from kinase to sirtuin inhibition. *Journal of Medicinal Chemistry*, **49**, 7307–7316.

77 Purandare, A.V., Chen, Z., Huynh, T., Pang, S., Geng, J., Vaccaro, W., Poss, M.A., Oconnell, J., Nowak, K. and Jayaraman, L. (2008) Pyrazole inhibitors of coactivator associated arginine methyltransferase 1 (CARM1). *Bioorganic & Medicinal Chemistry Letters*, **18**, 4438–4441.

78 Spannhoff, A., Machmur, R., Heinke, R., Trojer, P., Bauer, I., Brosch, G., Schule, R., Hanefeld, W., Sippl, W. and Jung, M. (2007) A novel arginine methyltransferase inhibitor with cellular activity. *Bioorganic & Medicinal Chemistry Letters*, **17**, 4150–4153.

79 Heinke, R., Spannhoff, A., Meier, R., Trojer, P., Bauer, I., Jung, M. and Sippl, W., (2008) Virtual Screening and Biological Characterisation of Novel Histone Arginine Methyltransferase PRMT1 Inhibitors. **3** (in press).

80 Osborne, T., Roska, R.L., Rajski, S.R. and Thompson, P.R. (2008) In Situ Generation of a Bisubstrate Analogue for Protein Arginine Methyltransferase 1. *Journal of the American Chemical Society* (in press).

81 Greiner, D., Bonaldi, T., Eskeland, R., Roemer, E. and Imhof, A. (2005) Identification of a specific inhibitor of the histone methyltransferase SU(VAR)3-9. *Nature Chemical Biology*, **1**, 143–145.

82 Kubicek, S., O'Sullivan, R.J., August, E.M., Hickey, E.R., Zhang, Q., Teodoro, M.L., Rea, S., Mechtler, K., Kowalski, J.A., Homon, C.A., Kelly, T.A. and Jenuwein, T. (2007) Reversal of H3K9me2 by a small-molecule inhibitor for the G9a histone methyltransferase. *Molecular Cell*, **25**, 473–481.

83 Frietze, S., Lupien, M., Silver, P.A. and Brown, M. (2008) CARM1 regulates estrogen-stimulated breast cancer growth through up-regulation of E2F1. *Cancer Research*, **68**, 301–306.

84 Hong, H., Kao, C., Jeng, M.H., Eble, J.N., Koch, M.O., Gardner, T.A., Zhang, S., Li, L., Pan, C.X., Hu, Z., MacLennan, G.T. and Cheng, L. (2004) Aberrant expression of CARM1, a transcriptional coactivator of androgen receptor, in the development of prostate carcinoma and androgen-independent status. *Cancer*, **101**, 83–89.

85 Lee, Y.H., Coonrod, S.A., Kraus, W.L., Jelinek, M.A. and Stallcup, M.R. (2005) Regulation of coactivator complex assembly and function by protein arginine methylation and demethylimination. *Proceedings of the National Academy of Sciences of the United States of America*, **102**, 3611–3616.

86 Le Guezennec, X., Vermeulen, M., Brinkman, A.B., Hoeijmakers, W.A., Cohen, A., Lasonder, E. and Stunnenberg, H.G. (2006) MBD2/NuRD and MBD3/NuRD, two distinct complexes with different biochemical and functional properties. *Molecular and Cellular Biology*, **26**, 843–851.

87 Verbiest, V., Montaudon, D., Tautu, M.T., Moukarzel, J., Portail, J.P., Markovits, J., Robert, J., Ichas, F. and Pourquier, P. (2008) Protein arginine (N)-methyl transferase 7 (PRMT7) as a potential target for the sensitization of tumor cells to camptothecins. *FEBS Letters*, **582**, 1483–1489.

88 Pogribny, I.P., Tryndyak, V.P., Muskhelishvili, L., Rusyn, I. and Ross, S.A. (2007) Methyl deficiency, alterations in global histone modifications, and carcinogenesis. *The Journal of Nutrition*, **137**, 216S–222.

89 McGarvey, K.M., Fahrner, J.A., Greene, E., Martens, J., Jenuwein, T. and Baylin, S.B. (2006) Silenced tumor suppressor genes reactivated by DNA demethylation do not return to a fully euchromatic chromatin state. *Cancer Research*, **66**, 3541–3549.

90 Aniello, F., Colella, G., Muscariello, G., Lanza, A., Ferrara, D., Branno, M. and Minucci, S. (2006) Expression of four histone lysine-methyltransferases in parotid gland tumors. *Anticancer Research*, **26**, 2063–2067.

91 Li, H., Rauch, T., Chen, Z.X., Szabo, P.E., Riggs, A.D. and Pfeifer, G.P. (2006) The histone methyltransferase SETDB1 and the DNA methyltransferase DNMT3A interact directly and localize to promoters silenced in cancer cells. *The Journal of Biological Chemistry*, **281**, 19489–19500.

92 Saigo, K., Yoshida, K., Ikeda, R., Sakamoto, Y., Murakami, Y., Urashima, T., Asano, T., Kenmochi, T. and Inoue, I. (2008) Integration of hepatitis B virus DNA into the myeloid/lymphoid or mixed-lineage leukemia (MLL4) gene and rearrangements of MLL4 in human hepatocellular carcinoma. *Human Mutation*, **29**, 703–708.

93 Hamamoto, R., Silva, F.P., Tsuge, M., Nishidate, T., Katagiri, T., Nakamura, Y. and Furukawa, Y. (2006) Enhanced SMYD3 expression is essential for the growth of breast cancer cells. *Cancer Science*, **97**, 113–118.

94 Hamamoto, R., Furukawa, Y., Morita, M., Iimura, Y., Silva, F.P., Li, M., Yagyu, R. and

Nakamura, Y. (2004) SMYD3 encodes a histone methyltransferase involved in the proliferation of cancer cells. *Nature Cell Biology*, **6**, 731–740.

95 Scoumanne, A. and Chen, X. (2008) Protein methylation: a new mechanism of p53 tumor suppressor regulation. *Histology and Histopathology*, **23**, 1143–1149.

13
Histone Demethylases[1)]

Rasmus P. Clausen, Marianne T. Pedersen, and Kristian Helin

13.1
Introduction

Regulation of gene expression is a dynamic process during which several different histone residues are covalently modified to affect the ability of RNA polymerase to access the transcriptional start site. Thus, histone modifications such as methylation are believed to constitute important regulatory marks involved in the control of gene transcription. Strict regulation of gene expression patterns is crucial during development and differentiation, and in these processes histone-modifying enzymes play a central role. In recent years, enzymes catalyzing histone modifications have attracted much interest as potential drug targets. This has been stimulated by several results showing deregulated expression of these enzymes in human diseases such as cancer [1–4].

13.2
Chromatin

The genetic information of all eukaryotic organisms – the DNA – is wrapped around histone proteins forming an organized structure called chromatin. Histones, especially their flexible tails extending from the nucleosomal core, are subjected to a number of posttranslational modifications. These include methylation of lysine (K) and arginine (R) residues, acetylation of lysines and phosphorylation of serines and threonines. Whereas histone acetylation generally is linked to gene activation, arginine and lysine methylation can lead to either activation or deactivation depending on the methylation state, the position of the methylation site at the histone and the context in which the mark is found. In general, methylation of H3K4, H3K36 and H3K79 are found in regions with transcriptional activity, whereas H3K9me2/me3, H4K20me3 and H3K27me2/me3 are associated with transcriptionally silenced chromatin [1–4].

1) RPC and MTP contributed equally to this chapter.

Epigenetic Targets in Drug Discovery. Edited by Wolfgang Sippl and Manfred Jung

ISBN: 978-3-527-32355-5

In current models for transcriptional regulation, covalent modifications of histones influence transcriptional competence by establishing a local environment, that is open or closed chromatin, regulating accessibility of the DNA. Unlike histone acetylation, methylation does not affect the net charge of the affected residue and is not believed to affect DNA–histone interactions *per se*. Histone modifications are suggested to be part of a "code" that is read by proteins via specific binding domains and in this way translated into a functional signal. Thus, histone methylation can prepare genes for either transcriptional activation or repression depending on the effector proteins that are recruited [1–4].

13.3
Histone Methylation and Demethylation

The histone proteins can be *N*-methylated sequentially, introducing up to two methyl groups at arginines and up to three methyl groups at lysines, as can be seen in a crystal structure of trimethyllysine 4 and dimethylarginine 2 at histone H3 (H3K4me3 and H3R2me2; Figure 13.1) [5]. These reactions are catalyzed by specific histone methyl transferases (HMTs) with the methylating agent *S*-adenosyl-L-methionine (1) as the methyl group donor (see Chapter 12). Dimethylation of arginines can lead to both asymmetric and symmetric methylation since two of the three nitrogens in the guanidinium group can be methylated (Figure 13.2).

Our current knowledge regarding histone methylation stems in large part from the study of histone methyltransferases. Several of these enzymes are essential for development, with deregulated expression being linked to human disorders such as cancer [4]. Whereas proteins responsible for methylation of histones have been known for almost a decade, enzymes with histone demethylase activity (HDM) have only recently been discovered. Here we summarize our current knowledge regarding histone demethylases with a focus on the demethylation mechanisms, potential roles

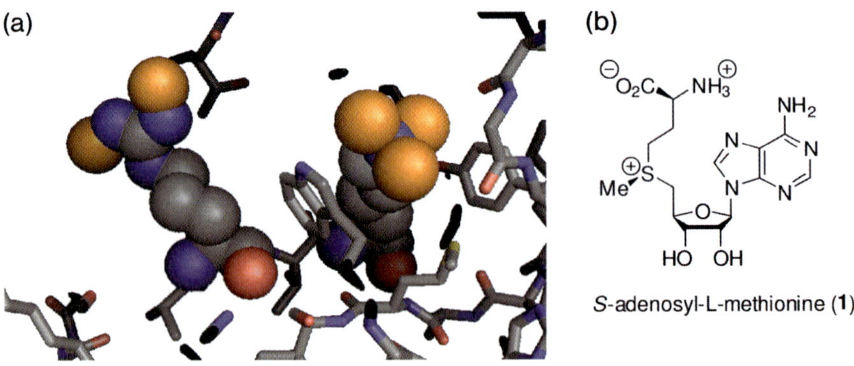

S-adenosyl-L-methionine (**1**)

Figure 13.1 (a) Trimethyllysine 4 and dimethylarginine 2 at histone H3 from X-ray structure [4]. (b) Chemical structure of the methylating agent *S*-adenosyl-L-methionine.

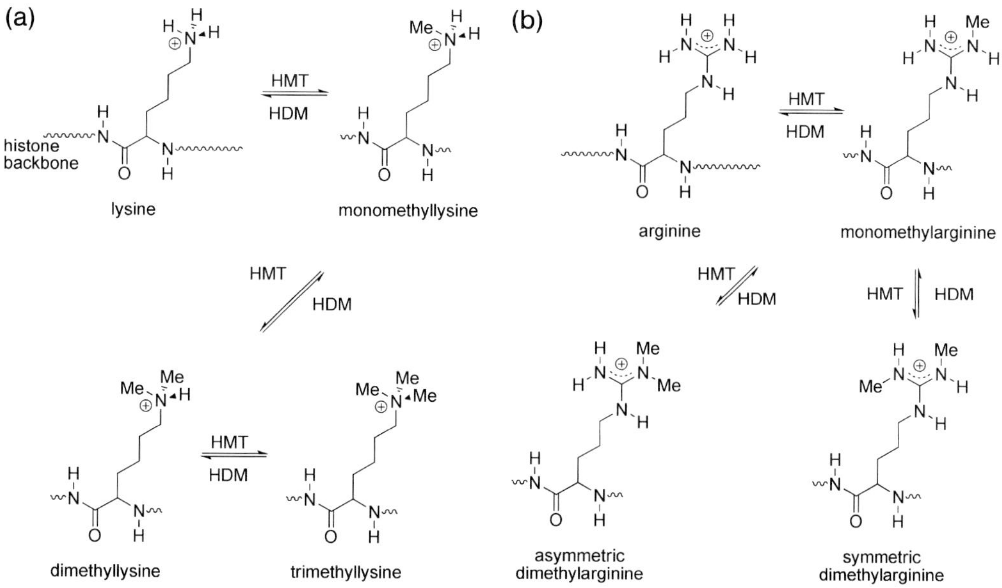

Figure 13.2 (a) Sequential methylation and demethylation of lysines catalyzed by histone methyl transferases (HMTs) and histone demethylases (HDMs), respectively. (b) Sequential methylation and demethylation of arginines catalyzed by HMTs and HDMs, respectively, leading to symmetric and asymmetric dimethylarginines.

in development and disease as well as the possibilities of developing specific inhibitors as pharmacological tools and therapeutic agents.

13.4 Histone Demethylases

As stated above, the first histone demethylases have been identified only recently. Although, peptidylarginine deaminase results in demethylation of the histone the products are citrulline and methylamine and not arginine [6, 7]. Thus, it is not a true demethylase catalyzing the reverse reaction of the HMTs. A purified enzyme capable of demethylating mono- and dimethylated lysine was first described in 1964 [8]. Detection of enzymic demethylation of methylated histone was reported in 1973, however no single protein performing the reaction was isolated [9, 10]. Nevertheless, until recently it was speculated whether methylation was a direct reversible process at all [11]. In 2004, Shi and co-workers discovered the first true demethylase specifically demethylating histone H3 at lysine 4 (H3K4) and termed it lysine-specific demethylase-1 (LSD1), providing strong evidence for a dynamic regulation of histone methylation [12]. It had already been suggested that demethylases were amine oxidases, based on the notion that a broad class of compounds are substrates for

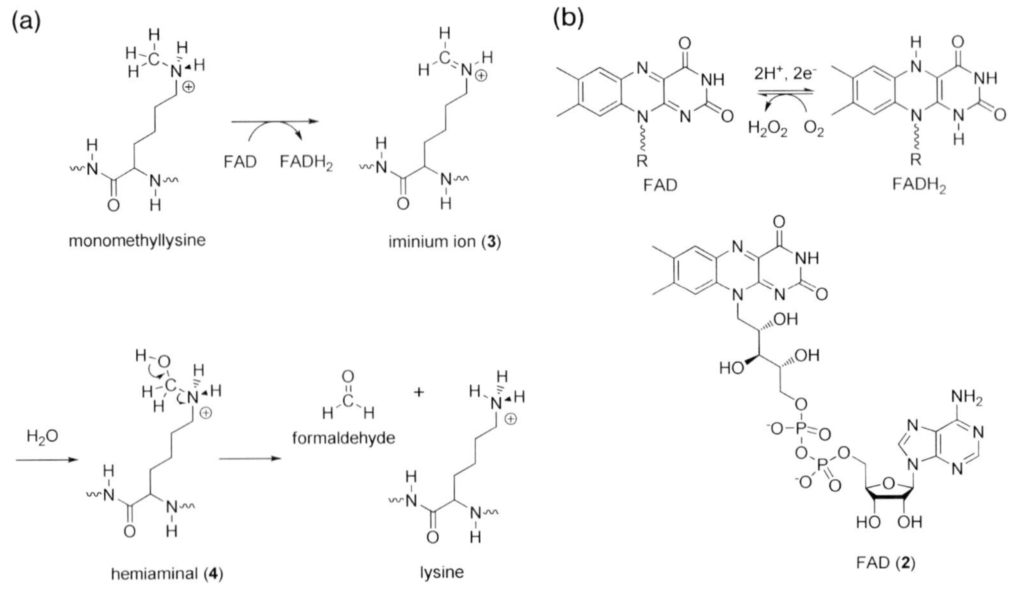

Figure 13.3 (a) Mechanism for demethylation catalyzed by LSD1. (b) Structures of the FAD redox pair.

amine oxidases [11]. The discovery was spurred by several reports noting that formaldehyde was produced in this process, suggesting an oxygenation reaction catalyzed by an oxygenase/hydroxylase or a dehydrogenation reaction by an amine oxidase. Dehydrogenation of the methyl amino group yields a methyl imino group that hydrolyzes to an instable hemiaminal followed by release of formaldehyde (Figure 13.3), whereas oxygenation forms the hemiaminal directly from the methyl amino group. The sequence homology with FAD-dependent amine oxidases and a strong indication of a transcriptional role suggested that the LSD1 gene could code for a demethylase. The characterization of LSD1 showed that histone demethylation indeed could occur via dehydrogenation.

Two years later it was shown that demethylation could also occur as a result of an oxygenation reaction with the purification of a novel JmjC domain-containing protein, termed JHDM1, that specifically demethylates histone H3 at lysine 36 (H3K36) in the presence of Fe(II) and α-ketoglutarate [13]. The discovery was inspired by studies demonstrating that the methyl groups of 1-methyladenine (1-meA) and 3-methylcytosine (3-meC) in DNA can be removed by the AlkB family of proteins via Fe(II) and α-ketoglutarate-dependent hydroxylation [14, 15]. In the same year several other oxygenases from the same family were reported to catalyze histone lysine demethylation [16–21].

Interestingly, since the expression levels of several of these demethylases are increased in primary tumors (Table 13.1) and it is speculated that the demethylases contribute to tumor formation and maintenance, they present strong candidate drug targets.

Table 13.1 Potential drug targets.

Name	Evidence for oncogenic potential
LSD1	• Overexpressed in prostate cancers correlating with relapse during therapy. • Depletion impairs androgen-dependent proliferation of a prostate cancer cell line.
FBXL10 FBXL11	• Overexpressed in lymphomas and mammary adenocarcinomas. • Inhibit replicative senescence in MEFs.
JMJD2A JMJD2B JMJD2C	• *JMJD2C* is amplified in esophageal squamous carcinomas and in desmoblastic medulloblastomas. • JMJD2A, JMJD2B and JMJD2C are overexpressed in prostate cancers. • Depletion of JMJD2C inhibits proliferation of various cancer cell lines.
JARID1B JARID1C	• JARID1B is overexpressed in breast and prostate cancers and JARID1C in prostate cancers. • Depletion of JARID1B inhibits proliferation of breast cancer cell lines and tumor growth in a syngeneic mouse mammary tumor model.

Note that some enzymes have important roles in nontransformed cells and/or tumor-suppressive activities. See text for details and references.

13.5
LSD1/KDM1

LSD1 (synonyms include AOF2, BHC110, p110b, KDM1) was the first histone demethylase to be isolated and characterized. LSD1 is a FAD-dependent amine oxidase that specifically demethylates H3K4 at histone substrates *in vitro* [12]. Like other FAD-dependent amine oxidase, LSD1 oxidizes the lysine methyl ammonium group by catalyzing the overall transfer of hydrogen from the methyl amino group to FAD (**2**), generating a methyliminium ion (3, Figure 13.3). Two mechanisms have been proposed for this oxidation step: a single-electron transfer (SET) and a polar nucleophilic covalent mechanism; however no definitive evidence for either mechanism has been disclosed [22, 23]. Both mechanisms involve a free lone pair on nitrogen offering a chemical explanation for the specificity for mono- and dimethylated lysine, since trimethylated lysines do not have a free lone pair. It has been shown that a trimethylated H3K4 peptide acts as a competitive inhibitor, which supports the argument that the trimethylated peptide readily binds in the active site but cannot be converted [24]. The generated methyliminium ion spontaneously hydrolyzes to formaldehyde and a demethylated lysine residue via an unstable hemiaminal (**4**).

LSD1 was initially demonstrated to demethylate H3K4me1/me2 as a component of the CoREST/Rcor1 co-repressor complex. In agreement with methylation of H3K4 being linked to activation of transcription, demethylation by LSD1 is associated with repression of CoREST target genes including neuronal genes in nonneuronal cells [12]. The catalytic activity is influenced by the other protein partners in the complex [24, 25]. Later, LSD1 was reported to be a co-activator for the androgen receptor (AR). The AR appears to change the specificity of LSD1 from H3K4 to H3K9, which activates the transcription of AR target genes [26]. Furthermore, evidence was recently provided that LSD1 demethylates the p53 tumor suppressor protein, thereby repressing transcriptional activity and the induction of apoptosis [27].

Several studies link LSD1 to both gene activation and repression programs working in concert with other co-activators and co-repressors. Among the transcription factors reported to interact with LSD1 are ERα, GFI1 and GFI1B, all suggested to have important roles in development and oncogenesis [28, 29]. LSD1 is essential for mouse development [30]; and deletion of the *Drosophila* homolog reduces viability and results in sterility and abnormal ovary development [31]. Specific deletion of *Lsd1* in the mouse pituitary demonstrated that LSD1 is required for late cell lineage determination [30], while depletion of LSD1 was found to either impair or promote differentiation of mammalian hematopoietic lineages *in vitro* [29]. Interestingly, LSD1 is downregulated in vascular smooth muscle cells derived from *db/db* mice, a mouse model for type 2 diabetes. The decreased levels of LSD1 could be linked to enhanced expression of inflammatory genes and to subsequent proatherogenic responses. These findings implicate dysregulation of LSD1 in vascular inflammation and diabetic complications [32].

Currently, LSD1 is considered to be an interesting target for anticancer therapies [33]. LSD1 is overexpressed in prostate cancers correlating with an aggressive biology; and downregulation of LSD1 impairs androgen stimulated proliferation of prostate cancer cells [26, 34].

Ten structures of LSD1 have been released so far [35–40]. Importantly, some of these contain inhibitors of LSD1. These reports suggest how the histone is recognized and how inhibitors may be designed.

13.5.1
Inhibitors of LSD1

Several potent inhibitors of LSD1 have already been reported. The mechanism for demethylation by LSD1 via a redox reaction catalyzed by FAD suggests that it is target for mechanism-based or suicide inactivators. This class of enzyme inhibitors is relatively inert until it is processed by the target enzyme resulting in covalent modification of residues or cofactors in the active site. Suicide inactivators may display high specificity and irreversible inhibition of the inactivated enzyme, so that the recovery of catalyst function requires *de novo* protein synthesis [41]. Several suicide inactivators have been developed for the monoamine oxidases MAO-A and MAO-B that has close homology to LSD1. Propargyl- and cyclopropylamine containing inhibitors are oxidized by the MAOs to generate electrophilic and radical species that covalently modify these enzymes [42]. They are used therapeutically in the treatment of cardiovascular and neuropsychiatric diseases and two of them, pargyline (5; Figure 13.4) and tranylcypromine (6) are also reported to inhibit LSD1 [26, 39, 43, 44]. Pargyline inhibits the demethylation of H3K9 by LSD1 and consequently blocks AR-dependent transcription [26]. The mechanism of LSD1 inactivation by 6 has been studied using kinetic and structural approaches. Radical ring opening of the cyclopropyl group has been proposed; however, differential adduct formation involves either C4a or N5 attack of the flavin on the radical

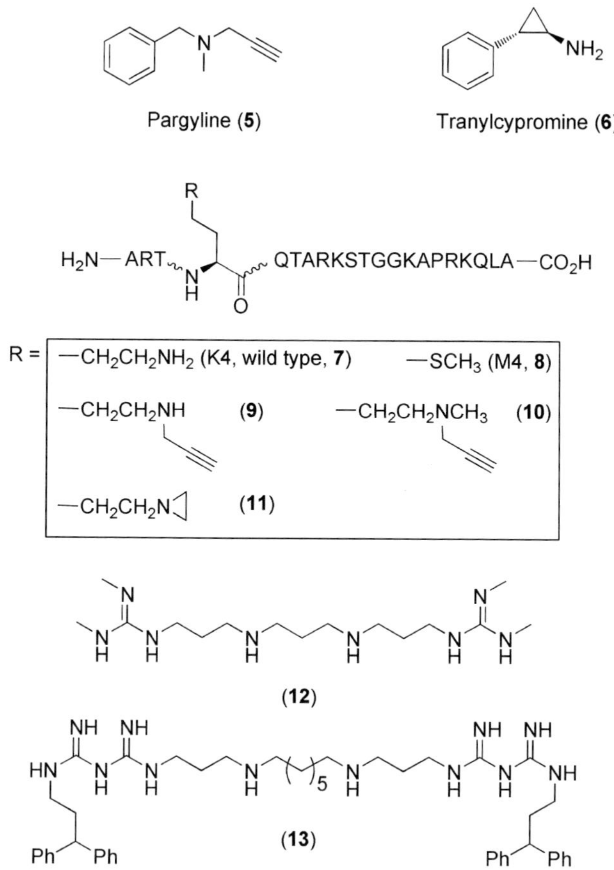

Figure 13.4 Various LSD1 inhibitors. Suicide inactivators pargyline 5 and tranylcypromine 6. Histone H3 tail 21-amino acid peptide analogs **7–11** as reversible and irreversible inibitors. Noncompetitive polyamine inhibitors **12** and **13**.

species [37, 39, 44]. Compound (**6**) shows a K_i of 500 μM and a k_{inact} of 0.67 min^{-1}, which is fast compared to the substrate turnover k_{cat} of 3–3.5 min^{-1} of LSD1 and 7 min^{-1} for the LSD1/CoREST complex.

Several analogs of a 21-amino-acid peptide of the H3 tail (**7**; Figure 13.4) have been shown to be inhibitors. Thus, the peptide consisting of the first 21 amino acids of H3 but with K4 exchanged for a methionine (**8**) is a potent inhibitor of LSD1 with a $K_i = 0.05$ μM [36]. The wild-type peptide has a $K_i = 1.8$ μM [45]. Truncation significantly reduces the affinity. *N*-Propargyl substitution of the distal amino group of K4 (**9**) and K4me1 (**9**) in the 21-amino-acid H3 peptide leads to potent suicide inactivators with K_i ranging from 0.1 to 0.6 μM and k_{inact} of 0.25 min^{-1} [39, 46, 47]. In contrast, the *N*-aziridine-modified H3K4 (**11**) is a reversible rather than time-dependent inhibitor of LSD1 [46, 47]. Covalent bond formation by the H3-propargylamines to N5 in FAD in LSD1 occurs as demonstrated by NMR spectrometry. To capture the structure of the inactivated LSD1 using X-ray crystallography, the H3-propargyl inactivated enzyme was reacted with sodium borohydride to reduce the linker double bonds before crystallization. This structure revealed the potential basis for K4 selectivity – the structure involved a series of three gamma turns over the first seven H3 amino acid residues [39]. It is possible that seven-membered ring gamma turn mimics may offer a new direction in designing LSD1 inhibitors [48]. Based on the considerable homology LSD1 shares with FAD-dependent polyamine oxidases, including spermine oxidase (SMO/PAOh1) and the fact that guanidines have been shown to inhibit both SMO/PAOh1 and other polyamine oxidases, a number of biguanide and bisguanidine polyamine analogs were tested as inhibitors of LSD1. Two of these (**12**, **13**) were potent inhibitors of LSD1 and displayed noncompetitive kinetics [49].

Since there are no proteins with extensive homology to LSD1 and the catalytic site is not very conserved amongst amine oxidases [40], it should be possible to exploit these differences, when developing an inhibitor of LSD1. Thus, even though the inhibitors described so far appear nonselective, it appears likely that elaborating the scaffold of the suicide inhibitors will lead to the development of selective inhibitors. It is difficult to assess whether the inhibitory peptides described are selective. But, the low affinity of the peptides towards LSD1 despite a relatively high number of amino acids suggests that these sequences can be improved and it is likely that shorter sequences, modified peptides or peptidomimetic compounds with higher affinity could lead to smaller molecules mimicking the histone tail, as seen for other targets [50].

13.6
JmjC Domain-Containing Demethylases

The jumonji protein family is characterized by the presence of the conserved JmjC domain that was first identified in the jumonji protein (JARID2). Jumonji means cruciform in Japanese and the gene was so named because mice with a genetrap inserted in the Jumonji locus develop an abnormal cross-like neural tube [51]. There are 27 different JmjC domain proteins (Figure 13.5) within the human genome, of which 15 so far have been published to demethylate specific lysines or arginines in the H3 tail.

Demethylation likely occurs via the same mechanism as for other Fe(II) and α-ketoglutarate-dependent hydroxylases established from crystallographic, spectroscopic and isotope incorporation studies [52]. As shown in Figure 13.6A, Fe is co-ordinated by water molecules, two histidines and a glutamate residue. These residues are highly conserved within the family of Fe(II) and α-ketoglutarate dependent hydroxylases, except that glutamate is exchanged for aspartate in some hydroxylases. Initially, two water molecules are exchanged for α-ketoglutarate (step I) and then the methylated lysine residue on the histone enters the active site. This intermediate step is visualized in a crystal structure of JMJ2DA containing Ni instead of Fe (Figure 13.6B) [53]. Water is replaced by oxygen (steps II, III). From this step less is known about the details of the mechanism, but presumably, an electron transfer from Fe to oxygen results in a reactive peroxide that can attack

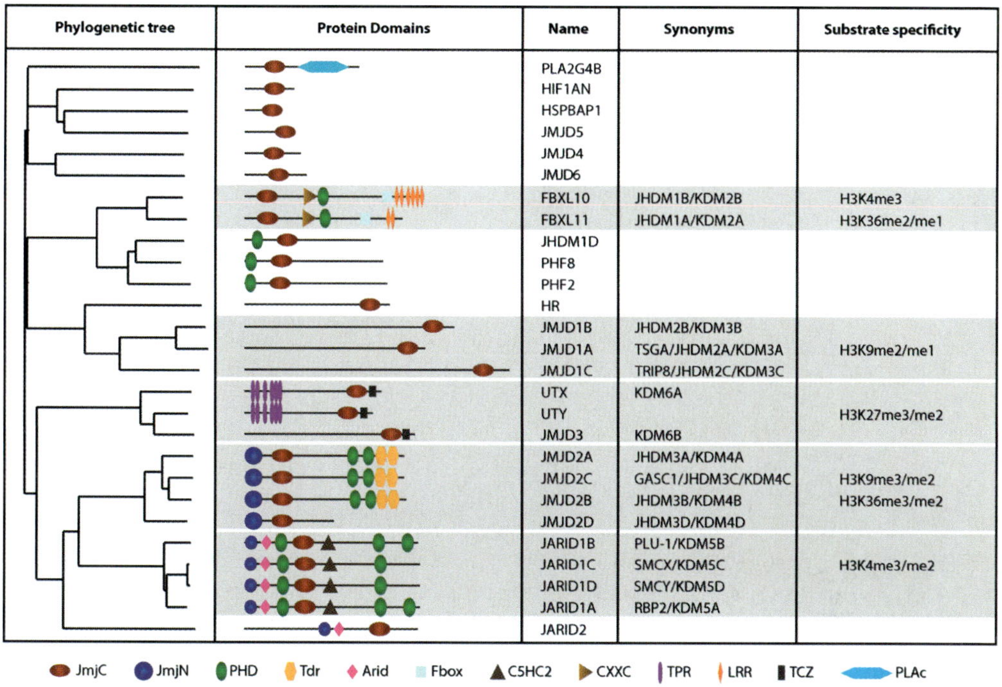

Figure 13.5 The human Jumonji C family. Phylogenetic tree of the human JmjC domain containing proteins modified from Cloos *et al.* [3]. The domain structures of the proteins are indicated. The clusters for which histone lysine demethylase activity have been published are shown in gray. See text for details and references. Jumonji C domain (JmjC); Jumonji N domain (JmjN); plant homeodomain (PHD); Tudor domain (Tdr); AT-rich interacting domain (Arid); F-box domain (Fbox); C5CH2 zinc-finger domain (C5HC2); CXXC zinc-finger domain (CXXC); tetratricopeptide domain (TPR); leucine-rich repeat domain (LRR); treble-clef zinc finger domain (TCZ); cytoplasmic phospholipase A2 (PLAc).

α-ketoglutarate (step IV, V). This is followed by insertion of an oxygen atom into the C1–C2 carbon–carbon bond of α-ketoglutarate leading to a carbonate–succinate mixed anhydride bound to an Fe(III)-hydroxyl radical anion (step VI). The activated oxygen species positioned near the substrate abstracts a hydrogen atom and forms a substrate radical plus an Fe(III)-hydroxide species (step VII). Subsequent recombination results in hydroxylated substrate and restores the Fe(II) form of the enzyme (step VIII). Finally, the products are exchanged by water molecules, leading to the starting species (step IX).

13.6.1 The FBXL/KDM2 Cluster

As mentioned above, the first JmjC domain containing demethylase described was FBXL11/JHDM1A/KDM2A, which catalyzes the demethylation of H3K36me2/me1 [13]. While the closely related protein FBXL10/JHDM1B/KDM2B initially

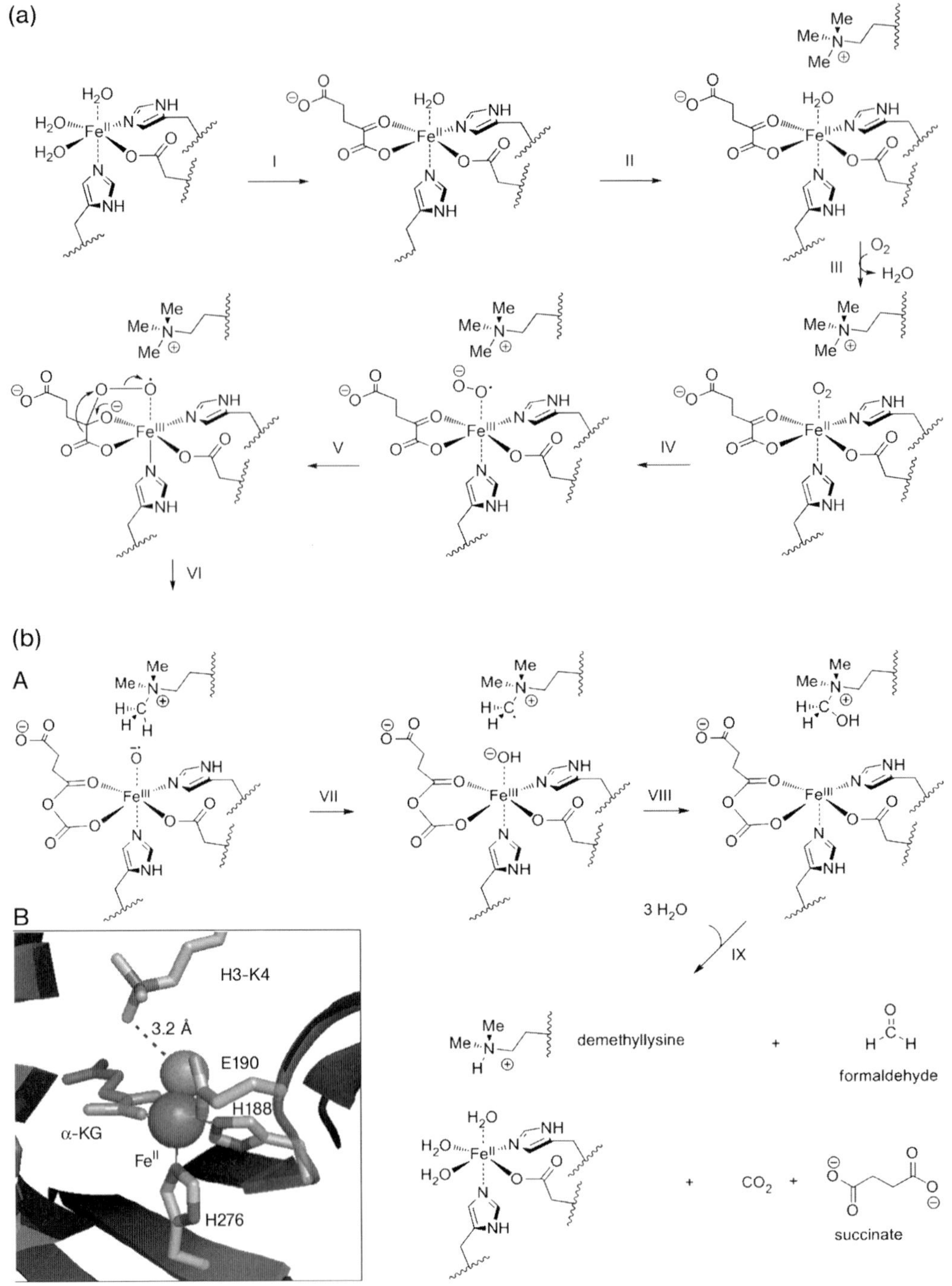

Figure 13.6 (a) Mechanism for the hydroxylation of lysine *N*-methyl group leading to dehydroxylation and release of formaldehyde, succinate and CO_2. (b) Active site from crystal structure of JMJD2A containing Ni instead of Fe and representing the state where α-ketoglutarate and the methylated lysine residue has entered (step I).

was reported also to be a H3K36 demethylase [13], a later study suggested it to be associated with H3K4me3 demethylase activity [54]. Intriguingly, insertional mutagenesis studies in rodents identified *FBXL10* as both a potential tumor suppressor gene [55] and – along with FBXL11 – as a putative proto-oncogene [56]. The oncogenic potential of FBXL10 could be linked to the finding that FBXL10 – dependent on the JmjC domain – inhibits replicative growth arrest (senescense) in mouse embryonic fibroblasts [56]. However, FBXL10 was also demonstrated to negatively regulate proliferation of HeLa cervical carcinoma cells correlating with demethylase-dependent repression of ribosomal RNA genes [54]. Further indicating diverse roles for FBXL10 in tumorigenesis, depletion of FBXL10 is associated with spontaneous mutagenesis [55] and FBXL10 has been shown to act as a repressor of the proto-oncogene c-Jun [57] and to be part of a co-repressor complex recruited by BCL6 – a transcription factor commonly translocated in lymphomas [58]. A role for the demethylase activity of FBXL10 in these contexts has so far not been described.

Taken together, the various observations suggest that FBXL10 has context-dependent pro- and anti-oncogenic activities. In line with this, FBXL10 expression was reported to be significantly decreased in human glioblastomas relative to normal brain tissue [54], while FBXL10 was found to be overexpressed in lymphomas and mammary adenocarcinomas [56].

13.6.2
The JMJD1/KDM3 Cluster

The JMJD1 or KDM3 cluster has three members in mammalian cells: JMJD1A/TSGA/JHDM2A/KDM3A, JMJD1B/JHDM2B/KDM3B and JMJD1C/TRIP8/JHDM2C/KDM3C. Of these, JMJD1A was shown to be a H3K9me2/me1 specific demethylase [20], while the demethylase activity of the other family members has not been published.

JMJD1A is highly expressed during spermiogenesis, and male *Jmjd1a* genetrap mice are infertile. This defect has been linked to JMJD1A removing repressive H3K9 marks from key genes involved in the final stages of sperm chromatin condensation and maturation. The phenotype of the *Jmjd1a* genetrap mice is similar to those observed in human syndromes such as azoospermia or globozospermia, indicating that JMJD1A could be involved in these infertility syndromes [59]. While no other defects were reported for the *Jmjd1a* genetrap mice, JMJD1A was implicated in the regulation of gene expression in smooth muscle cells and embryonic stem (ES) cells and further found to play an important role for ES cell self-renewal *in vitro* [60, 61]. Interestingly, JMJD1A was also demonstrated to interact with AR stimulating androgen dependent transcription in prostate cancer cells [20]. Although, no specific role for JMJD1A was demonstrated in human tumors, these results could imply that JMJD1A might be an interesting target for the treatment of androgen-dependent prostate cancers.

The other two JMJD1 family members are largely uncharacterized. A splice variant of JMJD1C is also suggested to be a co-activator for nuclear receptors including AR and reduced expression of this splice variant observed in breast cancer tissues [62]. Interestingly, human JMJD1B is located in a chromosomal area that is often deleted in malignant myeloid leukemias and myelodysplasias; and ectopic expression of JMJD1B has been shown to suppress clonogenic growth of a myelodysplastic cell line [63].

13.6.3 The JMJD2/KDM4 Cluster

There are four members of the JMJD2 cluster: JMJD2A/JHDM3A/KDM4A, JMJD2B/JHDM3B/KDM4B, JMJD2C/GASC1/JHDM3C/KDM4C and JMJD2D/JHDM3D/KDM4D. The JMJD2 proteins have demethylase activity towards H3K9me3/me2 and H3K36me3/me2 [17–19, 21]. The dual specificity means that many different functions could be envisioned for the JMJD2 proteins, but so far their cellular roles are largely uncharacterized.

Depletion of the JMJD2 homolog in *Caenorhabditis elegans* leads to alterations in both H3K9 and H3K36 trimethylation levels and causes germ cell apoptosis with altered progression of meiotic DNA double-stranded break repair [19]. Whether the observed phenotype is caused by deregulation of target genes or mediated through global effects on chromatin condensation is so far not known. In mammalian cells, forced expression of JMJD2 proteins can affect heterochromatic architecture and in this way potentially influence genomic stability [17, 18, 21].

While JMDJ2A initially was implicated in the repression of gene expression [18, 64], JMJD2C has been linked to gene activation correlating with H3K9 demethylation. Like other demethylases, JMJD2C was found to be a co-activator for AR and to play an important role for ES cell self-renewal *in vitro* through regulation of key target genes [67, 61].

Several lines of evidence suggest that members of the JMJD2 family could be involved in malignant transformation. JMJD2C was identified as a gene amplified in esophageal squamous carcinomas [65]. It is also amplified in some desmoblastic medulloblastomas [66] and expression levels of JMJD2A, JMJD2B, and JMJD2C are elevated in prostate cancers compared to normal tissues [17, 67]. Importantly, downregulation of JMJD2C inhibits proliferation of esophageal and osteosarcoma cell lines and androgen-stimulated growth of prostate cancer cells [17, 67]. The JMJD2 proteins therefore represent interesting drug targets for cancer treatments.

Several structures of the JMJD2A have been released, some in complex with histone tail peptides and/or inhibitors [16, 53, 68–71]

13.6.4 The JARID1/KDM5 Cluster

The JARID1 family is constituted by JARID1A/KDM5A/RBP2, JARID1B/PLU-1/KDM5B, JARID1C/SMCX/KDM5C and JARID1D/SMCY/KDM5D. The JARID1 proteins have demethylase activity towards H3K4me3/me2 linking them to transcriptional repression [72–77].

JARID1A was identified through its ability to bind the tumor suppressor protein pRB, a key regulator of cell cycle progression, apoptosis and cellular differentiation [78, 79]. A complex interplay between JARID1A and pRB has been suggested with JARID1A stimulating transcription of some pRB target genes through unknown mechanisms [80]. Interestingly, among the identified JARID1A interaction partners are components of the polycomb repressive complex 2 (PRC2) [81]. PRC2 harbors H3K27me3 methyltransferase activity and is critically involved in the regulation of cell fate decisions during embryogenesis. Along with PRC2, JARID1A was demonstrated to regulate and repress a number of developmentally important target genes in ES cells during proliferation and differentiation leading to coordinated effects on H3K4 and H3K27 methylation [72, 81].

In agreement with JARID1A playing an important role in differentiation, depletion of JARID1A can cause growth arrest and promote differentiation in various cell lines [80]. However, *Jarid1a−/−* mice are viable and display only minor defects in the hematopoietic system that could be linked to derepression of JARID1A cytokine target genes [74]. This might reflect redundancy in the functions of mammalian JARID1 proteins. A *C. elegans* line expressing a mutant version of the only Jarid1 homolog shows defects in vulva formation [72] and mutation of the *Drosophila* homolog, *Lid*, is fatal [82]. Interestingly, Lid was found to be a co-activator for the *Drosophila* homolog of the oncoprotein MYC being required for dMyc-induced cell growth. dMyc was shown to inhibit the demethylase activity of Lid; and an interaction between MYC and the mammalian JARID1A and JARID1B has also been suggested [83].

JARID1B displays a restricted expression pattern. It is dynamically expressed during development, but in adult tissues high expression levels are largely confined to testis [84, 85]. Overexpression of JARID1B affects proliferation and inhibits differentiation of ES cells [86] and JARID1B has been reported to interact with the developmental transcription factors and oncoproteins, brain factor-1 (BF-1) and paired box 9 (PAX9) [87]. Importantly, JARID1B is linked to malignant transformation. High levels of JARID1B expression are found in breast and prostate cancers [84, 88]. Correlating with derepression of cell cycle control genes, depletion of JARID1B inhibits the proliferation of breast cancer cell lines as well as tumor growth in a syngeneic mouse mammary tumor model [77]. JARID1B therefore appears to be an interesting target for the development of anticancer therapy. Surprisingly, however, a splice-variant of JARID1B demonstrates a progressive downregulation in advanced and metastatic melanomas [89].

The *JARID1C* and *JARID1D* genes are located on the X and Y chromosomes, respectively, with *JARID1C* escaping X-inactivation [90]. While JARID1C has been reported to be overexpressed in prostate tumors and seminomas [91], JARID1C has mostly been studied in relation to neurological disorders. Missense mutations in *JARID1C* are very frequently found in patients with X-linked mental retardation [92] and, notably, such mutations have been demonstrated to reduce the cellular demethylase activity of JARID1C [73, 76]. In addition several lines of evidence link JARID1C to neuronal development. JARID1C was found in complex with REST regulating genes implicated in neurological disorders [76] and downregulation of JARID1C in rat granule neurons was demonstrated to impair dendritic morphogenesis [73]. In zebrafish depletion of the JARID1C homolog was shown to cause brain-patterning defects and significant neuronal cell death [73].

JARID1D – the least characterized JARID1 protein – was described to interact with Ring6a, a polycomb-like protein regulating expression of a polycomb target gene [75]. This could suggest overlapping functions between JARID1A and JARID1D.

13.6.5
The UTX/JMJD3 (KDM6) Cluster

The KDM6 cluster consists of UTX/KDM6A, UTY and JMJD3/KDM6B. Whereas UTX and JMJD3 are histone demethylases specific for H3K27me3/me2 and in this way linked to transcriptional activation, no activity has so far been reported for UTY [98, 93–95].

UTX is located on the X chromosome and escapes X-inactivation [96]. Several studies have demonstrated UTX as part of multiprotein complexes containing H3K4 methyltransferase activity [98, 97]. This is analogous to the interaction between JARID1A and PRC2. Indeed UTX and H3K4 methyltransferases have been found to de-repress polycomb target genes during differentiation [98, 93, 95]. A similar role has been suggested for JMJD3 [94]. These findings underscore the importance of co-ordinated regulation of H3K4 and H3K27 methylation during development.

Unlike UTX, JMJD3 is highly regulated at the transcriptional level. In macrophages, *JMJD3* is induced by inflammatory stimuli [94], while JMJD3 is transiently expressed during differentiation of stem cells down the neuronal lineage [99]. Correlating with target gene regulation, functional studies have implicated JMJD3 in neuronal commitment and keratinocyte differentiation [99, 100].

In agreement with UTX and JMJD3 playing key roles in differentiation, deletion of one of the three *C. elegans* JMJD3 homologs causes abnormal gonadal development [93], while depletion of UTX homologs in zebrafish affects posterior development [95]. Importantly, UTX shows decreased expression in various human malignancies, while the gene encoding JMJD3 is located next to the p53 tumor suppressor locus and thus commonly deleted in cancers [3].

13.6.6
Inhibitors of JmjC Domain-Containing Demethylases

Since JmjC domain-containing demethylases have only recently been discovered, only very few inhibitors have been reported and those reported are already known to inhibit other Fe(II)- and α-ketoglutarate-dependent hydroxylases. Thus, oxalyl glycine (Figure 13.7) is a very well established inhibitor of Fe(II)- and α-ketoglutarate-dependent hydroxylases. A crystal structure has been deposited containing 2,4-pyridine dicarboxylic acid and JMJD2A. This compound was previously shown to inhibit other hydroxylases [53, 101–103]. Very recently, a publication appeared during the revision of this chapter describing several useful scaffolds with low activity

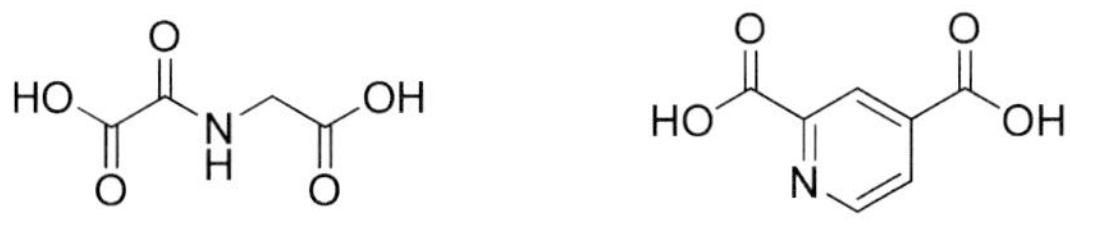

Oxalylglycine 2,4-Pyridine dicarboxylic acid

Figure 13.7 Chemical structures of JMJ2DA inhibitors.

at JMJD2E [104]. Elaboration on these structures may provide selective inhibitors. It is likely that selective inhibitors may be designed following the design strategies used for development of selective inhibitors of histone deacetylases. These inhibitors often consist of a metal-binding "warhead", a lipophilic stretch imitating the hydrophobic part of lysine and capped with a moiety inducing selectivity. Furthermore, it may be expected that many of the inhibitors consisting mainly of the metal-binding part may suffer from lack of selectivity.

13.7 Summary

Since the discovery of the first histone demethylase in 2004, a number of demethylases have been identified and implicated in the control of gene expression programs and cell fate decisions. The cellular functions of histone demethylases are only beginning to be deciphered, but many of these enzymes have nevertheless been found to play biologically important roles. Histone demethylases are linked to the regulation of for example stem cell self-renewal, differentiation, proliferation and hormone-dependent responses. These processes are critical for development and cellular homeostasis and their deregulation is implicated in pathological disorders.

From a therapeutic point of view it is interesting to note that several HDMs could be involved in malignant transformation, as indicated by their overexpression in human cancers and by their cellular roles. For the development of small molecule inhibitors, it will be of importance to determine whether inhibition of a tumor-promoting activity can be achieved without compromising vital roles in other cell types or for example promoting tumor-suppressive activities. However, LSD1, FBXL10, the JMJD2 proteins and JARID1B are interesting targets for the development of novel anticancer therapies.

Acknowledgements

In this work, R.P.C. and K.H. are supported by the University of Copenhagen Excellence Program. M.T.P. is supported by the P. Carl Petersen Foundation and the Danish Cancer Society. Work in the Helin laboratory is supported by grants from the Danish National Research Foundation, the Association for International Cancer Research, the Danish Cancer Society, the Danish Medical Research Council, the Danish Natural Science Research Council, the Benzon Foundation, the Lundbeck Foundation and the Novo Nordisk Foundation.

References

1 Jenuwein, T. and Allis, C.D. (2001) Translating the histone code. *Science*, **293**, 1074–1080.

2 Strahl, B.D. and Allis, C.D. (2000) The language of covalent histone modifications. *Nature*, **403**, 41–45.

3 Cloos, P.A., Christensen, J., Agger, K. and Helin, K. (2008) Erasing the methyl mark: histone demethylases at the center of cellular differentiation and disease. *Genes and Development*, **22**, 1115–1140.

4 Wang, G.G., Allis, C.D. and Chi, P. (2007) Chromatin remodeling and cancer, Part I: Covalent histone modifications. *Trends in Molecular Medicine*, **13**, 363–372.

5 Ramon-Maiques, S., Kuo, A.J., Carney, D., Matthews, A.G.W., Oettinger, M.A., Gozani, O. and Yang, W. (2007) The plant homeodomain finger of RAG2 recognizes histone H3 methylated at both lysine-4 and arginine-2. *Proceedings of the National Academy of Sciences of the United States of America*, **104**, 18993–18998.

6 Cuthbert, G.L., Daujat, S., Snowden, A.W., Erdjument-Bromage, H., Hagiwara, T., Yamada, M., Schneider, R., Gregory, P.D., Tempst, P., Bannister, A.J. and Kouzarides, T. (2004) Histone deimination antagonizes arginine methylation. *Cell*, **118**, 545–553.

7 Wang, Y., Wysocka, J., Sayegh, J., Lee, Y.H., Perlin, J.R., Leonelli, L., Sonbuchner, L.S., McDonald, C.H., Cook, R.G., Dou, Y., Roeder, R.G., Clarke, S., Stallcup, M.R., Allis, C.D. and Coonrod, S.A. (2004) Human PAD4 regulates histone arginine methylation levels via demethylimination. *Science*, **306**, 279–283.

8 Kim, S., Benoiton, L. and Paik, W.K. (1964) Epsilon-Alkyllysinase - Purification + Properties of Enzyme. *The Journal of Biological Chemistry*, **239**, 3790–3796.

9 Paik, W.K. and Kim, S. (1973) Enzymatic Demethylation of Calf Thymus Histones. *Biochemical and Biophysical Research Communications*, **51**, 781–788.

10 Paik, W.K. and Kim, S. (1974) Epsilon-Alkyllysinase New Assay Method, Purification, and Biological Significance. *Archives of Biochemistry and Biophysics*, **165**, 369–378.

11 Bannister, A.J., Schneider, R. and Kouzarides, T. (2002) Histone Methylation: Dynamic or Static? *Cell*, **109**, 801–806.

12 Shi, Y.J., Lan, F., Matson, C., Mulligan, P., Whetstine, J.R., Cole, P.A., Casero, R.A. and Shi, Y. (2004) Histone demethylation mediated by the nuclear arnine oxidase homolog LSD1. *Cell*, **119**, 941–953.

13 Tsukada, Y., Fang, J., Erdjument-Bromage, H., Warren, M.E., Borchers, C.H., Tempst, P. and Zhang, Y. (2006) Histone demethylation by a family of JmjC domain-containing proteins. *Nature*, **439**, 811–816.

14 Falnes, P.O., Johansen, R.F. and Seeberg, E. (2002) AlkB-mediated oxidative demethylation reverses DNA damage in Escherichia coli. *Nature*, **419**, 178–182.

15 Trewick, S.C., Henshaw, T.F., Hausinger, R.P., Lindahl, T. and Sedgwick, B. (2002) Oxidative demethylation by *Escherichia coli* AlkB directly reverts DNA base damage. *Nature*, **419**, 174–178.

16 Chen, Z.Z., Zang, J.Y., Whetstine, J., Hong, X., Davrazou, F., Kutateladze, T.G., Simpson, M., Mao, Q.L., Pan, C.H., Dai, S.D., Hagman, J., Hansen, K., Shi, Y. and Zhang, G.Y. (2006) Structural insights into histone demethylation by JMJD2 family members. *Cell*, **125**, 691–702.

17 Cloos, P.A.C., Christensen, J., Agger, K., Maiolica, A., Rappsilber, J., Antal, T., Hansen, K.H. and Helin, K. (2006) The putative oncogene GASC1 demethylates tri- and dimethylated lysine 9 on histone H3. *Nature*, **442**, 307–311.

18 Klose, R.J., Yamane, K., Bae, Y., Zhang, D., Erdjument-Bromage, H., Tempst, P., Wong, J. and Zhang, Y. (2006) The

transcriptional repressor JHDM3A demethylates trimethyl histone H3 lysine [thinsp]9 and lysine[thinsp]36. *Nature*, **442**, 312–316.
19 Whetstine, J.R., Nottke, A., Lan, F., Huarte, M., Smolikov, S., Chen, Z.Z., Spooner, E., Li, E., Zhang, G.Y., Colaiacovo, M. and Shi, Y. (2006) Reversal of histone lysine trimethylation by the JMJD2 family of histone demethylases. *Cell*, **125**, 467–481.
20 Yamane, K., Toumazou, C., Tsukada, Y., Erdjument-Bromage, H., Tempst, P., Wong, J.M. and Zhang, Y. (2006) JHDM2A, a JmjC-containing H3K9 dernethylase, facilitates transcription activation by androgen receptor. *Cell*, **125**, 483–495.
21 Fodor, B.D., Kubicek, S., Yonezawa, M., O'Sullivan, R.J., Sengupta, R., Perez-Burgos, L., Opravil, S., Mechtler, K., Schotta, G. and Jenuwein, T. (2006) Jmjd2b antagonizes H3K9 trimethylation at pericentric heterochromatin in mammalian cells. *Genes and Development*, **20**, 1557–1562.
22 Binda, C., Mattcvi, A. and Edmondson, D.E. (2002) Structure-function relationships in flavoenzyme-dependent amine oxidations. A comparison of polyamine oxidase and monoamine oxidase. *The Journal of Biological Chemistry*, **277**, 23973–23976.
23 Silverman, R.B. (1995) Radical Ideas About Monoamine-Oxidase. *Accounts of Chemical Research*, **28**, 335–342.
24 Stavropoulos, P., Blobel, G. and Hoelz, A. (2006) Crystal structure and mechanism of human lysine-specific demethylase-1. *Nature Structural & Molecular Biology*, **13**, 626–632.
25 Shi, Y.J., Matson, C., Lan, F., Iwase, S., Baba, T. and Shi, Y. (2005) Regulation of LSD1 histone demethylase activity by its associated factors. *Molecules and Cells*, **19**, 857–864.
26 Metzger, E., Wissmann, M., Yin, N., Muller, J.M., Schneider, R., Peters, A.H.F.M., Gunther, T., Buettner, R. and Schule, R. (2005) LSD1 demethylates repressive histone marks to promote androgen-receptor-dependent transcription. *Nature*, **437**, 436–439.
27 Huang, J., Sengupta, R., Espejo, A.B., Lee, M.G., Dorsey, J.A., Richter, M., Opravil, S., Shiekhattar, R., Bedford, M.T., Jenuwein, T. and Berger, S.L. (2007) p53 is regulated by the lysine demethylase LSD1. *Nature*, **449**, 105–108.
28 Garcia-Bassets, I., Kwon, Y.S., Telese, F., Prefontaine, G.G., Hutt, K.R., Cheng, C.S., Ju, B.G., Ohgi, K.A., Wang, J., Escoubet-Lozach, L., Rose, D.W., Glass, C.K., Fu, X.D. and Rosenfeld, M.G. (2007) Histone methylation-dependent mechanisms impose ligand dependency for gene activation by nuclear receptors. *Cell*, **128**, 505–518.
29 Saleque, S., Kim, J., Rooke, H.M. and Orkin, S.H. (2007) Epigenetic regulation of hematopoietic differentiation by Gfi-1 and Gfi-1b is mediated by the cofactors CoREST and LSD1. *Molecular Cell*, **27**, 562–572.
30 Wang, J., Scully, K., Zhu, X., Cai, L., Zhang, J., Prefontaine, G.G., Krones, A., Ohgi, K.A., Zhu, P., Garcia-Bassets, I., Liu, F., Taylor, H., Lozach, J., Jayes, F.L., Korach, K.S., Glass, C.K., Fu, X.D. and Rosenfeld, M.G. (2007) Opposing LSD1 complexes function in developmental gene activation and repression programmes. *Nature*, **446**, 882–887.
31 Di Stefano, L., Ji, J.Y., Moon, N.S., Herr, A. and Dyson, N. (2007) Mutation of Drosophila Lsd1 disrupts H3-K4 methylation, resulting in tissue-specific defects during development. *Current Biology*, **17**, 808–812.
32 Reddy, M.A., Villeneuve, L.M., Wang, M., Lanting, L. and Natarajan, R. (2008) Role of the lysine-specific demethylase 1 in the proinflammatory phenotype of vascular smooth muscle cells of diabetic mice. *Circulation Research*, **103**, 615–623.
33 Forneris, F., Binda, C., Battaglioli, E. and Mattevi, A. (2008) LSD1: oxidative chemistry for multifaceted functions in

chromatin regulation. *Trends in Biochemical Sciences*, **33**, 181–189.

34 Kahl, P., Gullotti, L., Heukamp, L.C., Wolf, S., Friedrichs, N., Vorreuther, R., Solleder, G., Bastian, P.J., Ellinger, J., Metzger, E., Schule, R. and Buettner, R. (2006) Androgen receptor coactivators lysine-specific histone demethylase 1 and four and a half LIM domain protein 2 predict risk of prostate cancer recurrence. *Cancer Research*, **66**, 11341–11347.

35 Chen, Y., Yang, Y., Wang, F., Wan, K., Yamane, K., Zhang, Y. and Lei, M. (2006) Crystal structure of human histone lysine-specific demethylase 1 (LSD1). *Proceedings of the National Academy of Sciences of the United States of America*, **103**, 13956–13961.

36 Forneris, F., Binda, C., Adamo, A., Battaglioli, E. and Mattevi, A. (2007) Structural Basis of LSD1-CoREST Selectivity in Histone H3 Recognition. *The Journal of Biological Chemistry*, **282**, 20070–20074.

37 Mimasu, S., Sengoku, T., Fukuzawa, S., Umehara, T. and Yokoyama, S. (2008) Crystal structure of histone demethylase LSD1 and tranylcypromine at 2.25 A. *Biochemical and Biophysical Research Communications*, **366**, 15–22.

38 Tochio, N., Umehara, T., Koshiba, S., Inoue, M., Yabuki, T., Aoki, M., Seki, E., Watanabe, S., Tomo, Y., Hanada, M., Ikari, M., Sato, M., Terada, T., Nagase, T., Ohara, O., Shirouzu, M., Tanaka, A., Kigawa, T. and Yokoyama, S. (2006) Solution structure of the SWIRM domain of human histone demethylase LSD1. *Structure*, **14**, 457–468.

39 Yang, M., Culhane, J.C., Szewczuk, L.M., Jalili, P., Ball, H.L., Machius, M., Cole, P.A. and Yu, H. (2007) Structural Basis for the Inhibition of the LSD1 Histone Demethylase by the Antidepressant trans-2-Phenylcyclopropylamine. *Biochemistry*, **46**, 8058–8065.

40 Yang, M.J., Gocke, C.B., Luo, X.L., Borek, D., Tomchick, D.R., Machius, M., Otwinowski, Z. and Yu, H.T. (2006) Structural basis for CoREST-dependent demethylation of nucleosomes by the human LSD1 histone demethylase. *Molecular Cell*, **23**, 377–387.

41 Walsh, C.T. (1984) Suicide Substrates, Mechanism Based Enzyme Inactivators - Recent Developments. *Annual Review of Biochemistry*, **53**, 493–535.

42 Edmondson, D.E., Mattevi, A., Binda, C., Li, M. and Hubalek, F. (2004) Structure and mechanism of monoamine oxidase. *Current Medicinal Chemistry*, **11**, 1983–1993.

43 Lee, M.G., Wynder, C., Schmidt, D.M., McCafferty, D.G. and Shiekhattar, R. (2006) Histone H3 lysine 4 demethylation is a target of nonselective antidepressive medications. *Chemistry & Biology*, **13**, 563–567.

44 Schmidt, D.M.Z. and McCafferty, D.G. (2007) trans-2-Phenylcyclopropylamine Is a Mechanism-Based Inactivator of the Histone Demethylase LSD1. *Biochemistry*, **46**, 4408–4416.

45 Forneris, F., Binda, C., Vanoni, M.A., Battaglioli, E. and Mattevi, A. (2005) Human Histone Demethylase LSD1 Reads the Histone Code. *The Journal of Biological Chemistry*, **280**, 41360–41365.

46 Culhane, J.C., Szewczuk, L.M., Liu, X., Da, G., Marmorstein, R. and Cole, P.A. (2006) A Mechanism-Based Inactivator for Histone Demethylase LSD1. *Journal of the American Chemical Society*, **128**, 4536–4537.

47 Szewczuk, L.M., Culhane, J.C., Yang, M., Majumdar, A., Yu, H. and Cole, P.A. (2007) Mechanistic Analysis of a Suicide Inactivator of Histone Demethylase LSD1. *Biochemistry*, **46**, 6892–6902.

48 Cole, P.A. (2008) Chemical probes for histone-modifying enzymes. *Nature Chemical Biology*, **4**, 590–597.

49 Huang, Y., Greene, E., Murray, S.T., Goodwin, A.C., Baylin, S.B., Woster, P.M. and Casero, R.A. Jr (2007) Inhibition of lysine-specific demethylase 1 by polyamine analogues results in reexpression of aberrantly silenced genes. *Proceedings of the National Academy of Sciences of the United States of America*, **104**, 8023–8028.

50 Bach, A., Chi, C.N., Olsen, T.B., Pedersen, S.W., Roder, M.U., Pang, G.F., Clausen, R.P., Jemth, P. and Stromgaard, K. (2008) Modified Peptides as Potent Inhibitors of the Postsynaptic Density-95/N-Methyl-d-Aspartate Receptor Interaction. *Journal of Medicinal Chemistry*, **51**, 6450–6459.

51 Takeuchi, T., Yamazaki, Y., Katoh-Fukui, Y., Tsuchiya, R., Kondo, S., Motoyama, J. and Higashinakagawa, T. (1995) Gene trap capture of a novel mouse gene, jumonji, required for neural tube formation. *Genes and Development*, **9**, 1211–1222.

52 Hausinger, R.P. (2004) Fe(II)/alpha-Ketoglutarate-Dependent Hydroxylases and Related Enzymes. *Critical Reviews in Biochemistry and Molecular Biology*, **39**, 21–68.

53 Couture, J.F., Collazo, E., Ortiz-Tello, P.A., Brunzelle, J.S. and Trievel, R.C. (2007) Specificity and mechanism of JMJD2A, a trimethyllysine-specific histone demethylase. *Nature Structural & Molecular Biology*, **14**, 689–695.

54 Frescas, D., Guardavaccaro, D., Bassermann, F., Koyama-Nasu, R. and Pagano, M. (2007) JHDM1B/FBXL10 is a nucleolar protein that represses transcription of ribosomal RNA genes. *Nature*, **450**, 309–313.

55 Suzuki, T., Minehata, K., Akagi, K., Jenkins, N.A. and Copeland, N.G. (2006) Tumor suppressor gene identification using retroviral insertional mutagenesis in Blm-deficient mice. *The EMBO Journal*, **25**, 3422–3431.

56 Pfau, R., Tzatsos, A., Kampranis, S.C., Serebrennikova, O.B., Bear, S.E. and Tsichlis, P.N. (2008) Members of a family of JmjC domain-containing oncoproteins immortalize embryonic fibroblasts via a JmjC domain-dependent process. *Proceedings of the National Academy of Sciences of the United States of America*, **105**, 1907–1912.

57 Koyama-Nasu, R., David, G. and Tanese, N. (2007) The F-box protein Fbl10 is a novel transcriptional repressor of c-Jun. *Nature Cell Biology*, **9**, 1074–1080.

58 Gearhart, M.D., Corcoran, C.M., Wamstad, J.A. and Bardwell, V.J. (2006) Polycomb group and SCF ubiquitin ligases are found in a novel BCOR complex that is recruited to BCL6 targets. *Molecular and Cellular Biology*, **26**, 6880–6889.

59 Okada, Y., Scott, G., Ray, M.K., Mishina, Y. and Zhang, Y. (2007) Histone demethylase JHDM2A is critical for Tnp1 and Prm1 transcription and spermatogenesis. *Nature*, **450**, 119–123.

60 Lockman, K., Taylor, J.M. and Mack, C.P. (2007) The histone demethylase, Jmjd1a, interacts with the myocardin factors to regulate SMC differentiation marker gene expression. *Circulation Research*, **101**, e115–e123.

61 Loh, Y.H., Zhang, W., Chen, X., George, J. and Ng, H.H. (2007) Jmjd1a and Jmjd2c histone H3 Lys 9 demethylases regulate self-renewal in embryonic stem cells. *Genes and Development*, **21**, 2545–2557.

62 Wolf, S.S., Patchev, V.K. and Obendorf, M. (2007) A novel variant of the putative demethylase gene, s-JMJD1C, is a coactivator of the AR. *Archives of Biochemistry and Biophysics*, **460**, 56–66.

63 Hu, Z., Gomes, I., Horrigan, S.K., Kravarusic, J., Mar, B., Arbieva, Z., Chyna, B., Fulton, N., Edassery, S., Raza, A. and Westbrook, C.A. (2001) A novel nuclear protein, 5qNCA (LOC51780) is a candidate for the myeloid leukemia tumor suppressor gene on chromosome 5 band q31. *Oncogene*, **20**, 6946–6954.

64 Gray, S.G., Iglesias, A.H., Lizcano, F., Villanueva, R., Camelo, S., Jingu, H., Teh, B.T., Koibuchi, N., Chin, W.W., Kokkotou, E. and Dangond, F. (2005) Functional characterization of JMJD2A, a histone deacetylase- and retinoblastoma-binding protein. *The Journal of Biological Chemistry*, **280**, 28507–28518.

65 Yang, Z.Q., Imoto, I., Fukuda, Y., Pimkhaokham, A., Shimada, Y., Imamura, M., Sugano, S., Nakamura, Y. and Inazawa, J. (2000) Identification of a novel gene, GASC1, within an amplicon at 9p23-24 frequently detected in esophageal cancer cell lines. *Cancer Research*, **60**, 4735–4739.

66 Ehrbrecht, A., Muller, U., Wolter, M., Hoischen, A., Koch, A., Radlwimmer, B., Actor, B., Mincheva, A., Pietsch, T., Lichter, P., Reifenberger, G. and Weber, R.G. (2006) Comprehensive genomic analysis of desmoplastic medulloblastomas: identification of novel amplified genes and separate evaluation of the different histological components. *The Journal of Pathology*, **208**, 554–563.

67 Wissmann, M., Yin, N., Muller, J.M., Greschik, H., Fodor, B.D., Jenuwein, T., Vogler, C., Schneider, R., Gunther, T., Buettner, R., Metzger, E. and Schule, R. (2007) Cooperative demethylation by JMJD2C and LSD1 promotes androgen receptor-dependent gene expression. *Nature Cell Biology*, **2007**, 347–353.

68 Chen, Z., Zang, J., Kappler, J., Hong, X., Crawford, F., Wang, Q., Lan, F., Jiang, C., Whetstine, J., Dai, S., Hansen, K., Shi, Y. and Zhang, G. (2007) Structural basis of the recognition of a methylated histone tail by JMJD2A. *PNAS*, **104**, 10818–10823.

69 Huang, Y., Fang, J., Bedford, M.T., Zhang, Y. and Xu, R.M. (2006) Recognition of Histone H3 Lysine-4 Methylation by the Double Tudor Domain of JMJD2A. *Science*, **312**, 748–751.

70 Lee, J., Thompson, J.R., Botuyan, M.V. and Mer, G. (2008) Distinct binding modes specify the recognition of methylated histones H3K4 and H4K20 by JMJD2A-tudor. *Nature Structural & Molecular Biology*, **15**, 109–111.

71 Ng, S.S., Kavanagh, K.L., McDonough, M.A., Butler, D., Pilka, E.S., Lienard, B.M.R., Bray, J.E., Savitsky, P., Gileadi, O., von Delft, F., Rose, N.R., Offer, J., Scheinost, J.C., Borowski, T., Sundstrom, M., Schofield, C.J. and Oppermann, U. (2007) Crystal structures of histone demethylase JMJD2A reveal basis for substrate specificity. *Nature*, **448**, 87–91.

72 Christensen, J., Agger, K., Cloos, P.A., Pasini, D., Rose, S., Sennels, L., Rappsilber, J., Hansen, K.H., Salcini, A.E. and Helin, K. (2007) RBP2 belongs to a family of demethylases, specific for tri-and dimethylated lysine 4 on histone 3. *Cell*, **128**, 1063–1076.

73 Iwase, S., Lan, F., Bayliss, P., de la Torre-Ubieta, L., Huarte, M., Qi, H.H., Whetstine, J.R., Bonni, A., Roberts, T.M. and Shi, Y. (2007) The X-linked mental retardation gene SMCX/JARID1C defines a family of histone H3 lysine 4 demethylases. *Cell*, **128**, 1077–1088.

74 Klose, R.J., Yan, Q., Tothova, Z., Yamane, K., Erdjument-Bromage, H., Tempst, P., Gilliland, D.G., Zhang, Y. and Kaelin, W.G. Jr (2007) The retinoblastoma binding protein RBP2 is an H3K4 demethylase. *Cell*, **128**, 889–900.

75 Lee, M.G., Norman, J., Shilatifard, A. and Shiekhattar, R. (2007) Physical and functional association of a trimethyl H3K4 demethylase and Ring6a/MBLR, a polycomb-like protein. *Cell*, **128**, 877–887.

76 Tahiliani, M., Mei, P., Fang, R., Leonor, T., Rutenberg, M., Shimizu, F., Li, J., Rao, A. and Shi, Y. (2007) The histone H3K4 demethylase SMCX links REST target genes to X-linked mental retardation. *Nature*, **447**, 601–605.

77 Yamane, K., Tateishi, K., Klose, R.J., Fang, J., Fabrizio, L.A., Erdjument-Bromage, H., Taylor-Papadimitriou, J., Tempst, P. and Zhang, Y. (2007) PLU-1 is an H3K4 demethylase involved in transcriptional repression and breast cancer cell proliferation. *Molecular Cell*, **25**, 801–812.

78 Defeo-Jones, D., Huang, P.S., Jones, R.E., Haskell, K.M., Vuocolo, G.A., Hanobik, M.G., Huber, H.E. and Oliff, A. (1991) Cloning of cDNAs for cellular proteins that bind to the retinoblastoma gene product. *Nature*, **352**, 251–254.

79 Fattaey, A.R., Helin, K., Dembski, M.S., Dyson, N., Harlow, E., Vuocolo, G.A., Hanobik, M.G., Haskell, K.M., Oliff, A., Defeo-Jones, D. *et al.* (1993) Characterization of the retinoblastoma binding proteins RBP1 and RBP2. *Oncogene*, **8**, 3149–3156.

80 Benevolenskaya, E.V., Murray, H.L., Branton, P., Young, R.A. and Kaelin, W.G. Jr (2005) Binding of pRB to the PHD protein RBP2 promotes cellular differentiation. *Molecular Cell*, **18**, 623–635.

81 Pasini, D., Hansen, K.H., Christensen, J., Agger, K., Cloos, P.A. and Helin, K. (2008) Coordinated regulation of transcriptional repression by the RBP2 H3K4 demethylase and Polycomb-Repressive Complex 2. *Genes and Development*, **22**, 1345–1355.

82 Gildea, J.J., Lopez, R. and Shearn, A. (2000) A screen for new trithorax group genes identified little imaginal discs, the Drosophila melanogaster homologue of human retinoblastoma binding protein 2. *Genetics*, **156**, 645–663.

83 Secombe, J., Li, L., Carlos, L. and Eisenman, R.N. (2007) The Trithorax group protein Lid is a trimethyl histone H3K4 demethylase required for dMyc-induced cell growth. *Genes and Development*, **21**, 537–551.

84 Lu, P.J., Sundquist, K., Baeckstrom, D., Poulsom, R., Hanby, A., Meier-Ewert, S., Jones, T., Mitchell, M., Pitha-Rowe, P., Freemont, P. and Taylor-Papadimitriou, J. (1999) A novel gene (PLU-1) containing highly conserved putative DNA/chromatin binding motifs is specifically up-regulated in breast cancer. *The Journal of Biological Chemistry*, **274**, 15633–15645.

85 Madsen, B., Spencer-Dene, B., Poulsom, R., Hall, D., Lu, P.J., Scott, K., Shaw, A.T., Burchell, J.M., Freemont, P. and Taylor-Papadimitriou, J. (2002) Characterisation and developmental expression of mouse Plu-1, a homologue of a human nuclear protein (PLU-1) which is specifically up-regulated in breast cancer. *Mechanisms of Development*, **119** (Suppl 1), S239–S246.

86 Dey, B.K., Stalker, L., Schnerch, A., Bhatia, M., Taylor-Papidimitriou, J. and Wynder, C. (2008) The histone demethylase KDM5b/JARID1b plays a role in cell fate decisions by blocking terminal differentiation. *Molecular and Cellular Biology*, **28**, 5312–5327.

87 Tan, K., Shaw, A.L., Madsen, B., Jensen, K., Taylor-Papadimitriou, J. and Freemont, P.S. (2003) Human PLU-1 Has transcriptional repression properties and interacts with the developmental transcription factors BF-1 and PAX9. *The Journal of Biological Chemistry*, **278**, 20507–20513.

88 Xiang, Y., Zhu, Z., Han, G., Ye, X., Xu, B., Peng, Z., Ma, Y., Yu, Y., Lin, H., Chen, A.P. and Chen, C.D. (2007) JARID1B is a histone H3 lysine 4 demethylase up-regulated in prostate cancer. *Proceedings of the National Academy of Sciences of the United States of America*, **104**, 19226–19231.

89 Vogt, T., Kroiss, M., McClelland, M., Gruss, C., Becker, B., Bosserhoff, A.K., Rumpler, G., Bogenrieder, T., Landthaler, M. and Stolz, W. (1999) Deficiency of a novel retinoblastoma binding protein 2-homolog is a consistent feature of sporadic human melanoma skin cancer. *Laboratory Investigation; A Journal of Technical Methods and Pathology*, **79**, 1615–1627.

90 Wu, J., Ellison, J., Salido, E., Yen, P., Mohandas, T. and Shapiro, L.J. (1994) Isolation and characterization of XE169, a novel human gene that escapes X-inactivation. *Human Molecular Genetics*, **3**.

91 Kim, T.D., Shin, S. and Janknecht, R. (2008) Repression of Smad3 activity by histone demethylase SMCX/JARID1C.

Biochemical and Biophysical Research Communications, **366**, 563–567.

92 Jensen, L.R., Amende, M., Gurok, U., Moser, B., Gimmel, V., Tzschach, A., Janecke, A.R., Tariverdian, G., Chelly, J., Fryns, J.P., Van Esch, H., Kleefstra, T., Hamel, B., Moraine, C., Gecz, J., Turner, G., Reinhardt, R., Kalscheuer, V.M., Ropers, H.H. and Lenzner, S. (2005) Mutations in the JARID1C gene, which is involved in transcriptional regulation and chromatin remodeling, cause X-linked mental retardation. *American Journal of Human Genetics*, **76**, 227–236.

93 Agger, K., Cloos, P.A.C., Christensen, J., Pasini, D., Rose, S., Rappsilber, J., Issaeva, I., Canaani, E., Salcini, A.E. and Helin, K. (2007) UTX and JMJD3 are histone H3K27 demethylases involved in HOX gene regulation and development. *Nature*, **449**, 731–734.

94 De Santa, F., Totaro, M.G., Prosperini, E., Notarbartolo, S., Testa, G. and Natoli, G. (2007) The histone H3 lysine-27 demethylase Jmjd3 links inflammation to inhibition of polycomb-mediated gene silencing. *Cell*, **130**, 1083–1094.

95 Lan, F., Bayliss, P.E., Rinn, J.L., Whetstine, J.R., Wang, J.K., Chen, S., Iwase, S., Alpatov, R., Issaeva, I., Canaani, E., Roberts, T.M., Chang, H.Y., Shi, Y. (2007) A histone H3 lysine 27 demethylase regulates animal posterior development. *Nature*, **449**, 689–694.

96 Greenfield, A., Carrel, L., Pennisi, D., Philippe, C., Quaderi, N., Siggers, P., Steiner, K., Tam, P.P., Monaco, A.P., Willard, H.F. and Koopman, P. (1998) The UTX gene escapes X inactivation in mice and humans. *Human Molecular Genetics*, **7**, 737–742.

97 Issaeva, I., Zonis, Y., Rozovskaia, T., Orlovsky, K., Croce, C.M., Nakamura, T., Mazo, A., Eisenbach, L. and Canaani, E. (2007) Knockdown of ALR (MLL2) reveals ALR target genes and leads to alterations in cell adhesion and growth. *Molecular and Cellular Biology*, **27**, 1889–1903.

98 Lee, M.G., Villa, R., Trojer, P., Norman, J., Yan, K.P., Reinberg, D., Di Croce, L. and Shiekhattar, R. (2007) Demethylation of H3K27 regulates polycomb recruitment and H2A ubiquitination. *Science*, **318**, 403–404.

99 Jepsen, K., Solum, D., Zhou, T., McEvilly, R.J., Kim, H.J., Glass, C.K., Hermanson, O. and Rosenfeld, M.G. (2007) SMRT-mediated repression of an H3K27 demethylase in progression from neural stem cell to neuron. *Nature*, **450**, 415–419.

100 Sen, G.L., Webster, D.E., Barragan, D.I., Chang, H.Y. and Khavari, P.A. (2008) Control of differentiation in a self-renewing mammalian tissue by the histone demethylase JMJD3. *Genes and Development*, **22**, 1865–1870.

101 Franklin, T.J., Morris, W.P., Edwards, P.N., Large, M.S. and Stephenson, R. (2001) Inhibition of prolyl 4-hydroxylase in vitro and in vivo by members of a novel series of phenanthrolinones. *The Biochemical Journal*, **353**, 333–338.

102 Halbwirth, H., Fischer, T.C., Schlangen, K., Rademacher, W., Schleifer, K.J., Forkmann, G. and Stich, K. (2006) Screening for inhibitors of 2-oxoglutarate-dependent dioxygenases: Flavanone 3[beta]-hydroxylase and flavonol synthase. *Plant Science*, **171**, 194–205.

103 Tschank, G., Brocks, D.G., Engelbart, K., Mohr, J., Baader, E., Gunzler, V. and Hanauskeabel, H.M. (1991) Inhibition of Prolyl Hydroxylation and Procollagen Processing in Chick-Embryo Calvaria by A Derivative of Pyridine-2,4-Dicarboxylate - Characterization of the Diethyl Ester As A Proinhibitor. *The Biochemical Journal*, **275**, 469–476.

104 Rose, N.R., Ng, S.S., Mecinović, J., Liénard, B.M., Bello, S.H., Sun, Z., McDonough, M.A., Oppermann, U. and Schofield, C.J. (2008) Inhibitor Scaffolds for 2-Oxoglutarate-Dependent Histone Lysine Demethylases. *Journal of Medicinal Chemistry*, **51**, 7053–7056.

Index

Epigenetic Targets in Drug Discovery. Edited by Wolfgang Sippl and Manfred Jung

ISBN: 978-3-527-32355-5